Understanding Neurology

Understanding Neurology

Edited by Steven Graham

AMERICAN
MEDICAL PUBLISHERS
www.americanmedicalpublishers.com

American Medical Publishers,
41 Flatbush Avenue,
1st Floor, New York,
NY 11217, USA

Visit us on the World Wide Web at:
www.americanmedicalpublishers.com

ISBN: 978-1-63927-334-8

Cataloging-in-Publication Data

Understanding neurology / edited by Steven Graham.
p. cm.
Includes bibliographical references and index.
ISBN 978-1-63927-334-8
1. Neurology. 2. Nervous system--Diseases. 3. Nervous system--Diseases--Treatment. I. Graham, Steven.
RC346 .U53 2022
616.8--dc23

Table of Contents

Preface

Every book is initially just a concept; it takes months of research and hard work to give it the final shape in which the readers receive it. In its early stages, this book also went through rigorous reviewing. The notable contributions made by experts from across the globe were first molded into patterned chapters and then arranged in a sensibly sequential manner to bring out the best results.

Neurology is a sub-field of medical science that deals with the disorders of the nervous system. Neurology applies neuroscience to study the nervous system. It focuses on the diagnosis and treatment of all the conditions and diseases of the central nervous system and peripheral nervous system. The central nervous system consists of the brain and spinal cord, whereas the peripheral nervous system includes the nerves and ganglia present outside the brain and spinal cord. This discipline also studies their coverings, blood vessels, and all the effector tissue like muscle. The treatment of diseases depends on the neurological problem. Certain neurological disorders are diagnosed by using EEG and intraoperative monitoring. This book consists of contributions made by international experts. It strives to provide a fair idea about this discipline and to help develop a better understanding of the latest advances within this field. It will provide comprehensive knowledge to the readers.

It has been my immense pleasure to be a part of this project and to contribute my years of learning in such a meaningful form. I would like to take this opportunity to thank all the people who have been associated with the completion of this book at any step.

Editor

1

Non-neuronal cholinergic activity is potentiated in myasthenia gravis

Bin Han[1], Chao Zhang[1], Shoufeng Liu[2], Yiping Xia[3], Hao Sun[4], Zhongying Gong[5], Alain R. Simard[6], Qiang Liu[1,7] and Junwei Hao[1*]

Abstract

Background: Non–neuronal acetylcholine (ACh) restricts autoimmune responses and attenuates inflammation by cholinergic anti-inflammation pathway. To date, the implication of ACh in myasthenia gravis (MG) remained unexplored. This study aimed to investigate the possible relationship between ACh levels, anti–muscle-specific tyrosine kinase (MuSK) antibody titers, main clinical features and outcomes of MG patients.

Methods: We successfully measured ACh levels in human peripheral blood mononuclear cells (PBMCs) from 125 MG patients and 50 matched healthy controls by using ultra-performance liquid chromatography-tandem mass spectrometry (UPLC-MS/MS). We assessed the quantitative MG (QMG) scores for each patient and titered anti-MuSK antibody.

Results: We found that PBMC-derived ACh level was significantly higher in MG patients, especially in patients of class III, IV-V, compared with that in controls (0.142 ± 0.108 vs. 0.075 ± 0.014 ng/million cells, $p = 0.0003$) according to the Myasthenia Gravis Foundation of America clinical classification. Importantly, we also found that ACh levels were positively correlated with QMG scores ($r = 0.83$, $p < 0.0001$) and anti–MuSK Ab levels ($r = 0.85$, $p < 0.0001$).

Conclusions: Our demonstration of elevated ACh levels in PBMCs of MG patients foreshadows potential new avenues for MG research and treatment.

Keywords: Acetylcholine, Myasthenia gravis, Inflammation, Cholinergic anti-inflammatory pathway

Background

Myasthenia gravis (MG) is a well-recognized autoimmune disorder affecting neuromuscular junction [1, 2]. Inflammatory environment plays a crucial role in the progress of this disease [3], appropriate interference with inflammation is a very promising therapeutic strategy and requires further research.

Recently, studies regarding the immune-modulating properties of acetylcholine (ACh) derived from non-neuronal cells has prompted an increasing interest in the field of the cholinergic anti-inflammatory pathway. Interestingly, non-neuronal ACh and main components of the cholinergic system, such as choline acetyltransferase (ChAT), acetylcholinesterase (AChE), vesicular acetylcholine transporter (VAChT) and high-affinity choline transporter (ChT1), are expressed in multiple human cell types, including keratinocytes [4], pancreatic cells [5] and immune cells [6]. For instance, ACh released by $ChAT^{+}$ B cells limits local neutrophil recruitment to modulate innate immunity during sterile endotoxemia [7]. Additionally, ACh-producing T cells in the spleen, induced by vagus nerve stimulation, are known to decrease the intensity of inflammatory responses through the inhibition of TNF–α production [8]. Lymphocyte-derived ACh may thus play a key role in the interaction between the nervous system and immune system to restore homeostasis, a mechanism called the 'cholinergic anti-inflammatory pathway' [9, 10]. Targeting this pathway, which reduces pro-inflammatory cytokine secretion, was effective in many experimental animal models, including inflammatory bowel disease [11], experimental autoimmune encephalomyelitis (EAE) [12–16], arthritis [17], ischemia-reperfusion injury [18], sepsis [19, 20], pancreatitis [21], myocardial ischemia [22] and hemorrhagic shock [23].

* Correspondence: hjw@tmu.edu.cn
[1]Department of Neurology, Tianjin Neurological Institute, Tianjin Medical University General Hospital, Tianjin 300052, China
Full list of author information is available at the end of the article

These studies suggest a tight inter-relationship between non-neuronal ACh and inflammatory reactions. However, peripheral cholinergic function related to ACh has not been investigated in MG till now.

These observations brought us to question whether human PBMC-derived ACh play a critical role in the process of MG. Here, we described a simple and stable ultra-performance liquid chromatography-tandem mass spectrometry (UPLC-MS/MS) method of our design for quantifying ACh levels in peripheral blood mononuclear cells (PBMCs). In addition, we investigated the relationships between ACh levels and MG severity.

Methods

Subjects

This study was approved by institutional review boards from Tianjin Medical University General Hospital, Tianjin Huanhu Hospital, Shandong Provincial Hospital Affiliated to Shandong University and Tianjin First Center Hospital. Informed consent was obtained from all participants prior to inclusion. For this study, 125 eligible patients diagnosed with MG for the first time and 50 matched healthy individuals were enrolled from April 2015 to May 2016. The optimum diagnosis of MG was based on a combination of patients' clinical manifestations, abnormal electrodiagnostic studies on single-fiber electromyography testing, abnormal repetitive nerve stimulation and previous response to treatment. Aberrant levels of anti-acetylcholine receptor (AChR) and anti–muscle-specific tyrosine kinase (MuSK) antibodies supported the diagnosis; however, a seronegative antibody titer was considered insufficient to refute the diagnosis of MG. All the patients received no cholinesterase inhibitors and immunosuppressive agents before definite diagnosis of MG. Exclusion criteria included patients with cardiovascular and cerebrovascular diseases, coagulation disorders, pregnancy, other disorders causing weakness or fatigue, combined with other autoimmune diseases, history of malignant disease except for thymus, inability to provide informed consent. MG subtyping followed the Myasthenia Gravis Foundation of America (MGFA) clinical classification, and the severity of disease and effectiveness of treatment were assessed by a validated quantitative MG Scoring system (QMG Score) [24].

Isolation of human PBMCs

Before patients receiving treatment, venous blood samples were extracted into ice-cold tubes containing EDTA and centrifuged immediately thereafter at 3000 rpm for 10 min, separating the samples into two layers. The upper layer, plasma, was subpackaged and stored at -80 °C for further analysis. The lower layer, precipitated blood cells, was the source of PBMCs isolated with Ficoll density gradients.

Detection of PBMC-derived intracellular ACh by UPLC–MS/MS

A stable method developed by our team was used to detect ACh levels [25]. Briefly, the fresh PBMCs were separated from blood and added to 100 μL deionized H_2O/ 0.1% formic acid (vol:vol), and vortexed for 15 s to make homogenate, which was de-proteined by adding 300 μL acetonitrile containing isotope internal standard (D9-ACh, C/D/N, Quebec, Canada). The sample was vortexed again for 1 min then centrifuged at 15000 rpm for 10 min. The supernatant was transferred to a sterile autosampler glass vials for measurement. The recovery of ACh following the sample cleanup procedure, as estimated from the pre and post cleanup standard curves, was 96.5%.

For highly specific and sensitive measurement of intracellular ACh, we used an Acquity UPLC system coupled to a Xevo TQ-S (Waters Corporation, Milford, MA, USA). ACh was separated by liquid chromatography using a CORTECS HILIC column (1.7 μm, 100 mm × 2.1 mm). Serially diluted ACh was used to construct a standard curve. All standards and samples received a uniform aliquot of D9-ACh internal standard to correct for variations in extraction efficiency.

Anti-AChR and anti–MuSK Ab titering

Anti-AChR and anti–MuSK Ab levels in the blood plasma were determined in duplicates, and mean values calculated, by ELISA (Trust Specialty Zeal, USA [AChR Ab assay range: 6 pmol/L-1200 pmol/L; MuSK Ab assay range: 2 U/L-400 U/L]) according to the manufacturer's instructions.

Quantitative real-time PCR (qRT-PCR)

Total RNA was extracted from fresh human PBMCs with the TRIzol reagent (Invitrogen, USA) according to the manufacturer's protocol. Reverse transcription reactions were carried out with TransScript First-Strand cDNA Synthesis Super Mix (TransGen Biotech, China) according to the supplied protocol. qPCR reactions were all performed in triplicate. FastStart Universal SYBR Green Master (Roche, Germany) was used as the detection dye. We used β-actin as an internal reference gene to normalize the expression level for AChE, ChAT, ChT1 and VAChT. The amplification and detection of specific products were performed with the CFX Connect^{TM} Real-Time System (Bio-Rad, USA). PCR conditions were the following: denaturation at 95 °C for 10 min, followed by 39 cycles of 95 °C for 15 s, 58-61 °C for 30 s, 72 °C for 20 s, and a final extension step of 72 °C for 10 min. The mean value was calculated by plotting Ct, and then used for further calculation. The mean relative expression was gained by the $2^{-\Delta\Delta Ct}$ comparative method. The primers for amplification were the following: 5′-GGGTGGTAGACGCTACAACC-3′ (forward) and

5′-GTGCCCTCAAAACCTGGGTAT-3′ (reverse) for AChE, 5′- AACCACGGAGATGTTCTGCTGCTAT-3′ (forward) and 5′- TTGTTGCCAATGGCTTGCTCTC AG-3′ (reverse) for ChAT, 5′-ATCCCAGCCATACT-CATTGG-3′ (forward) and 5′-CAGAAACTGCACCAA GACCA-3′ (reverse) for ChT1, 5′- GGCATAGCCCTAG TCGACAC-3′ (forward) and 5′-CGTAGGCCACCGAA TAGGAG-3′ (reverse) for VAChT.

Western blot analysis

Human PBMCs were lysed in RIPA (Solarbio) coupled with PMSF, a protease inhibitor. Afterward, we detected protein concentrations using BCA protein assay reagent; the equal protein samples were then mixed with 4 × sample buffer and boiled for 10 min. The samples were separated by 10% SDS-PAGE gel and transferred onto PVDF membranes (Millipore, USA) by the semi-dry transfer method. After blocking in 5% nonfat dried milk in TBST for 2 h at room temperature, the blots were incubated with specific antibodies overnight at 4 °C. After washing, the membranes were incubated with secondary antibodies for 1 h at room temperature. The specific protein bands were detected using a Bio-Rad Gel Doc Imager. The specific antibodies (Santa Cruz, CA, USA) included were mouse anti-AChE (1:100), mouse anti-ChAT (1:100) and goat anti-VAChT (1:1000). The relative amounts of proteins were normalized against GAPDH.

Determination of cholinergic components in PBMCs by ELISA

Human PBMCs were lysed, and total protein concentration of the lysates was determined by BCA method. The levels of AChE, VAChT and ChAT proteins were then measured by ELISA (Shanghai Yuanye biological technology co., LTD, Shanghai, China) according to the manufacturers' instructions. All samples and standards were determined in duplicate. All data were calculated and normalized to the total protein concentration in each sample.

Statistical analysis

Statistical analysis was performed using SPSS Statistics 20.0 (IBM Corp, USA. Released 2011). Data are expressed as means ± SD. For data with normal distribution, one-way analysis of variance with Dunnet test was used to assess the differences among groups. An independent-sample t test was used to compare differences between two groups. For data with nonnormal distribution, the Mann–Whitney U tests to compare differences between two groups. Kruskal-Wallis test was applied to test for mutiple groups. Repeated measures ANOVA was used to compare differences before and after treatment. Regression analysis was conducted to test for associations between parameters (ACh, QMG scores and anti–MuSK Ab concentrations). Values of $p < 0.05$ were considered to be statistically significant.

Results

Baseline characteristics

The characteristics of all participants enrolled in this study were shown in Table 1. There were no statistically significant differences in age, or gender in the MG patients as compared with healthy controls. In addition, we have shown the treatment plan after blood drawing in this table.

PBMC-derived ACh content changed in MG patients compared with controls

We first established that UPLC-MS/MS was a precise, stable and available technique to detect intracellular ACh then used this method routinely to determine the PBMC-derived ACh content of our MG patients. To eliminate the influence of cholinesterase inhibitors, we assessed ACh levels by preprocessing PBMCs with eserine, a cholinesterase inhibitor, for 30 min in the vacuette blood collection tubes once blood samples were drawn and compared MG patients untreated or treated with pyridostigmine (Additional file 1). We did not find statistically significant differences ($p > 0.05$). Eight patients were in each group, and the two groups showed no significant differences in QMG score (2.00 ± 1.604 vs. 1.75 ± 1.488, $p = 0.7513$). Subsequently, we recorded significantly higher levels of ACh per million cells in MG patients compared with controls (0.142 ± 0.108 vs. 0.075 ± 0.014 ng/million cells, $p = 0.0003$) (Fig. 1a). Similarly, amount of relative mRNA expression for ChT1, the rate-limiting enzyme for ACh, was higher in samples from MG patients than those from controls ($p = 0.0449$) (Fig. 1b). However, there was no statistical significance for ChAT, a direct synthetase for ACh, mRNA expression ($p = 0.9061$) (Fig. 1c). The MG group contained dramatically less AChE, a degrading enzyme for ACh, mRNA than in controls ($p = 0.0011$) (Fig. 1d).

Intracellular ACh levels in relation to MG severity

Based on these findings, we further defined whether ACh levels differ in patients with varied subtypes of MG as classified by the MGFA. ACh content was significantly elevated in patients with class III-V MG ($p < 0.0001$), but not those in class I-II, compared with controls (Fig. 2a). In support, a positive correlation was found between ACh levels and QMG scores in our cohort ($r = 0.83$, $p < 0.0001$) (Fig. 2b). Meanwhile, correlation between MGFA classification and the QMG score in MG patients ($n = 125$) was assessed using the Spearman rank correlation analysis, and positive correlation was observed between them ($r = 0.874$, $p < 0.001$). Also, we observed that ACh

Table 1 Comparative demographics of patients with MG and controls

Characteristics	MGFA Classification				Control
	I	II	III	IV-V	
NO. of samples(n)	58	30	24	13	50
Age (years)	46.10 ± 9.45	43.80 ± 10.83	45.63 ± 10.94	48.23 ± 9.65	46.14 ± 9.89
Female n (%)	28 (48.3)	15 (50.0)	10 (54.2)	5 (45.5)	26 (52.0)
AChR Ab pos n (%)	42 (72.4)	20 (66.7)	17 (70.8)	7 (53.8)	NA
MuSK Ab pos n (%)	3 (5.2)	3 (10.0)	4 (16.7)	5 (38.5)	NA
Double negative n (%)	13 (22.4)	7 (23.3)	3 (12.5)	1 (7.7)	
Treatment	Pyridostigmine, 23 of 58 added oral Prednisone	Pyridostigmine, 25 of 28 added oral Prednisone	Pyridostigmine, IVIG, Subsequent oral prednisone	Pyridostigmine, IVIG, IV methylprednisolone	NA

MG myasthenia gravis, *AChR Ab* acetylcholine receptor antibody, *MuSK Ab* muscle-specific tyrosine kinase antibody, I to V according to Myasthenia Gravis Foundation of America (MGFA) clinical classification; *NA* not available

levels had declined significantly in patients two weeks after the initial treatment (0.286 ± 0.077 vs. 0.167 ± 0.064, $p < 0.0001$) (Fig. 2c). Eighteen of these patients were treated with pyridostigmine, IVIG and oral prednisone, while others were treated with pyridostigmine, IVIG and IV methylprednisolone. Further, disease severity evaluated by QMG scores before and after treatment with immunological therapy decreased at the post-treatment period to the level of statistical significance (14.20 ± 5.176 vs. 9.07 ± 3.562, $p < 0.0001$) (Fig. 2d). Therefore, our data showing that immunological therapy was effective treatment is consistent with previous studies [26, 27]. We also quantified the anti-AChR and anti–MuSK Ab levels in the plasma of MG patients. No significant association was found between anti-AChR Ab levels and ACh levels ($r = 0.22$, $p = 0.1673$) (Fig. 3a), however, the ACh levels correlated positively with anti–MuSK Ab levels ($r = 0.85$, $p < 0.0001$ by regression analysis) (Fig. 3b). In our cohort, the anti–MuSK Ab concentrations increased as MG worsened ($p = 0.0135$ by Kruskal-Wallis) (Fig. 3c). Meanwhile, a positive correlation was found between the anti–MuSK Ab levels and QMG scores ($r = 0.69$, $p = 0.0046$ by regression analysis) (Fig. 3d). In addition, we found that the ACh levels are significantly elevated in anti-MuSK Ab positive group compared with double-negative and anti-AChR Ab-positive groups ($p < 0.001$, $p < 0.01$, respectively). However, there was no significant statistical differ ence between double-negative and anti-AChR Ab-positive groups

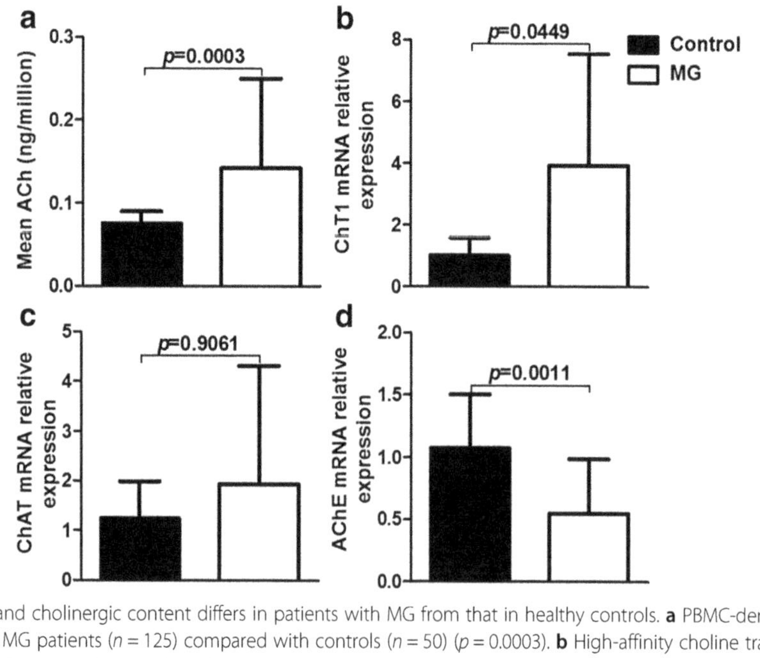

Fig. 1 PBMC-derived ACh and cholinergic content differs in patients with MG from that in healthy controls. **a** PBMC-derived ACh per million cells was obviously increased in MG patients ($n = 125$) compared with controls ($n = 50$) ($p = 0.0003$). **b** High-affinity choline transporter (ChT1) mRNA expression was higher in MG patients ($n = 15$) than that in control ($n = 6$) ($p = 0.0449$). **c** Choline acetyltransferase (ChAT) mRNA relative expression showed no obvious change ($p = 0.9061$). **d** A sharp decrease in acetylcholinesterase (AChE) mRNA expression was observed between MG patients and controls ($p = 0.0011$). (**c-d**; $n = 10$ for control, $n = 36$ for MG)

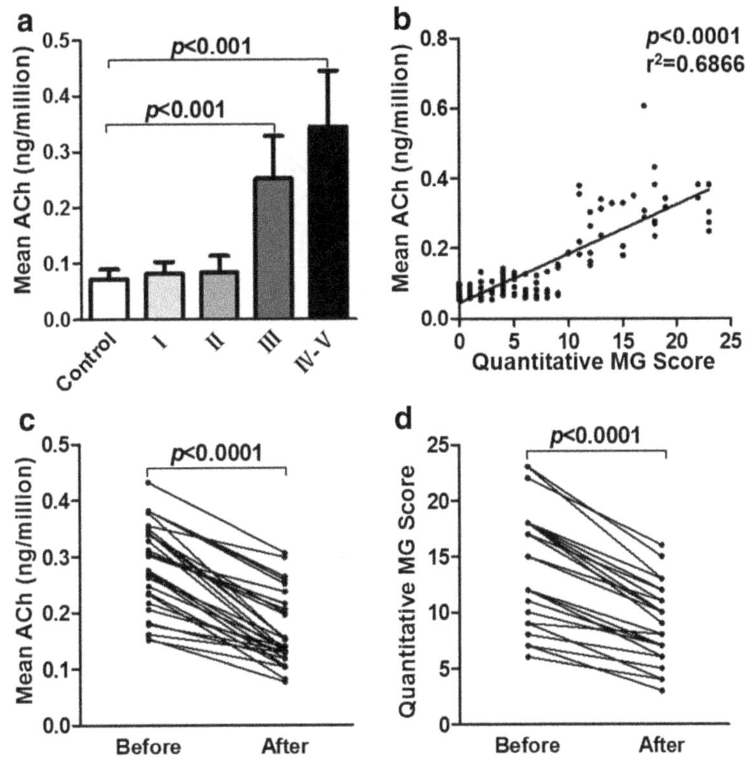

Fig. 2 PBMC-derived ACh levels correlate positively with MG severity. **a** Histogram shows that ACh concentrations per million cells increased along with MG severity according to the MGFA clinical classification ($n = 50$ for control, $n = 58$ for class I, $n = 30$ for class II, $n = 24$ for class III, $n = 13$ for class IV-V) ($p < 0.0001$). **b** ACh level distribution relative to QMG scores ($n = 125$) ($p < 0.0001$). **c** ACh content decreased in patient's blood drawn before treatment and 2 weeks after initial treatment, respectively ($p < 0.0001$). **d** QMG scores also decreased in patients ($p < 0.0001$). (**c-d**; $n = 30$ in each group)

($p > 0.05$) (Fig. 3e). Overall, some of our findings are in accord with those from previous studies [28–30]. The increased ACh levels denoted that cholinergic activity is potentiated and increased ACh levels may reflect an inflammatory status in patients with MG.

Cholinergic components in PBMCs

When we further explored discrepancies of cholinergic components in PBMCs from MG patients and controls, the relative expression of intracellular AChE and VAChT mRNA had decreased significantly in class III-V patients ($p = 0.0130$, $p = 0.0091$, respectively) (Fig. 4a-b). Yet we did not observe a statistically significant increase in ChAT mRNA expression ($p = 0.2175$) (Fig. 4c). These mRNA levels were similar to the corresponding proteins assessed by Western blotting (Fig. 4d). In addition, the levels of these three proteins in PBMCs were also measured by ELISA. The protein concentrations conformed to the show in Western blotting (Fig. 4e-g). These data thus indicate that the cholinergic activity was changed and the higher ACh levels observed in MG patients perhaps resulted from lower AChE expression.

Discussion

Our principal findings in this study are that ACh levels increase prominently in PBMCs from patients with MG exceeding those from healthy individuals and ACh likely correlates with the severity of MG. The up-regulated ACh may enhance the lymphocytes' ability to counteract inflammation via cholinergic signaling to restore homeostasis. Moreover, we observed elevations of circulating anti-MuSK Ab concentrations in MG patients with more serious clinical symptoms, which was accordance with a previous study [29]. Since non-neuronal ACh play an important role in immune regulation, an outcome that likely designates ACh as a possible homeostatic marker induced by the inflammatory reaction in MG.

Experimental evidence indicates that non-neuronal ACh profoundly modulates the innate immune system [7, 31] by binding to nicotinic AChRs such as those that inhibit cytokine release, ameliorate tissue injury and attenuate cytokine-mediated effects in experimental sepsis, endotoxemia and other inflammatory syndromes [8, 32, 33]. On the other hand, the cholinergic anti-inflammatory pathway may be activated by an inflammatory response [10]. Since the roles of PBMC-derived ACh in MG were not previously studied, our study may help to explore the

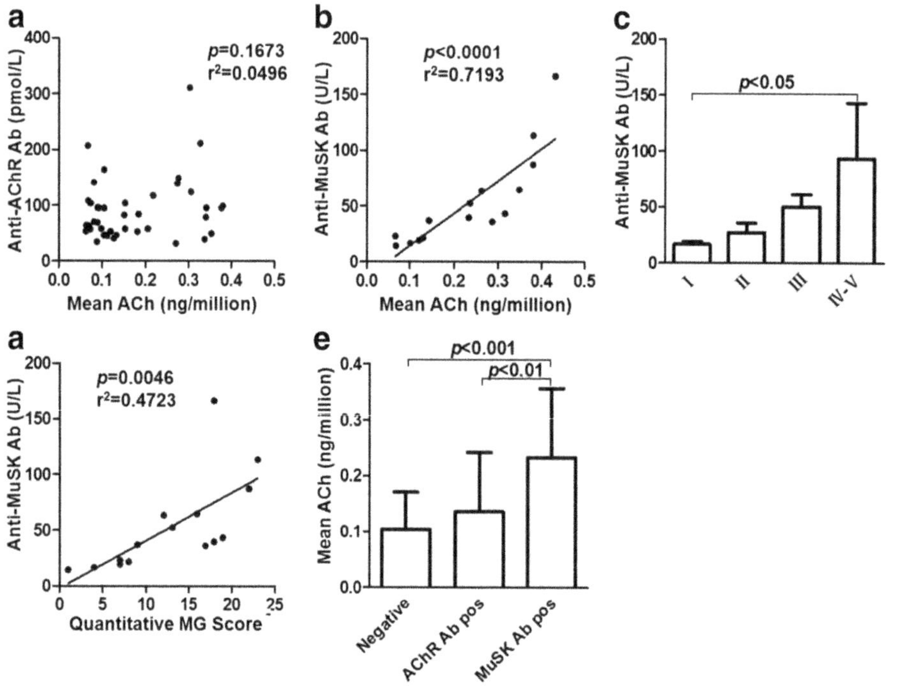

Fig. 3 PBMC-derived ACh is positively associated with anti-MuSK Ab concentrations. **a** No correlation was found between ACh levels and anti-AChR antibodies ($n = 40$) ($p = 0.1673$). **b** A positive correlation was found between ACh levels and anti-MuSK antibodies ($n = 15$) ($p < 0.0001$ by regression analysis). **c** Histogram shows that anti-MuSK Ab concentrations relative to MG severity ($n = 3$ for class I and II, $n = 4$ for class III, $n = 5$ for class IV-V) ($p = 0.0135$ by Kruskal-Wallis). **d** Anti-MuSK Ab distributions in relation to QMG scores ($n = 15$) ($p = 0.0046$ by regression analysis). **e** The ACh levels were higher in anti-MuSK Ab-positive group than that in double-negative and anti-AChR Ab-positive groups ($n = 24$ in double-negative group, $n = 86$ in anti-AChR Ab-positive group, $n = 15$ in anti-MuSK Ab-positive group) ($p < 0.001$, $p < 0.01$, respectively)

mechanism of MG from a different aspect. Indeed, PBMC-derived ACh levels were significantly higher in MG patients compared with those in healthy controls, particularly higher in class III-V patients according to the MGFA clinical classification. These differences may be caused by the extent of disease, since anti-inflammatory responses are usually determined by the magnitude of the inflammatory response [10]. Under inflammatory conditions in MG, the vagus nerve may be activated by pro-inflammatory cytokines, which could potentiate ACh production by splenic lymphocytes. Therefore, increasing ACh levels in PBMCs likely reflects MG-induced cholinergic hyperexcitation, which potentially serves as endogenous protection from excessive inflammatory reactions. Activation of ACh, therefore, represents a promising therapeutic strategy to improve cholinergic anti-inflammatory function and combat inflammation.

In humans, accumulating evidence indicates that AChE is directly or indirectly involved in the regulation of inflammatory responses or functions as a predictor of inflammation, usually correlated with multiple inflammatory markers, such as those in patients with inflammatory bowel disease [34] or stroke [35]. Presently, AChE inhibitors are used to interfere with the breakdown of ACh and impact the cholinergic system, such as in MG patients. In this current study, AChE expression was significantly lower in patients with MG than in their healthy counterparts, indicating a possible role of ACh content and AChE in regulating inflammation in MG patients.

To explore the potential relevance of ACh levels in the regulation of inflammation in MG, we further conducted a correlation analysis. Surprisingly, we found that ACh levels correlated positively with QMG scores as well as anti-MuSK Ab titers of MG patients. Actually, anti-MuSK-positive patients have a higher frequency of severe clinical symptoms [29]. As previously reported, quantities of anti-MuSK antibodies increased along with MG severity according to the MGFA clinical classification, and correlated with QMG scores in our cohort. As also demonstrated here, the more severe states of disease paralleled the higher PBMC-derived ACh concentrations. We then found that the trend of PBMC-derived ACh content and QMG scores declined in patients after treatment with immunotherapy, which maybe result from the declined cholinergic excitation when patients were in a relatively stable state after treatment. On the other hand, the immunotherapy may influenced the synthesis, storage and degradation of ACh. We therefore speculate that an endogenous ACh-mediated

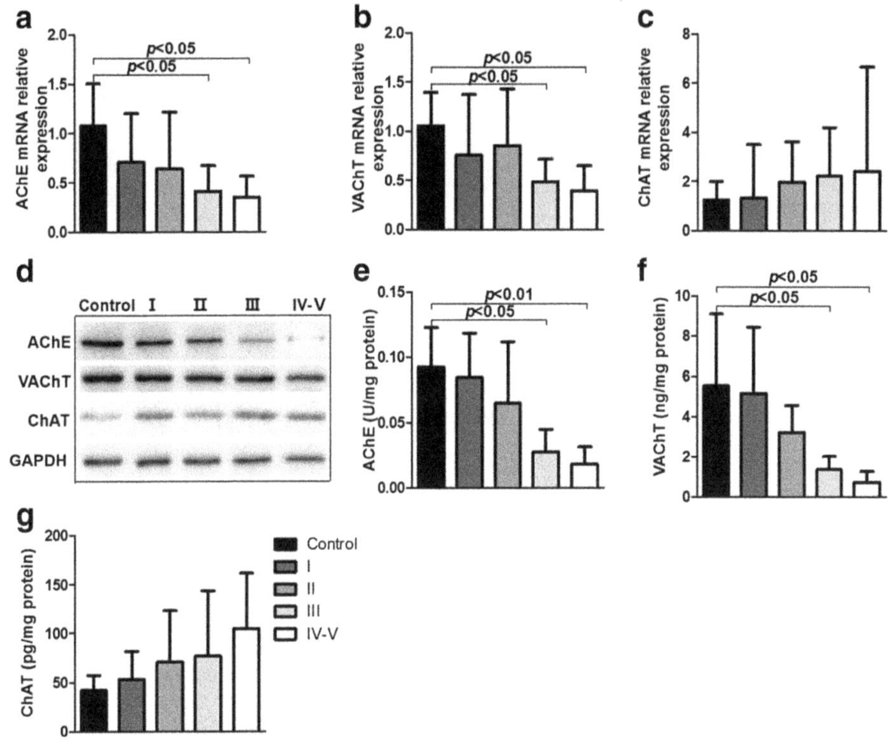

Fig. 4 Cholinergic components change in MG patients versus controls. **a** The expression of AChE mRNA was significantly declined in MG patients, especially class III-V, compared with controls ($p = 0.0130$ by Kruskal-Wallis). **b** The VAChT mRNA expression also decreased in MG patients ($p = 0.0091$ by Kruskal-Wallis). **c** There was no obvious change about the ChAT mRNA expression ($p = 0.2175$ by Kruskal-Wallis). **d** Western blots were used to assess levels of the corresponding proteins showing a similar tendency. **e** AChE protein expression in PBMCs detected by ELISA was significantly decreased in class III and class IV-V groups compared with control ($p < 0.05$, $p < 0.01$, respectively). The data were presented as U of AChE per mg protein. **f** VAChT expression was also reduced, especially in class III-V group ($p < 0.05$), compared with control. The data were presented as ng of VAChT per mg protein. **g** The level of ChAT in PBMCs was not significantly different among these groups ($p = 0.3271$). The data were presented as pg of ChAT per mg protein. (**a-c**; $n = 10$ in the control, class I, class II and class III groups, $n = 6$ in the class IV-V group) (**d-g**; $n = 5$ in each group)

anti-inflammatory pathway may be launched in an attempt to restore homeostasis in MG patients. However, the fact that anti-MuSK Ab levels remained high suggests that, despite higher levels of ACh, this pathway is not sufficient to reverse disease pathology, possibly due to their limited number [19].

Some limitations of our study must be addressed. First, studies *in vivo* and *in vitro* are still necessary to determine the relationships among all these components. Second, the changes of ACh might result from other factors that influence the cholinergic system, such as infection, age or emotion. Further studies should determine their contributions, if any.

Conclusions

Accumulating evidence suggests that non-neuronal ACh has immunomodulatory effects. Interestingly, we found that elevations in PBMC-derived ACh levels accompanied increasingly severe MG, which may be induced by inflammatory reflex and depend on the magnitude of the inflammatory response. Intervention in cholinergic activity may change the course of this disease. The decline of disease severity after treatment with immunotherapy indicates that ACh levels may be valuable for monitoring the progression or treatment efficacy of MG, which larger and well- defined cohort studies should confirm.

Abbreviations

ACh: Acetylcholine; AChE: Acetylcholinesterase; AChR: Acetylcholine receptor; ChAT: Choline acetyltransferase; ChT1: High-affinity choline transporter; MG: Myasthenia gravis; MGFA: Myasthenia Gravis Foundation of America; MuSK: Muscle-specific tyrosine kinase; QMG: Quantitative MG; UPLC-MS/MS: Ultra-performance liquid chromatography-tandem mass spectrometry; VAChT: Vesicular acetylcholine transporter

Acknowledgements

We wish to thank all participants in this study. We thank Yaowen Zhang, Chao Gao, Yali Bu and Hongwei Yang for the recruitment of subjects.

Funding

This work was financially supported by the National Natural Science Foundation of China (81571600, 81322018, 81273287 and 81100887 to JWH), the Youth Top-notch Talent Support Program, and the National Key Clinical Specialty Construction Project of China.

Authors' contributions

JH, BH, CZ, ARS and QL conceived and designed the project. BH, SL, YX, HS and ZG executed the experimental work. JH, BH, CZ and YX analyzed the data. JH, BH, CZ, ARS and QL wrote the manuscript. All authors read and approved the final manuscript.

Competing interests

The authors declare that they have no competing interests.

Author details

[1]Department of Neurology, Tianjin Neurological Institute, Tianjin Medical University General Hospital, Tianjin 300052, China. [2]Department of Neurology, Tianjin HuanHu Hospital, Tianjin 300060, China. [3]Laboratory of Physical and Chemical Research, Tianjin Centers for Disease Control and Prevention, Tianjin 300011, China. [4]Department of Neurology, Shandong Provincial Hospital Affiliated to Shandong University, Jinan, Shandong 250021, China. [5]Department of Neurology, Tianjin First Center Hospital, Tianjin Medical University, Tianjin 300192, China. [6]Département de chimie et biochimie, Université de Moncton, Moncton, New Brunswick E1A 3E9, Canada. [7]Department of Neurology, Barrow Neurological Institute, St. Joseph's Hospital and Medical Center, Phoenix, AZ 85013, USA.

References

1. Vincent A, Palace J, Hilton-Jones D. Myasthenia gravis. The Lancet. 2001; 357(9274):2122–8.
2. Meriggioli MN, Sanders DB. Autoimmune myasthenia gravis: emerging clinical and biological heterogeneity. The Lancet Neurology. 2009;8(5):475–90.
3. Berrih-Aknin S, Le Panse R. Myasthenia gravis: a comprehensive review of immune dysregulation and etiological mechanisms. J Autoimmun. 2014;52:90–100.
4. Grando SA, Kist DA, Qi M, Dahl MV. Human keratinocytes synthesize, secrete, and degrade acetylcholine. J Invest Dermatol. 1993;101(1):32–6.
5. Rodriguez-Diaz R, Dando R, Jacques-Silva MC, Fachado A, Molina J, Abdulreda MH, Ricordi C, Roper SD, Berggren PO, Caicedo A. Alpha cells secrete acetylcholine as a non-neuronal paracrine signal priming beta cell function in humans. Nat Med. 2011;17(7):888–92.
6. Fujii T, Yamada S, Watanabe Y, Misawa H, Tajima S, Fujimoto K, Kasahara T, Kawashima K. Induction of choline acetyltransferase mRNA in human mononuclear leukocytes stimulated by phytohemagglutinin, a T-cell activator. J Neuroimmunol. 1998;82(1):101–7.
7. Reardon C, Duncan GS, Brustle A, Brenner D, Tusche MW, Olofsson PS, Rosas-Ballina M, Tracey KJ, Mak TW. Lymphocyte-derived ACh regulates local innate but not adaptive immunity. Proc Natl Acad Sci U S A. 2013;110(4):1410–5.
8. Rosas-Ballina M, Olofsson PS, Ochani M, Valdes-Ferrer SI, Levine YA, Reardon C, Tusche MW, Pavlov VA, Andersson U, Chavan S, et al. Acetylcholine-synthesizing T cells relay neural signals in a vagus nerve circuit. Science (New York, NY). 2011;334(6052):98–101.
9. Steinman L. Elaborate interactions between the immune and nervous systems. Nat Immunol. 2004;5(6):575–81.
10. Tracey KJ. The inflammatory reflex. Nature. 2002;420(6917):853–9.
11. Ji H, Rabbi MF, Labis B, Pavlov VA, Tracey KJ, Ghia JE. Central cholinergic activation of a vagus nerve-to-spleen circuit alleviates experimental colitis. Mucosal Immunol. 2014;7(2):335–47.
12. Nizri E, Irony-Tur-Sinai M, Lory O, Orr-Urtreger A, Lavi E, Brenner T. Activation of the cholinergic anti-inflammatory system by nicotine attenuates neuroinflammation via suppression of Th1 and Th17 responses. J Immunol. 2009;183(10):6681–8.
13. Shi FD, Piao WH, Kuo YP, Campagnolo DI, Vollmer TL, Lukas RJ. Nicotinic attenuation of central nervous system inflammation and autoimmunity. J Immunol. 2009;182(3):1730–9.
14. Hao J, Simard AR, Turner GH, Wu J, Whiteaker P, Lukas RJ, Shi FD. Attenuation of CNS inflammatory responses by nicotine involves alpha7 and non-alpha7 nicotinic receptors. Exp Neurol. 2011;227(1):110–9.
15. Simard AR, Gan Y, St-Pierre S, Kousari A, Patel V, Whiteaker P, Morley BJ, Lukas RJ, Shi FD. Differential modulation of EAE by alpha9*- and beta2*-nicotinic acetylcholine receptors. Immunol Cell Biol. 2013;91(3):195–200.
16. Jiang W, St-Pierre S, Roy P, Morley BJ, Hao J, Simard AR. Infiltration of CCR2 + Ly6Chigh Proinflammatory Monocytes and Neutrophils into the Central Nervous System Is Modulated by Nicotinic Acetylcholine Receptors in a Model of Multiple Sclerosis. J Immunol. 2016;196(5):2095–108.
17. van Maanen MA, Lebre MC, van der Poll T, LaRosa GJ, Elbaum D, Vervoordeldonk MJ, Tak PP. Stimulation of nicotinic acetylcholine receptors attenuates collagen-induced arthritis in mice. Arthritis Rheum. 2009;60(1):114–22.
18. Bernik TR, Friedman SG, Ochani M, DiRaimo R, Susarla S, Czura CJ, Tracey KJ. Cholinergic antiinflammatory pathway inhibition of tumor necrosis factor during ischemia reperfusion. J Vasc Surg. 2002;36(6):1231–6.
19. Borovikova LV, Ivanova S, Zhang M, Yang H, Botchkina GI, Watkins LR, Wang H, Abumrad N, Eaton JW, Tracey KJ. Vagus nerve stimulation attenuates the systemic inflammatory response to endotoxin. Nature. 2000;405(6785):458–62.
20. Huston JM, Gallowitsch-Puerta M, Ochani M, Ochani K, Yuan R, Rosas-Ballina M, Ashok M, Goldstein RS, Chavan S, Pavlov VA, et al. Transcutaneous vagus nerve stimulation reduces serum high mobility group box 1 levels and improves survival in murine sepsis. Crit Care Med. 2007;35(12):2762–8.
21. van Westerloo DJ, Giebelen IA, Florquin S, Bruno MJ, Larosa GJ, Ulloa L, Tracey KJ, van der Poll T. The vagus nerve and nicotinic receptors modulate experimental pancreatitis severity in mice. Gastroenterology. 2006;130(6):1822–30.
22. Mioni C, Bazzani C, Giuliani D, Altavilla D, Leone S, Ferrari A, Minutoli L, Bitto A, Marini H, Zaffe D, et al. Activation of an efferent cholinergic pathway produces strong protection against myocardial ischemia/reperfusion injury in rats. Crit Care Med. 2005;33(11):2621–8.
23. Guarini S, Altavilla D, Cainazzo MM, Giuliani D, Bigiani A, Marini H, Squadrito G, Minutoli L, Bertolini A, Marini R, et al. Efferent vagal fibre stimulation blunts nuclear factor-kappaB activation and protects against hypovolemic hemorrhagic shock. Circulation. 2003;107(8):1189–94.
24. Jaretzki A, Barohn RJ, Ernstoff RM, Kaminski HJ, Keesey JC, Penn AS, Sanders DB. Myasthenia gravis: Recommendations for clinical research standards. Neurology. 2000;55(1):16–23.
25. Zhang C, Xia Y, Jiang W, Wang C, Han B, Hao J. Determination of non-neuronal acetylcholine in human peripheral blood mononuclear cells by use of hydrophilic interaction ultra-performance liquid chromatography-tandem mass spectrometry. J Chromatogr B Analyt Technol Biomed Life Sci. 2016;1022:265–73.
26. Barth D, Nabavi Nouri M, Ng E, Nwe P, Bril V. Comparison of IVIg and PLEX in patients with myasthenia gravis. Neurology. 2011;76(23):2017–23.
27. Zinman L, Ng E, Bril V. IV immunoglobulin in patients with myasthenia gravis: a randomized controlled trial. Neurology. 2007;68(11):837–41.
28. Vincent A, Bowen J, Newsom-Davis J, McConville J. Seronegative generalised myasthenia gravis: clinical features, antibodies, and their targets. The Lancet Neurology. 2003;2(2):99–106.
29. Bartoccioni E, Scuderi F, Minicuci GM, Marino M, Ciaraffa F, Evoli A. Anti-MuSK antibodies: correlation with myasthenia gravis severity. Neurology. 2006;67(3):505–7.
30. Gilhus NE, Verschuuren JJ. Myasthenia gravis: subgroup classification and therapeutic strategies. The Lancet Neurology. 2015;14(10):1023–36.
31. Kawashima K, Fujii T, Moriwaki Y, Misawa H, Horiguchi K. Reconciling neuronally and nonneuronally derived acetylcholine in the regulation of immune function. Ann N Y Acad Sci. 2012;1261:7–17.
32. Sternberg EM. Neural regulation of innate immunity: a coordinated nonspecific host response to pathogens. Nat Rev Immunol. 2006;6(4):318–28.
33. Tracey KJ. Physiology and immunology of the cholinergic antiinflammatory pathway. J Clin Invest. 2007;117(2):289–96.
34. Maharshak N, Shenhar-Tsarfaty S, Aroyo N, Orpaz N, Guberman I, Canaani J, Halpern Z, Dotan I, Berliner S, Soreq H. MicroRNA-132 modulates cholinergic signaling and inflammation in human inflammatory bowel disease. Inflamm Bowel Dis. 2013;19(7):1346–53.
35. Ben Assayag E, Shenhar-Tsarfaty S, Ofek K, Soreq L, Bova I, Shopin L, Berg RM, Berliner S, Shapira I, Bornstein NM, et al. Serum cholinesterase activities distinguish between stroke patients and controls and predict 12-month mortality. Molecular medicine (Cambridge, Mass). 2010;16(7-8):278–86.

2

Outcome of neurological early rehabilitation patients carrying multi-drug resistant bacteria

J. D. Rollnik[1*], M. Bertram[2], C. Bucka[3], M. Hartwich[4], M. Jöbges[5], G. Ketter[6], B. Leineweber[7], M. Mertl-Rötzer[8], D. A. Nowak[9], T. Platz[10], K. Scheidtmann[11], R. Thomas[12], F. von Rosen[13], C. W. Wallesch[14], H. Woldag[15], P. Peschel[16], J. Mehrholz[17] and M. Pohl[18]

Abstract

Background: Colonization or infection with multi-drug resistant (MDR) bacteria is considered detrimental to the outcome of neurological and neurosurgical early rehabilitation patients.

Methods: In a German multi-center study, 754 neurological early rehabilitation patients were enrolled and and reviewed in respect to MDR status, length of stay (LOS) and the following outcome variables: Barthel Index (BI), Early Rehabilitation Index (ERI), Glasgow Outcome Score Extended (GOSE), Coma Remission Scale (CRS), Functional Ambulation Categories (FAC).

Results: The mean age of the study population was 68.0 ± 14.8 years. Upon admission, the following prevalence for MDRs was observed: MRSA (methicillin resistant staphylococcus aureus) 7.0% (53/754), ESBL- (extended spectrum beta-lactamase) producing bacteria strains 12.6% (95/754), VRE (vancomycin resistant enterococci) 2.8% (21/754). Patients colonized or infected with MDR bacteria (MDR+) were significantly more frequently diagnosed with a critical illness polyneuropathy – CIP – than non-colonized (MDR-) patients: 29.0% vs. 14.8%. In addition, they were more frequently mechanically ventilated (MDR+: 55/138, 39.9%; MDR- 137/616, 22.2%). MDR+ patients were referred to rehabilitation earlier, had a longer LOS in early rehabilitation, lower BI on admission and at discharge, lower ERI on admission and lower CRS at discharge than MDR- patients. There was a highly significant correlation of the BI upon admission with the BI at discharge ($r_s = 0.492$, $p < 0.001$). GOSE at discharge differed significantly between both groups (χ^2-test, $p < 0.01$). Perhaps of greatest importance, mortality among MDR+ was higher in comparison to MDR- (18.1% vs. 7.6%).

Conclusions: The outcome of neurological early rehabilitation patients colonized or infected with MDR bacteria including MRSA or ESBL producing strains is significantly poorer than by non-colonized patients. There is some evidence that the poor outcome could be related to the higher morbidity and lower functional status upon admission.

Keywords: MRSA, ESBL, Early rehabilitation, Outcome

* Correspondence: prof.rollnik@bdh-klinik-hessisch-oldendorf.de
[1]Institute for Neurorehabilitation Research (InFo), BDH-Klinik Hessisch Oldendorf, Hannover Medical School (MHH), Greitstr. 18-28, 31840 Hess. Oldendorf, Germany
Full list of author information is available at the end of the article

Background

In Germany, there exist an increasing number of specialized hospitals for early neurological and neurosurgical rehabilitation. These hospitals continue intensive and intermediate care treatment of patients who have been treated in intensive care units of acute-care facilities, who do not require specialized interventions but are still dependent on an intensive care setting. Many patients cared for in neurological and neurosurgical early rehabilitation facilities were previously treated in non-neurological/non-neurosurgical clinics, most of them suffering from neurological complications including critical illness polyneuropathy (CIP), hypoxic or septic encephalopathy [1].

Colonization and/or infection with multi-drug resistant (MDR) bacteria including methicillin resistant Staphylococcus aureus (MRSA) or extended spectrum beta-lactamase (ESBL) producing gram-negative strains is a challenge in neurological and neurosurgical early rehabilitation. To date, it has been shown that MRSA prevalence upon admission ranges from 7.0 to 14.5% [1–3], whereas colonization with ESBL producing bacteria from 12.6 to 14.0% [1, 3, 4]. Other MDR strains including vancomycin-resistant enterococci (VRE) play a minor role, being present in only approximately 2.8% of cases [1].

This means that almost every fourth patient entering neurological early rehabilitation is either colonized or infected with multi-drug resistant bacteria [1–4].

When a patient with MRSA or ESBL-producing bacteria is admitted, contact precautions (isolation) are recommended in Germany, in particular on intensive or intermediate care units [5, 6]. Obviously, isolation measures in rehabilitation facilities raise ethical concerns [7], due to their being responsible for symptoms of psychological distress including depression and anxiety [8]. Isolation measures interfere with the traditional rehabilitative approach and may cause poorer outcomes [7].

The impact of contact precautions on the outcome of neurological early rehabilitation patients was recently investigated in two single-center studies [9, 10]. It was shown that functional recovery of patients colonized or infected with either MRSA or ESBL-producing bacteria was poorer than in non-colonized patients [9, 10]. However, the poorer outcome was not a result of less therapy (due to isolation) but due to the lower functional status and higher morbidity upon admission [9, 10].

The present paper is based upon data from a 2014 German multi-center study on neurological and neurosurgical early rehabilitation [1]. The focus of the present investigation was to analyze the influence of multi-drug resistant bacteria upon the outcome of the rehabilitation measure.

Methods

The multi-center study collected data prospectively from 754 patients admitted to 16 German neurological early rehabilitation centers in March, 2014 [1]. Prevalence of patients carrying MDR bacteria (colonization or infection) on admission was documented.

Age, gender, primary diagnosis, medical devices, Glasgow Coma Scale (GCS) [11], Coma Remission Scale (CRS) [12], Barthel Index (BI) [13], Early Rehabilitation Index (ERI) [14] and FAC (Functional Ambulation Categories) [15] on admission and at discharge were documented. In addition, Glasgow Outcome Scale-Extended (GOSE) [16] was obtained at discharge.

Statistics: Since main variables such as BI on admission and at discharge were not normally distributed, non-parametric testing was performed. Statistical analyses included χ^2-, Mann-Whitney-U-tests for independent samples and Spearman-Rho correlations. Differences were regarded as significant with $p < 0.05$. Nonetheless, in the results section, mean values and standard deviations are displayed.

Results

The mean age of the whole study sample was 68.0 ± 14.8 years; 297 (39.4%) subjects were female. On admission, MRSA prevalence was 7.0% (53/754), ESBL-producing bacteria were present in 12.6% (95/754), while VRE were found in only 2.8% (21/754) of cases. Carriers of MRSA, ESBL-producing germs or VRE were assigned to the multi-drug resistant positive (MDR+) group (138/754, 18.3%), all other patients were regarded as MDR negative (MDR-). 31 MDR+ patients were colonized with more than one MDR strain.

Primary diagnoses and characteristics of MDR+ and MDR- patients are to be found in Tables 1 and 2.

Diagnoses were unequally distributed between MDR+ and MDR- (χ^2-test, $p < 0.001$), Table 1. The

Table 1 Primary diagnoses of early rehabilitation patients with (MDR+) and without (MDR-) multi-drug resistant (MDR) bacteria

	MDR+	MDR-	Sum
Polyneuropathy or other peripheral nerve impairment	40 (29.0%)	91 (14.8%)	131
Ischemic stroke	32 (23.2%)	207 (33.6%)	239
Intracranial hemorrhage	22 (15.9%)	132 (21.4%)	154
Traumatic brain injury	14 (10.1%)	73 (11.9%)	87
Hypoxia	9 (6.5%)	38 (6.2%)	47
Spinal cord injury	9 (6.5%)	19 (3.1%)	28
Brain tumor	3 (2.2%)	18 (2.9%)	21
Other primary diagnosis	9 (6.5%)	38 (6.2%)	47
Sum	138 (100%)	616 (100%)	754

Table 2 Characteristics of MDR+ and MDR- neurological early rehabilitation patients

	MDR+	MDR-	*p*-value*
N	138	616	-
Sex (m/w)	90/48	367/249	n.s.**
Age [years]	67.9 (13.7)	68.0 (15.0)	n.s.
Disease onset [days prior to admission]	51.5 (59.9)	75.1 (557.8)	<0.001
Length of stay in neurological early rehabilitation [days]	69.0 (64.7)	54.3 (46.3)	<0.01
Barthel Index (BI) on admission [0 to 100]	4.7 (7.3)	9.3 (11.9)	<0.001
BI at discharge [0 to 100]	20.0 (22.4)	26.2 (22.8)	<0.01
Λ BI (discharge-admission)	15.3 (21.5)	16.8 (19.5)	n.s.
Early Rehabilitation Index (ERI) on admission [−325 to 0]	−129.0 (86.6)	−108.8 (84.3)	<0.05
ERI at discharge [−325 to 0]	−62.5 (75.4)	−53.5 (63.8)	n.s.
Λ ERI (discharge-admission)	55.3 (74.0)	66.5 (82.5)	n.s.
Coma Remission Scale (CRS) on admission [0 to 24]	17.8 (7.8)	18.4 (7.4)	n.s.
CRS at discharge [0 to 24]	18.1 (9.2)	20.3 (7.4)	<0.05
Λ CRS (discharge-admission)	0.0 (9.5)	1.6 (7.3)	n.s.
Glasgow Coma Scale (GCS) on admission [3 to 15]	11.5 (3.8)	11.8 (3.6)	n.s.
GCS at discharge [3 to 15]	11.7 (4.7)	12.9 (3.6)	n.s.
Λ GCS (discharge-admission)	0.1 (4.9)	1.1 (3.4)	n.s.

Mean and standard deviation are displayed
* Mann-Whitney-*U*-test, ** χ^2-test, n.s. = not significant ($p > 0.05$)

most frequent diagnosis among MDR+ was critical-illness polyneuropathy (CIP) and a higher proportion of MDR+ patients suffered from CIP compared to MDR- (29.0% vs. 14.8%). This finding could be explained by the fact that relatively more MDR+ were mechanically ventilated on admission (MDR+: 55/138, 39.9%; MDR- 137/616, 22.2%) and CIP was the leading diagnosis among ventilated patients (71/192, 37.0%). Ventilated patients had a significantly lower BI on admission ($p < 0.001$) and at discharge ($p < 0.001$) than spontaneously breathing patients.

MDR+ patients were referred to rehabilitation earlier, had a longer length of stay (LOS) in early rehabilitation, lower BI on admission and at discharge, lower ERI on admission and lower CRS at discharge, Table 2. BI upon admission correlated significantly with BI at discharge ($r_s = 0.492$, $p < 0.001$). The older the patients, the lower the BI at discharge was documented ($r_s = -0.174$, $p < 0.001$). However, MDR+ and MDR- did not differ significantly with respect to age (Table 2).

GOSE at discharge differed significantly between both groups (χ^2-test, $p < 0.01$), in particular mortality among MDR+ was higher compared to MDR- (18.1% vs. 7.6%), Table 3.

Table 3 Glasgow Outcome Scale - Extended (GOSE) at discharge

GOSE	MDR+	MDR-	Sum
1 death	25 (18.1%)	47 (7.6%)	72 (9.5%)
2 vegetative state	12 (8.7%)	45 (7.3%)	57 (7.6%)
3 lower severe disability	41 (29.7%)	246 (39.9%)	287 (38.1%)
4 upper severe disability	58 (42.0%)	257 (41.7%)	315 (41.8%)
5 lower moderate disability	2 (1.4%)	21 (3.4%)	23 (3.1%)
6 upper moderate disability	0	0	0
7 lower good recovery	0	0	0
8 upper good recovery	0	0	0
Sum	138 (100%)	616 (100%)	754 (100%)

Neither FAC on admission (Table 4) nor at discharge (Table 5) differed significantly between both groups (χ^2-test, n.s.).

Discussion

The high prevalence of MDR bacteria is an emerging challenge in neurological and neurosurgical early rehabilitation. In the present study, 18.3% of all patients were either colonized or infected with MDR bacteria upon admission. While MRSA prevalence (7.0%) was lower than reported before [2, 3], colonization with MDR gram negative strains (12.6%) was in line with previous studies [2, 4]. MRSA and ESBL producing bacteria proved to be quite common, whereas the VRE prevalence was less than 3%.

It has previously been shown in a single-center study that patients with MRSA or ESBL-producing germs are at risk for a poor outcome [9, 10]. The present multi-center

Table 4 Functional Ambulation Categories (FAC) upon admission

FAC	MDR+	MDR-	Sum
0 - patient cannot walk	128 (92.8%)	541 (88.1%)	669 (89.0%)
1 - patients needs firm continuous support from 1 person who helps carrying weight and with balance	6 (4.3%)	45 (7.3%)	51 (6.8%)
2 - patient needs continuous or intermittent support of one person to help with balance and coordination.	2 (1.4%)	18 (2.9%)	20 (2.7%)
3 - patient requires verbal supervision or stand-by help from one person without physical contact	2 (1.4%)	9 (1.5%)	11 (1.5%)
4 - patient can walk independently on level ground, but requires help on stairs, slopes or uneven surfaces	0	1 (0.2%)	1 (0.1%)
5 - patient can walk independently anywhere	0	0	0
Sum	138 (100%)	614 (100%)	752 (100%)

Table 5 Functional Ambulation Categories (FAC) at discharge

FAC	MDR+	MDR-	Sum
0 - patient cannot walk	88 (65.2%)	336 (56.0%)	424 (57.7%)
1 - patients needs firm continuous support from 1 person who helps carrying weight and with balance	16 (11.9%)	69 (11.5%)	85 (11.6%)
2 - patient needs continuous or intermittent support of one person to help with balance and coordination.	12 (8.9%)	85 (14.2%)	97 (13.2%)
3 - patient requires verbal supervision or stand-by help from one person without physical contact	10 (7.4%)	64 (10.7%)	74 (10.1%)
4 - patient can walk independently on level ground, but requires help on stairs, slopes or uneven surfaces	8 (5.9%)	37 (6.2%)	45 (6.1%)
5 - patient can walk independently anywhere	1 (0.7%)	9 (1.5%)	10 (1.4%)
Sum	135 (100%)	600 (100%)	735 (100%)

data support this hypothesis. MDR+ had a significantly worse functional status – as measured with the BI – at discharge. While FAC did not show significant differences between MDR+ and MDR-, the GOS was poorer among carriers of MDR bacteria.

How are these data to be interpreted? First of all, functional status on admission was lower among MDR+ patients. Some authors have suggested that low a functional status upon admission may be one of the most important predictors for a poor outcome [9, 10]. There was a clear, highly significant correlation between BI on admission and at discharge in the present study sample. Furthermore, ERI on admission was lower in the MDR+ group. The ERI provides a good estimate of early rehabilitation patients' morbidity [14, 17]. In addition, we found that among patients on mechanical ventilation, a significantly higher proportion of patients were MDR+. It is well known that mechanically ventilated patients have a higher morbidity, mortality and poorer outcome in neurological early rehabilitation [1, 18, 19].

In addition, improvements in the assessments (ERI, CRS and GCS) from admission to discharge were not differing between MDR+ and MDR- groups. As far as the changes in BI (discharge minus admission) are concerned, it has to be pointed out that there were no significant differences between the groups, either. So, MDR+ patients benefitted from neurological early rehabilitation, despite lower functional status on admission and contact precautions.

Another finding was that MDR+ patients were referred earlier to rehabilitation from acute-care hospitals than MDR-. One possible explanation for this finding is the fact that colonization with MDR bacteria pose a significant economic burden, since patients colonized with MRSA and ESBL producing bacteria have to be frequently isolated, thus occupying hospital beds [3]. This might contribute to earlier transfers to rehabilitation facilities in order to minimize financial losses in acute-care hospitals. In addition, patients requiring prolonged weaning from mechanical ventilation are steadily increasing in early rehabilitation facilities [1, 18, 19]. Overall, this is a welcome trend since neurologically impaired patients, e.g., following stroke, may profit from an early transfer [20]. Further studies are required on the impact of MDR bacteria on the outcome of neurological and neurosurgical early rehabilitation patients.

Conclusions

The outcome of neurological early rehabilitation patients with multi-drug resistant (MDR) bacteria such as MRSA or ESBL producing strains is poorer than by non-colonized patients. There is some evidence that the poor outcome may be explained by higher morbidity and lower functional status on admission.

Abbreviations

BI: Barthel Index; CIP: Critical illness polyneuropathy; CRS: Coma remission scale; ERI: Early rehabilitation index; ESBL: Extended spectrum beta-lactamase; FAC: Functional ambulation categories; GCS: Glasgow coma scale; GOSE: Glasgow outcome scale extended; LOS: Length of stay; MDR: Multi-drug resistant; MRSA: Methicillin resistant staphylococcus aureus; VRE: Vancomycin resistant enterococci

Acknowledgements

The authors are thankful for the support by the Dept. of Public Health, University of Dresden, Germany.

Funding

Not applicable.

Authors' contributions

JDR as the first author made statistical analyses, drafted and wrote the paper. MP as senior author was director of the multi-center study on neurological early rehabilitation [1] and approved the final version of this paper. All other authors contributed data, read and approved the paper.

Competing interests

The authors declare that they have no competing interests.

Author details

[1]Institute for Neurorehabilitation Research (InFo), BDH-Klinik Hessisch Oldendorf, Hannover Medical School (MHH), Greitstr. 18-28, 31840 Hess. Oldendorf, Germany. [2]Kliniken Schmieder Heidelberg, Heidelberg, Germany. [3]Neurologische Klinik Westend, Bad Wildungen, Germany. [4]Asklepios Schlossberg Klinik Bad König, Bad König, Germany. [5]Brandenburg Klinik Bernau, Berlin, Germany. [6]Neurologisches Rehabilitationszentrum "Godeshöhe" Bonn, Bonn, Germany. [7]Neurologische Klinik GmbH Bad Neustadt, Bad Neustadt an der Saale, Germany. [8]Schön Klinik Bad Aibling, Bad Aibling, Germany. [9]Helios Klinik Kipfenberg, Kipfenberg, Germany. [10]BDH-Klinik Greifswald, Greifswald, Germany. [11]Hegau-Jugendwerk Gailingen, Gailingen, Germany. [12]Asklepios Kliniken Schildautal Seesen, Seesen,

Germany. [13]Schön Klinik Bad Staffelstein, Bad Staffelstein, Germany. [14]BDH-Klinik Elzach, Elzach, Germany. [15]Neurologisches Rehabilitationszentrum Leipzig, Bennewitz, Germany. [16]Department of Public Health, University of Dresden, Dresden, Germany. [17]Department of Public Health, University of Dresden, Dresden, Germany. [18]Klinik Schloss Pulsnitz, Pulsnitz, Germany.

References

1. Pohl M, Bertram M, Bucka C, Hartwich M, Jöbges M, Ketter G, Leineweber B, Mertl-Rötzer M, Platz T, Rollnik JD, Scheidtmann K, Thomas R, von Rosen F, Wallesch C, Woldag H, Peschel P, Mehrholz J. Course of Rehabilitation in the Early Neurological/Neurosurgical Rehabilitation: Results of a Multi-Centre Evaluation in Germany 2014. Nervenarzt. 2016, in press.
2. Thomas R. MRSA in early rehabilitation – incidence, prevalence and morbidity. Neurol Rehabil. 2013;19:118–22.
3. Rollnik JD, Samady AM, Grüter L. Multidrug-resistant germs in neurological early rehabilitation (2004–2013). Rehabilitation (Stuttg). 2014;53:346–50.
4. Thomas R, Zimmermann O. In-hospital rehabilitation: bacterial spectrum and resistance development in a German institution. Neurol Rehabil. 2013;19:321–6.
5. Commission for Hospital Hygiene and Infection Prevention at the Robert Koch-Institute. Recommendations for the prevention and control of methicillin-resistant Staphylococcus aureus isolates (MRSA) in hospitals and other healthcare facilities. GMS Krankenhhyg Interdiszip. 2009;4:Doc01.
6. Commission for Hospital Hygiene and Infection Prevention at the Robert Koch-Institute. Hygiene measures for infection or colonization with multidrug-resistant gram-negative bacilli. Commission recommendation for hospital hygiene and infection prevention (KRINKO) at the Robert Koch Institute (RKI). Bundesgesundheitsbl. 2012;55:1311–54.
7. Pike JH, McLean D. Ethical concerns in isolating patients with methicillin-resistant Staphylococcus aureus on the rehabilitation ward: a case report. Arch Phys Med Rehabil. 2002;83:1028–30.
8. Tarzi S, Kennedy P, Stone S, Evans M. Methicillin-resistant Staphylococcus aureus: psychological impact of hospitalization and isolation in an older adult population. J Hosp Infect. 2001;49:250–4.
9. Rollnik JD. Outcome of MRSA carriers in neurological early rehabilitation. BMC Neurol. 2014;14:34.
10. Rollnik JD. Outcome of neurological early rehabilitation patients colonized with extended-spectrum beta-lactamase (ESBL) producing bacteria. Open J Ther Rehabil. 2015;3:1–8.
11. Teasdale G, Jennett B. Assessment of coma and impaired consciousness. A practical scale. Lancet. 1974;2:81–3.
12. Ortega-Suhrkamp E, von Wild KR. Standards of neurologic-neurosurgical early rehabilitation–a concept of the study group neurological-neurosurgical early rehabilitation. Acta Neurochir Supp. 2002;79:11–9.
13. Mahoney FI, Barthel DW. Functional evaluation: the Barthel index. Md State Med J. 1965;14:61–5.
14. Rollnik JD. The Early Rehabilitation Barthel Index (ERBI). Rehabilitation (Stuttg). 2011;50:408–11.
15. Lord SE, McPherson K, McNaughton HK, Rochester L, Weatherall M. Community ambulation after stroke: how important and obtainable is it and what measures appear predictive? Arch Phys Med Rehabil. 2004;8:234–9.
16. Wilson JTL, Pettigrew LEL, Teasdale GM. Structured interviews for the Glasgow outcome scale and the extended Glasgow outcome scale: guidelines for their use. J Neurotrauma. 1997;15:573–85.
17. Rollnik JD, Janosch U. Current trends in the length of stay in neurological early rehabilitation. Dtsch Arztebl Int. 2010;107:286–92.
18. Oehmichen F, Ketter G, Mertl-Rötzer M, Platz T, Puschendorf W, Rollnik JD, Schaupp M, Pohl M. Weaning from prolonged mechanical ventilation in neurological weaning units: an evaluation of the German Working Group for early Neurorehabilitation. Nervenarzt. 2012;83:1300–7.
19. Rollnik JD, Berlinghof K, Lenz O, Bertomeu AM. Mechanical ventilation in neurological early rehabilitation. Akt Neurol. 2010;37:316–8.
20. Musicco M, Emberti L, Nappi G, Caltagirone C. Italian Multicenter Study on Outcomes of Rehabilitation of Neurological Patients. Early and long-term outcome of rehabilitation in stroke patients: the role of patient characteristics, time of initiation, and duration of interventions. Arch Phys Med Rehabil. 2003; 84:551–8.

3

A diagnostic biomarker profile for fibromyalgia syndrome based on an NMR metabolomics study of selected patients and controls

Bontle G. Malatji[1], Helgard Meyer[2], Shayne Mason[1], Udo F.H. Engelke[3], Ron A. Wevers[3], Mari van Reenen[1] and Carolus J. Reinecke[1*]

Abstract

Background: Fibromyalgia syndrome (FMS) is a chronic pain syndrome. A plausible pathogenesis of the disease is uncertain and the pursuit of measurable biomarkers for objective identification of affected individuals is a continuing endeavour in FMS research. Our objective was to perform an explorative metabolomics study (1) to elucidate the global urinary metabolite profile of patients suffering from FMS, and (2) to explore the potential of this metabolite information to augment existing medical practice in diagnosing the disease.

Methods: We selected patients with a medical history of persistent FMS (n = 18), who described their recent state of the disease through the Fibromyalgia Impact Questionnaire (FIQR) and an in-house clinical questionnaire (IHCQ). Three control groups were used: first-generation family members of the patients (n = 11), age-related individuals without any indications of FMS or related conditions (n = 10), and healthy young (18–22 years) individuals (n = 20). All subjects were female and the biofluid under investigation was urine. Correlation analysis of the FIQR showed the FMS patients represented a well-defined disease group for this metabolomics study. Spectral analyses of urine were conducted using a 500 MHz ^{1}H nuclear magnetic resonance (NMR) spectrometer; data processing and analyses were performed using Matlab, R, SPSS and SAS software.

Results and discussion: Unsupervised and supervised multivariate analyses distinguished all three control groups and the FMS patients, and significant increases in metabolites related to the gut microbiome (hippuric, succinic and lactic acids) were observed. We have developed an algorithm for the diagnosis of FMS consisting of three metabolites — succinic acid, taurine and creatine — that have a good level of diagnostic accuracy (Receiver Operating Characteristic (ROC) analysis — area under the curve 90%) and on the pain and fatigue symptoms for the selected FMS patient group.

Conclusion: Our data and comparative analyses indicated an altered metabolic profile of patients with FMS, analytically detectable within their urine. Validation studies may substantiate urinary metabolites to supplement information from medical assessment, tender-point measurements and FIQR questionnaires for an improved objective diagnosis of FMS.

Keywords: Fibromyalgia syndrome, Proton nuclear magnetic resonance (^{1}H–NMR) spectroscopy, Metabolomics, Metabolite markers, Pain

* Correspondence: carools.reinecke@nwu.ac.za
[1]Centre for Human Metabolomics, Faculty of Natural Sciences, North-West University (Potchefstroom Campus), Private Bag X6001, Potchefstroom, South Africa
Full list of author information is available at the end of the article

Background

Fibromyalgia syndrome (FMS) is a common chronic pain syndrome characterized by widespread musculo-skeletal pain and associated with multiple other symptoms such as cognitive impairment, disrupted sleep and chronic fatigue. The American College of Rheumtology (ACR) first published criteria for FMS in 1990 [1] which emphasized chronic widespread musculo-skeletal pain (including pain in the axial skeleton) in the presence of pain on at least 11 of 18 specified tender point sites with digital palpation of 4 kg/cm2.

The 2010 ACR updated criteria for FMS [2] are applied in a 2-part, self-administered questionnaire and do not require a tender point assessment. The first part assesses the presence of pain at 19 sites on a body diagram (widespread pain index) and part 2 measures the symptom severity score (0–3) of 3 core symptoms (insomnia, fatigue and cognitive impairment) and an average score (0–3) for additional somatic symptoms. FMS is the most common cause of widespread or generalized musculo-skeletal pain and affects 2–8% of the adult population with the highest prevalence in women between 30 and 55 years. [3, 4].

FMS is currently viewed as a central sensitivity syndrome associated with abnormal pain processing. It is regarded as a "pain amplification syndrome" associated with increased sensitivity of the nervous system and decreased anti-nociception which results in the clinical phenomena of hyperalgesia and allodynia. Dysfunction in central mono-aminergic neurotransmission which involves serotonin, norepinephrine, nerve growth factor, substance P and others have been implicated in the patho-physiology of FMS. [5–8] FMS patients often have associated comorbidities such as irritable bowel syndrome, interstitial cystitis and mood disorders [9, 10].

In the absence of an objective biomarker, the diagnosis of FMS is based on a comprehensive clinical assessment. Before 2010, the diagnosis was principally based on the 1990 ACR criteria of widespread pain (including in the axial skeleton) > 3 months and at least 11 painful "tender points" with digital palpation. Although the 2010 ACR criteria do not include a "tender point" count, a musculo-skeletal clinical examination remains mandatory, to exclude other couses of widespread pain and also to identify peripheral pain generators e.g. myofascial trigger points. Selective use of laboratory testing is used to exclude other causes of widespread pain such as polymyalgia rheumatica and hypothyroidism.

The pursuit of specific and measurable biomarkers that may assist in objectively identifying susceptible individuals, confirming disease diagnosis and facilitating treatment, is a continuing endeavour in FMS research. The development of high-throughput metabolic profiling and the study of the metabolome have proven to be particularly applicable in neurological research where small molecules are key in neurochemical metabolism and in performing a role as neurotransmitters, signalling modulators and osmolytes. It is now generally anticipated that metabolomics profiling methods, linked to systems biology approaches, will emerge with well-defined metabolic phenotypes, enhancing the understanding of brain metabolism in health and disease. Recently, a few metabolomics studies have been reported on fibromyalgia, potentially disclosing novel insights into metabolic perturbations in the brain that go brain metabolic homeostasis beyond alterations of neurotransmission variations associated with neurological disorders [11].

In a pilot study, presented only as a poster at an Annual Meeting of the Rheumatologic Society of the UK [12], Richards and co-workers (2001) reported that muscle metabolites detected in the urine of fibromyalgia patients may suggest a prevailing muscle damage. Although not by definition a metabolomics study, their targeted metabolite analysis of urine by nuclear magnetic resonance (NMR) spectroscopy revealed significant levels of creatine in FMS patients and elevated (t-test $p < 0.05$) urinary excretion of choline, taurine, citrate and trimethylamine N-oxide (TMAO) relative to matched controls.

The first metabolomics study on FMS, reported in 2013 [13], used 50 μl blood samples collected on blood spot cards (Whatman 903 Protein Saver Snap Apart Card, GE Healthcare, Westborough, MA, USA) from patients diagnosed with FMS (n = 14), osteoarthritis (OA; n = 15) and rheumatoid arthritis (RA; n = 12). Samples were dried and then transported to the laboratory for mid-infrared micro-spectroscopy (IRMS) and other analyses. The RA and OA groups appeared to be metabolically similar, but different from the metabolite profile of FMS. The IRMS approach did not conclusively identify the metabolites responsible for the diagnostic spectral differentiation, although changes in tryptophan catabolism seemed to be involved.

Another metabolomics approach to FMS involved liquid chromatography/quadrupole–time-of-flight/mass spectrometry (LC/Q-TOF/MS) with multivariate statistical analysis aimed at discriminating FMS patients (n = 22) and controls (n = 21) from blood plasma analysis [14]. Lysophosphocholine (lysoPCs), phosphocholine and ceramide lipids dominated the metabolite profile. The metabolites that discriminated the most between FMS patients and controls were identified as 1-tetradecanoyl-sn-glycero-3-phosphocholine [PC(14:0/0:0)] and 1-hexadecanoyl-sn-glycero-3-phosphocholine [PC(16:0/0:0)] — suggesting that lysoPCs may be potential biomarkers for FMS.

In addition to these metabolomics findings, a recent review on biomarkers of FMS included contributions from genetic and proteomic studies [15]. Although genetic factors have been shown to influence predisposition to FMS, no specific genes have been confirmed as being involved in this disease [16]. The review also listed several proteins of the immune response, cytoskeleton remodelling and the inflammatory process in FMS. Their role in FMS, however, is still controversial.

Thus the availability of biomarkers for unequivocal and objective diagnosis of FMS remains elusive in clinical practice. Yet, metabolites identified as being involved in the aetiology and pathogenesis of FMS could meanwhile contribute to insights into various presentations of FMS and provide ancillary diagnostic testing criteria to complement general diagnostic procedures. We thus present here the outcomes of a ^{1}H NMR metabolomics study on FMS. All experimental subjects were females and provided urine samples for the study. The investigation was designed as an untargeted approach and revealed metabolite information with predictive potential to discriminate between FMS patients and healthy young controls. The outcomes thus underscore the versatility of metabolomics to provide insights into disease pathophysiology, furthering potential novel approaches to supplement existing protocols proposed for the practising clinician to assess FMS and monitor its treatment [17].

Methods

Experimental subjects, physical characteristics, symptoms and clinical profiles

All the patients that were included in this study were previously diagnosed with FMS by the same specialist pain clinician from his chronic pain practice in Pretoria. This practice manages the full spectrum of chronic pain disorders, with a special interest in FMS and related pain disorders. The diagnosis was based on a comprehensive clinical assessment using the 1990 criteria. All patients in the study were confirmed with FMS before 2010 and all were on a comprehensive evidence-based management programme according to international guidelines. They were only included if they continued to complain of widespread musculo-skeletal pain (including in the axial skeleton) in the presence of >11 painful tender points with musculo-skeletal assessment.

Informed consent was obtained from all the participants in this study by means of a voluntarily completed consent form; ethical approval for the study was obtained as specified under Declarations. All participants in the study were female and the sample material investigated was urine. The experimental subjects consisted of one FMS patient group (Group 1) and three control groups (Groups 2 to 4). Clinical description and serum and urine sample collection on all experimental groups commenced from 2009 to 2011. Case definition and selection for the eventual study was done by clinical and scientific group of co-workers in 2010. Following scrutinizing of the records of patients with a medical history of FMS, a group of 18 FMS patients eventually selected based on the above selection criteria as well as after excluding outliers based on statistical analysis [(S5 in the Additional file 1: Supplementary Information (SI)].

The socio-demographic, tender point and myofascial pain experience, awareness of gastro-intestinal symptoms, pain-specific medication and levels of emotional experience associated with FMS for the 18 patients was obtained through the FIQR [17] and the IHCQ. The questionnaires are presented in Table S1 and the response to the IHCQ are summarised in Table S2 of the SI. The IHCQ included 18 items that could be extended to a total of 30 sub-items. The questionnaire provided socio-demographic information on the patients (3 items), personal clinical experience of pain and their FMS condition (5 items) and use of medication against pain (2 questions), emotional experience (7 questions) and digestive functioning (1 item). The urine samples were provided by the patients prior to application of pressure to the tender-points (TPs). For a total of 16 of these FMS patients a complete set of data was available for the comparative analysis of the FIQR and metabolomics data, as some information on some patients had to be excluded because the data were incomplete. Some degree of comorbidity of conditions that overlap with FMS (e.g. chronic fatigue syndrome) could not be excluded, as the mean level of energy in the FIQR was rated at 7,0 and according to responses to the IHCQ, 94% of the patients experienced sleep disturbances and did not awoke refreshed. The responses to an experience of mood disturbances (58% answered "Yes") and anxiety (52% answered "Yes") for the FMS patients as a group were moderate. Responses on depression was inconsistent (mean FIQR-score = 5.1 with 84% "Yes" answers on the IHCQ) but 88% indicated discomforts with their gastrointestinal functions (Indicated as Irritable Bowel Syndrome (IBS) in the IHCQ). These scores were accepted as indications of the mental and physical profile of the FMS patient group and were not further clinically verified.

Three control groups were used: (1) a group of 11 subjects that were first-degree relatives of the patients, meaning that they were a mother, sister or daughter relation (Group 2: CF); (2) a group of 10 unrelated subjects, selected by physicians and defined as unrelated and age matched controls to the patients (Group 3: CO); (3) a control group of young and healthy individuals, comprising 20 randomly selected students (aged 18–22 years) of North-West University (NWU) (Group 4: CN). All individuals in the control groups showed no indications of FMS or related conditions and was not required to complete the FIQR or IHCQ.

This investigation used availability sampling on the clinically selected FMS patients and controls (CO, CF and CN). However, statistical analyses indicated that the sample sizes provided sufficient power to detect large effects at a univariate level.in the FMS and CN comparison.

Sample preparation and ^{1}H NMR analysis

Spectral analyses were conducted according to the protocol at the NMR facility of the Translational Metabolic Laboratory at Radboud University Medical Centre in Nijmegen, the Netherlands [18, 19]. The urine samples were collected in South Africa, stored at –80 °C and transported to the Netherlands before being thawed at room temperature for analysis. A 1 ml volume of each sample was centrifuged at 3000 rpm for 10 min to remove any sediments or debris. A 70 µl volume of a deuterated solution containing 20.2 mM of trimethyl-2,2,3,3-tetradeuteropropionic acid (TSP, sodium salt; Sigma Aldrich) was added to 700 µl of the supernatant and vortexed. This internal standard (IS) solution served to lock the signal during analysis and to provide a chemical shift reference of $\delta = 0.00$. The sample was then acidified to pH 2.5 ± 0.05, with 37% concentrated hydrochloric acid (HCl). A 650 µl aliquot of the acidified sample was then transferred to a 5 mm NMR tube (Wilmad Royal Imperial; Wilmad LabGlass, USA) and analysed on a 500 MHz Bruker Avance spectrometer (Bruker Analytische Messtechnik, Karlsruhe, Germany) (pulse angle 90°, delay time 4 s, number of scans 256, temperature 298 K). Water suppression was achieved by using gated irradiation focused on the water frequency. All samples were automatically shimmed prior to acquisition of data, using topshim from Bruker BioSpin. The resultant raw spectral data, in the form of free induction decay, were Fourier transformed. These transformed spectra were then manually corrected for phase and baseline. All the samples were normalized with reference to the creatinine CH_3 peak at 3.13 ppm. We opted for two methods of spectral analysis. The first method entailed equidistant binning [20] using a bin width of 0.02 ppm applied to the selected region of 0.5–10 ppm, which gave a total of 461 integrated units per NMR spectrum, excluding the water region, for each individual of the four experimental groups. The second method entailed variable-sized binning. The equal-binning procedure masks subtle chemical shift differences, hides potentially significant changes of low-intensity peaks and incurs the risk of splitting peaks or spectral features between bins [21]. To avoid these problems we also used variable bin sizes in areas of peaks above the noise level, preventing peak division between multiple bins. This approach was specifically applied for the identification and quantification of discernible and important known metabolites, generating data for univariate analysis.

Data and statistical analysis

The original normalized spectral data (presented in Additional file 1 as Table S4 in S1 – Supplementary information (SI) or Additional file 2 – Raw data matrix) were pre-processed by performing log transformation and auto-scaling. Outliers were detected through Hotelling's T^2 and PCA scores (using a 90% confidence region) analysis and resulted in the exclusion of 4 outliers from further analysis. Univariate statistical analyses, specifically the Mann–Whitney test *p*-values (MW) and associated effect sizes (ES), were generated for each feature. Multivariate analyses were performed using cluster analysis (Euclidean distance and Ward linkage) principal components analysis (PCA) and partial least squares discriminant analysis (PLS-DA), using a 90% confidence interval (CI). Data processing and analyses were performed using Matlab (MATLAB with Statistics and PLS Toolbox Release 2012b, The MathWorks, Inc., Natick, MA, USA); R (R version 3.2.3 downloaded from https://www.R-project.org with the corrplot package downloaded from https://cran.r-project.org/web/packages/corrplot); the SPSS software package (SPSS Inc. (2015). IBM SPSS Statistics Version 22, Release 22.0.0, © IBM Corporation and its licensors - http://www-01.ibm.com/software/analytics/spss/) and SAS (SAS Institute Inc. 2016 The SAS System for Windows Release 9.4 TS Level 1 M3, SAS Institute Inc., Cary, NC, USA). A table containing all discriminant information, i.e. the power and VIP values as generated from the PCA and PLS-DA analyses, respectively, as well as the ES and MW *p*-values, was constructed.

We did not test for a normal distribution of the data, given the small number of cases and used Pearson's r and Spearman's rho to assess correlations, analysed through SPSS version 12.0 (SPSS, Inc., Chicago, IL). All tests were one-tailed, given the positive fold changes (FC) observed for all metabolites.

Results

Characteristics of the FMS patient group

The age profile of the patients concurs with the general agreement of FMS being uncommon in young subjects (<25–30 years), increasing with age towards the prevalence peak in middle-aged individuals, and then declines [3, 4]. According to the feedback, 88% of our patients had stable relationships with a male partner, 89% had one form or another of day-filling or employment activities, and their emotional experience was not severely affected by their disease. The pain experience and medication used resembled that generally prescribed for FMS. The mean scores and ranges of the 21 FIQR questions obtained for our patient group and those (designated as the reference group) used for the standardization of the questionnaire [17] are compared in Table S3.

To characterize further the relationship between questions or variables making up the FIQR questionnaire, we calculated Kendall's tau correlation coefficients for the FMS patient group (Fig. 1). The correlation coefficients along with their associated significance levels are indicated in Table S3. The highest correlation (r = 0.817) was indicated for the relationship between pain and the symptoms for FMS. The function domain contains 9 physical functioning items related to the ability to perform relatively demanding but regular daily muscle tasks. Apart from the low score for 'brushing hair', all remaining items showed high correlation coefficients among each other, ranging from 0.399 to 0.778. These high values collectively substantiate the major signs and symptoms experienced by the FMS patients. The 'overall impact' domain contained 2 items that asked about the number of days individuals felt well (could reach their goals) and the corresponding number they were unable to work because of FMS symptoms. These again showed high correlation coefficients, ranging from 0.421 to 0.686, with the 8 items in the functional domain indicating the underlying negative impact of the FMS symptoms on the daily routine of the FMS patients. The symptoms domain contained 9 items on which patients had to rate work and physiological, psychological and environmental difficulties related to FMS. Lower correlations, ranging from 0.076 to 0.499 (mean = 0.25), were found between the 8 functional items and sleep patterns, memory, anxiety and depression, indicating little overlap within the patient group with other FMS-related conditions. Taking everything into account, we conclude the FMS patients represent a well-defined group for this explorative metabolomics study.

Data generation and case selection

Representative scaled NMR spectra from an FMS patient and from the young control group (CN) is shown in Fig. 2 to illustrate some of the discernible qualitative NMR differences observed in these selected examples. Close inspection of the spectra indicates that there were no immediately discernible qualitative differences between the two representative examples, suggesting that FMS is not associated with distinctive metabolic aberrations, as otherwise observed in monogenetic disorders such as inborn errors of metabolism. Using the equal-bins spectral data, case reduction was first applied to all four experimental groups (Additional file 1: Figure S2). Four outliers were identified using a 95% confidence region in a Hotelling's T^2 test in conjunction with the respective PCA score plots with 90% confidence regions. Cases that were identified as outliers by either method were removed. The outliers were: group 1 (FMS patients) – one outlier; group 2 (CF; family controls) – two outliers; group 3 (CO; matched controls) – no outliers; group 4 (CN; young controls) – one outlier.

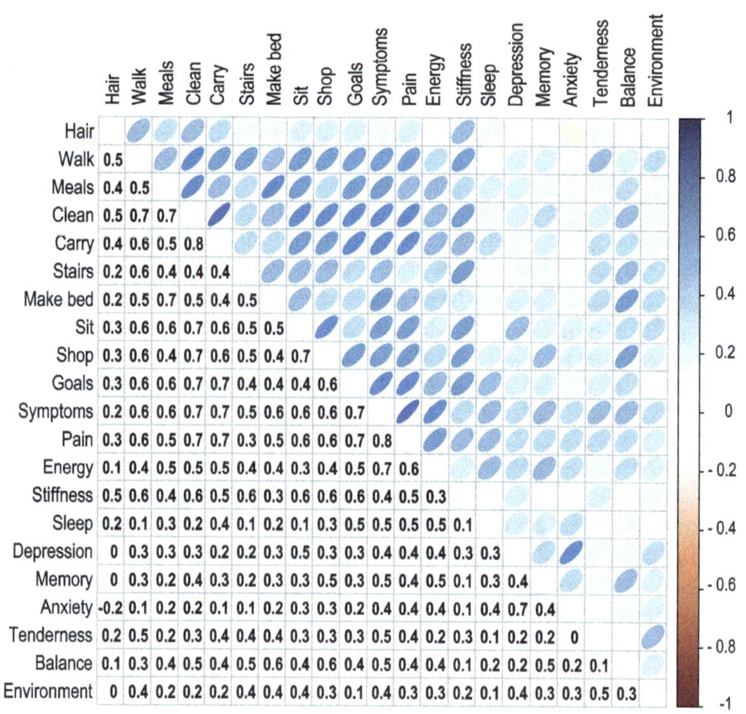

Fig. 1 Correlation matrix for all items on the FIQR questionnaire. Full details on the data analysis are included in the SI

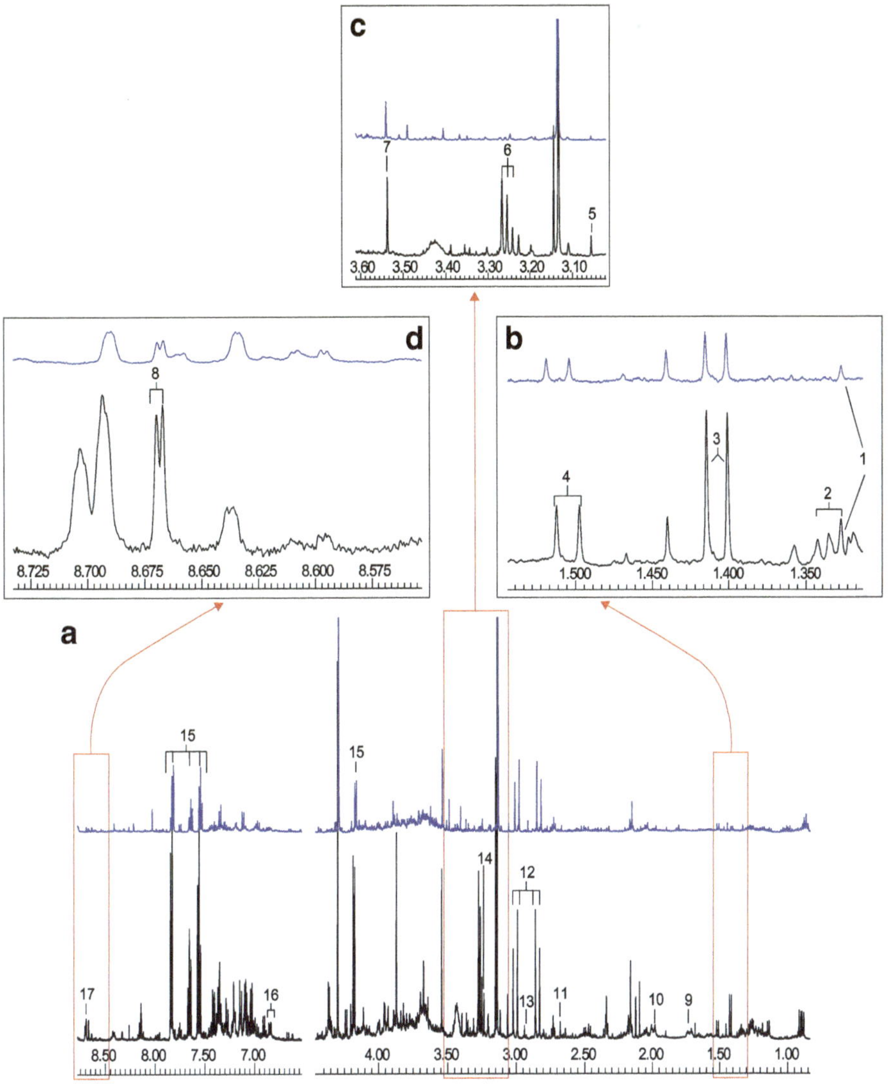

Fig. 2 Representative spectra from one FMS patient (**b**, *black*) and one young control subject (**a**, *blue*), both scaled according to the creatinine CH3 peak at 3.13 ppm. Expanded regions (**c-e**), framed in *red* in the spectra, are the regions where variables important in projection (VIP) through the supervised PLS-DA are located. The labelled metabolites with their chemical shift (in ppm) and multiplicity, respectively, indicated in brackets are given numerically as follows: 1, 3-hydroxyisovaleric acid (1.33 s); 2, threonine (1.33 d); 3, lactic acid (1.41 d); 4, alanine (1.50 d); 5, creatine (3.05 s); 6, taurine (3.25 t, 3.42 s – *broad line*); 7, trimethylamineN-oxide (TMAO) (3.54 s); 8, histidine (8.68 d); 9, 2-hydroxyisobutyric acid (1.44 s); 10, N-acetyl-X (2.03 s); 11, succinic acid (2.67 s); 12, citric acid (2.91 AB); 13, N,N-dimethylglycine (2.93 s); 14, carnitine (3.22 s); 15, hippuric acid (4.18 d, 7.55 t, 7.64 t, 7.83 d); 16, tyrosine (6.89 d); 17, histamine (8.70 d); 18, creatinine (3.13 s, 4.29 s)

Group characteristics

Supposed changes in metabolite profiles from the FMS patients and the three control groups (excluding outliers) were established through three multivariate approaches: unsupervised Euclidian and Ward hierarchical cluster analyses presented as dendrograms, unsupervised PCA, and supervised PLS-DA models, applied to the original 461 ^{1}H NMR profiled bins for the four experimental groups.

Figure 3 shows the group separations based on the unsupervised cluster analysis, indicating the perceived closeness of spectral data encapsulated in the NMR bins. The main clusters formed between the CF family members group (Fig. 3a) and the CO age-matched group (Fig. 3b) relative to the FMS patients are heterogeneous in terms of case distribution. In contrast, two well-defined clusters were formed between the FMS patients and CN young controls (Fig. 3c), suggesting distinct differences in the spectral fingerprints between these two groups.

Next, group separations based on unsupervised PCA and supervised PLS-DA were performed. The data were log transformed and auto-scaled. The PCA between the CF family members (Fig. 3d), CO

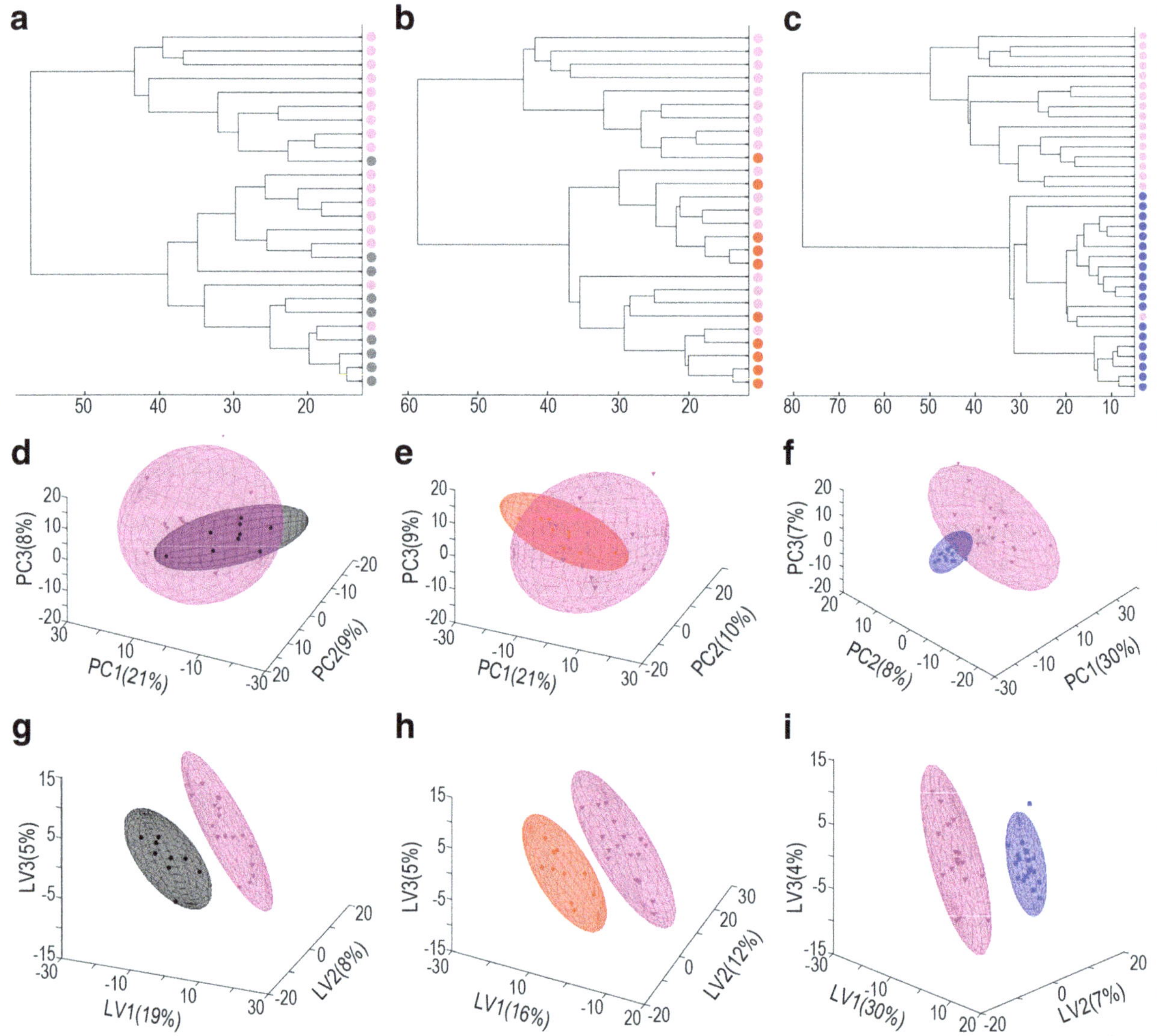

Fig. 3 Group separation between experimental groups through cluster and multivariate analysis based on equidistant binning data. (**a–c**): Dendrograms from cluster analysis are shown for the CF (**a**), CO (**b**) and CN (**c**) groups relative to FMS patients. Cases from the FMS patients are shown as *pink dots*, CF as *black*, CO as *red* and CF controls as *blue*. (**d–f**): PCA indicating the group separation between the FMS patients and CF (**d**), CO (**e**), and CN (**f**) groups respectively, with areas using the same colour code as the *dots* in the dendrograms. (**g–i**): PLS-DA indicating the separation between the FMS patients and CF (**g**), CO (**h**), and CN (**i**) groups respectively, with areas using the same colour code as in the PCA

matched controls (Fig. 3e) and FMS patients complemented results from the cluster analyses. A complete separation was obtained between all three control groups and the FMS patients (Fig. 3f–i) through supervised PLS-DA. Evaluation of the PLS-DA model shown in Fig. 3i (FMS vs CN) was performed by calculating the goodness-of-fit (R^2) and predictive ability (Q^2) parameters. These metrics confirmed the complete separation between the FMS and CN young control groups, with good model fit (R^2 = 0. 96), however this model may not generalize well (Q^2 = 0.29).

From the equal binning analysis it is evident that there are bins or combinations of bins that can discriminate between our patient and control groups. However, since it is not clinically practical to measure bins, we did not investigate this data further. Instead, the metabolites potentially responsible for the separation of the FMS patients and the CN young controls were subsequently identified by analyzing variable bins from the NMR spectra and converting these measures to concentration values of the identified metabolites.

Metabolite profile of the FMS patient group

Twenty-one metabolites could be identified and quantified from the NMR spectra. From this list we selected twenty endogenous metabolites (listed in Table 1), and also included 2-hydroxyisobutyric acid of exogenous

Table 1 Univariate, multivariate and descriptive statistics for the 20 bins, comparing FMS and CN

Variable	CS and M[Ps]	VIP	Mann-Whitney		Fold Change	Mean		StDev	
		3 LV	*p*-value	Effect size		CN	FMS	CN	FMS
2-Hydroxyisobutyric acid	1.44 s [CH3]	6.26	0.0001	0.72	−1.56	0.01	0.02	0.0	0.00
Succinic acid	2.66 s [(CH2)2]	0.25	0.0001	0.61	−1.63	0.02	0.03	0.01	0.01
Taurine	3.25 t [CH2]	5.21	0.0007	0.52	−2.29	0.20	0.45	0.05	0.57
Tyrosine	6.89 dd [(CH)2]	0.37	0.0029	0.45	−1.70	0.03	0.06	0.03	0.06
Lactic acid	1.41 d [CH3]	2.83	0.0044	0.42	−1.81	0.06	0.11	0.03	0.07
Creatine	3.05 s [CH3]	4.40	0.0053	0.41	−2.08	0.05	0.09	0.04	0.08
TMAO	3.54 s [(CH3)3]	2.21	0.0062	0.41	−2.10	0.06	0.14	0.06	0.23
Dimethylglycine	2.93 s [(CH3)2]	0.00	0.0127	0.36	−1.29	0.01	0.01	0.00	0.00
Leucine	0.95 t [(CH3)2]	0.00	0.0136	0.36	−1.11	0.01	0.02	0.00	0.00
Formic acid	8.25 s [CH]	0.01	0.0361	0.29	−1.15	0.03	0.03	0.01	0.01
Valine	1.04 d [CH3]	0.00	0.0436	0.28	−1.24	0.01	0.01	0.00	0.00
Histamine	8.70 d [CH]	0.08	0.0436	0.28	−1.29	0.06	0.07	0.06	0.05
N-acetyl-X	2.03 s [CH3]	0.02	0.0464	0.27	−1.28	0.01	0.02	0.00	0.01
Lysine	1.73 m [CH2]	0.61	0.0739	0.23	−1.03	0.11	0.12	0.03	0.06
Hippuric acid	4.18 d [CH2]	1.61	0.0966	0.21	−1.55	0.22	0.35	0.10	0.24
Citric acid	2.89 AB [(CH)4]	1.36	0.1070	0.20	−1.21	0.39	0.47	0.16	0.17
Alanine	1.51 d [CH3]	0.13	0.1785	0.15	−1.16	0.06	0.07	0.02	0.03
Histidine	8.68 d [CH]	0.85	0.1942	0.14	1.19	0.07	0.06	0.04	0.04
Carnitine	3.22 s [(CH3)3]	0.02	0.2107	0.13	−1.24	0.02	0.02	0.01	0.01
Threonine	1.33 d [CH3]	0.04	0.2648	0.10	−1.28	0.03	0.04	0.01	0.04
3-Hydroxyisovaleric acid	1.33 s [(CH3)2]	0.00	0.4942	0.00	−1.02	0.00	0.00	0.00	0.00

origin [22], with high VIP, ES and ES values, despite being present in low concentrations. The endogenous metabolites include seven amino acids (tyrosine, leucine, valine, histidine, alanine, threonine and lysine), seven metabolites directly or indirectly associated with energy metabolism (lactic acid, succinic acid, citric acid, 3-hydroxyisovaleric acid, creatine, carnitine and formic acid), three osmolytes (taurine, TMAO and dimethylglycine), a major mammalian detoxification product (hippuric acid), histamine and an N-acetyl-derivative. The N-acetyl-derivative showed a singlet at 2.03 ppm, possibly indicative of an N-acetyl group. One-dimensional spectral data suggested that aspartic acid (multiplet at 4.70 ppm) could be the moiety linked to the N-acetyl group, which, however, could not be substantiated as N-acetyl-aspartic acid by two-dimensional NMR spectral analysis Additional file 1: Figure S4). We thus designated the variable as an N-acetyl derivative (N-acetyl-X).

We subsequently performed multivariate (log and centred concentration values) and univariate (unscaled concentration values) analyses on the reduced bins (endogenous metabolites, converted to their respective metabolite concentrations) to refine our identification of the key variables that discriminate between the FMS patients and the controls. All cases were retained for this analysis as none were identified as outliers based on the concentrations. Multivariate PCA (Fig. 4a) and PLS-DA (Fig. 4b) both indicated that the 20 metabolites contained information that differentiates, but did not separate, the FMS patients from the young controls. Model performance was evaluated using the goodness of fit (R^2) and goodness of prediction (Q^2) parameters, which were $R^2(X) = 0.52$ and $Q^2(Y) = 0.05$, respectively, indicating a reasonable (R^2) but not necessarily reproducible (Q^2) fit between the variation in the data and the components (quantified metabolites) comprising the model for the present FMS group. It thus appears that some metabolites below the sensitivity range for quantification from the NMR spectra might be required for reproducibility (Q^2) and for further differentiation between the FMS patients and young controls.

Univariate analyses using Mann–Whitney *p*-values and fold changes, as summarized in a volcano plot (Fig. 5a), point to important substances that cause group differentiation. The outcome of this analysis of the data set of 20 variables is presented in Fig. 5a, indicating which large-magnitude changes (fold change: $|\log_2 FC|$ 1.5) are also statistically significant (Mann–Whitney test: $p < 0.05$). Six informative metabolites complied with these measures,

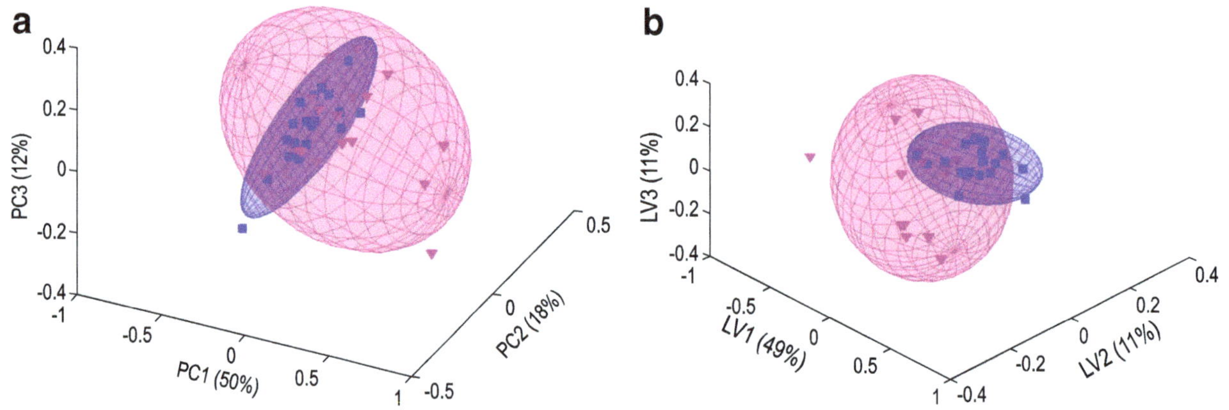

Fig. 4 PCA (**a**) and PLS-DA (**b**) for the FMS patients relative to the young controls, based on the quantified 20 metabolites

with their respective VIP values shown in brackets: succinic acid (0.246), taurine (5.214), tyrosine (0.365), lactic acid (2.832), creatine (4.402) and trimethylamine N-oxide (TMAO; 2.209).

Important endogenous metabolites in the FMS patient group

A summary of the results for the univariate and multivariate statistical analyses is presented in Table 1, nine of which could be related to physiological functions that could be related to FMS.

The neurological functions of succinic acid, tyrosine and lactic acid are well known: the aerobic mitochondrial energy regeneration function, a precursor for neurotransmitters and a key metabolite in the astrocyte-neuron lactate shuttle [23], respectively. Taurine is an abundant β-amino acid in the mammalian brain [24] and has been shown to be a neurotransmitter in the substantia nigra (SN). It has been suggested from micro-dialysis experiments on Sprague-Dawley rats that osmoregulation of the nonsynaptic taurine pool of the SN could influence the nigral cell vulnerability, seen in the pathogenesis of Parkinson's disease [25]. Likewise, nutritional studies [26] suggest that TMAO may be involved in diet-induced variations in the balance of several osmolytes, including betaine, choline, creatinine and creatine, whereas creatine has also been proposed as being involved in pain experienced in FMS [25]. Thus, we subsequently evaluated the potential diagnostic value of these six metabolites on FMS by means of a logistic regression analysis, as indicated below.

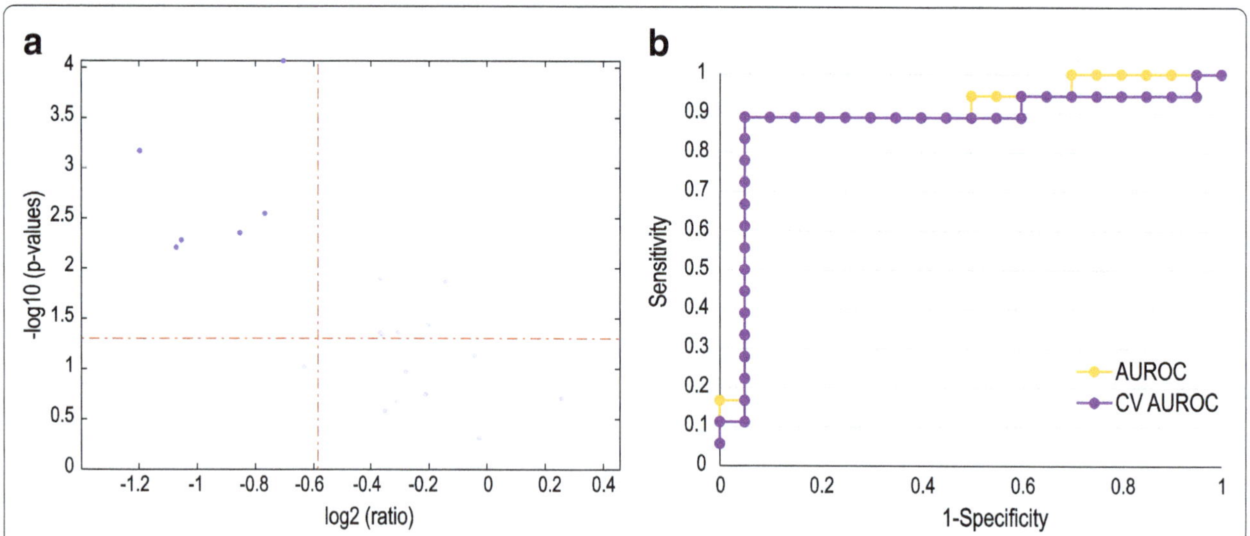

Fig. 5 Statistical assessments of three metabolites indicative of FMS: (**a**) Volcano plot mapped by the scaled fold change and *p*-values for the 20 metabolites observed for FMS patients and young controls. Metabolites with high FC and significant *p*-values among patients are indicated by *black squares*. (**b**) ROC analyses for discriminating FMS patients from controls (AUROC) as well as leave-one-out crossvalidated ROC analysis (CV AUROC). The discriminator consisted of the three informative metabolites (succinic acid, taurine and creatine) identified by multivariate, univariate and metabolic pathway analyses

Important exogenous metabolites in the FMS patient group

The pain intensity of patients with FMS has been reported to correlate with the degree of small intestinal bacterial overgrowth [9, 10]. This clinical observation may have pathogenetic relevance for FMS, because bacterial overgrowth leads to the exposure of immune cells to luminal antigens and consequent immune modulation. An untargeted NMR metabolomics study of celiac disease, a multifactorial immune-mediated enteropathy [27], suggested alterations of energy metabolism - a clinical characteristic in FMS - while urine data pointed to alterations of gut microbiota. At least three metabolites observed in the urine samples of our FMS patient group suggest perturbations in their gut metabolome (Fig. 6): (1) Hippuric acid is a normal and major component of urine and appear in humans as an increased excretory product from unnatural (detoxification) and natural (gastroesophageal reflux disease in children) sources. (2) 2-Hydroxyisobutyric acid, the most discriminatory variable between our FMS group and controls (VIP = 6.2 – Table 1), is an apparent catabolic from gut microbiotica and was shown to be statistically linked to *Faecalibacterium prausnitzii* [28] an important commensal bacterium of the human gut flora proposed to be an indicator of the dynamic basis of host–microbiome symbiosis. (3) Lactic acid is a key intermediate in many biochemical processes and is a measure of critical illness in patients with poor prognosis. It may be of endogenous (L-lactate) or exogenous (D-lactate) origin and we recently proposed that the determination of its enantiomers in infectious conditions may provide a basis for substantiating the clinical significance of disease markers [29]. The presence of these exogenous markers of gut origin provides further indications of the connectivity between disturbances in the gut microbial populations and the metabolic consequences of the altered microbial–mammalian metabolic balance influencing host disease, which will be discussed below in the context of FMS.

A putative biosignature for FMS

A combination of three selection methods (Forward, Backward and Step-wise selection) was used to identify the best metabolite predictors. Instead of using one selection method, a combined approach was chosen since each method has its advantages and disadvantages [30, 31]. Although our aim was to explore a small set of highly discriminatory endogenous metabolites, we also investigated the potential of a combination of these metabolites to function as a biosignature for the FMS patient group. We followed a forced entry approach to evaluate the combination of metabolites. Table 2 lists the methods used as well as the preferred metabolite predictors selected from the six informative metabolites. The last model (Forced entry) entered succinic acid, taurine and creatine, and produced the best model based on −2 Log Likelihood (−2LL) from the present data. Table 2 also reports other model performance measures, but -2LL was used to select the best model as it gives an indication of the variation not explained in the data, and gave the lowest -2LL value compared to the other models. The Forced entry model was also well calibrated since the Hosmer Lemeshow (HL) statistic was not significant. The model fit is reported by using the Max Rescaled R-squared value and only the Forced entry model had a satisfactory value of above 0.6.

Finally, the classification ability of each model was assessed by using a Receiver Operating Characteristic (ROC) analysis to the data mentioned. The values of the

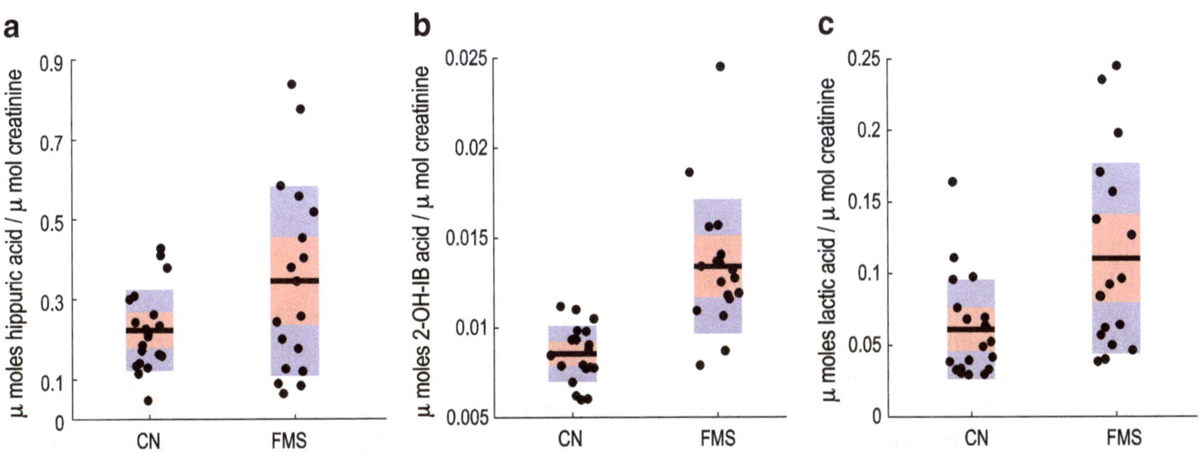

Fig. 6 Graphs showing important urinary metabolites related to the gut microbiome. Indicated in the figure are: FMS patients relative to young controls for hippuric (**a**), 2-hydroxyisobutyric (**b**) and lactic (**c**) acids. Values for all individual cases are shown as *dots*, while the squared area represents the 95% confidence interval (*orange*) and 1 standard deviation (*blue*) of the mean (*red line*)

Table 2 Summary of logistic regression results for the six informative metabolites. The predictors used or selected by the logistic regression model are listed as *Predictors selected*. Other columns report the model fit results (Max Rescaled R-squared), the relative variance explained (−2LL), the calibration (HL *p*-value), and the classification ability (AUC and AUC (LOO CV)) of each model

Selection method	Predictors selected	-2LL	HL *p*-value	Max rescaled R-squared	AUC	AUC (LOO CV)
Forward	Creatine & succinic acid	36.15	0.0273	0.47	0.8917	0.8583
Backward	Taurine	40.16	0.6336	0.37	0.8056	0.7556
Stepwise	Succinic acid	40.87	0.5496	0.35	0.8583	0.8306
Forced Entry	Creatine; succinic acid & taurine	29.66	0.0932	0.60	0.8972	0.875

area under the ROC curve (AUC) provide a measure of how well this combination could distinguish between the two groups. A value of AUC = 1 represents a perfect test, while a cursory guide for classifying the accuracy of a diagnostic test is given by: AUC = 0.90–1 (excellent, i.e. high sensitivity and high specificity); 0.80–0.90 (good); 0.70–0.80 (fair); 0.60–0.70 (poor); 0.50–0.60 (fail). To provide some indication of how well the model would potentially generalize, the last column in Table 2 reports the classification ability when one sample is left out repeatedly — in other words, based on a leave-one-out cross-validation strategy (AUC (LOO CV)). Again the Forced entry model performed the best (AUC = 90% [0.8972]; AUC (LOOCV) = 88% [0.8750]).

Correlation between clinical and metabolic indicators

Pearson and Spearman correlation analysis was done to compare the bivariate relationships between responses to the FIQR and the three endogenous variables defining the biosignature of FMS. Specifically, correlations were assessed between the sum of all three FIQR domains as well as the sum of the functional, impact and symptoms domains and SUM-3, SUM-2, creatine, succinic acid and taurine. Finally we inspected the data for symptoms related to metabolism to be included in the bivariate correlation analysis. In this regard it should be noted: (1) The scores of the 21 questions of the FIQR corresponds to an average based on the subjective self-assessment of the FMS patients as used in the behavioural sciences (i.e., it is not empirically based). We therefore used the mean scores of fibromyalgia patients on the symptoms for experience of pain, low energy levels and tenderness to touch only as a directive to include these symptoms in the bivariate correlation analysis [30]. Their mean values did not differed in practice from the data of a reference group of the revised FIQR (Additional file 1: Figure S1). (2) The number of FMS cases is relatively small for assessment of normality in the data distribution. We therefore included the Pearson and Spearman correlations in Table 3, but used only the Spearman's correlations for the interpretation of the bivariate correlation analyses, with guideline values for "small"($r \geq 0.1$), "medium" ($r \geq 0.3$) and "large" ($r \geq 0.5$) as operational convention for the correlation coefficients [32].

The results shown indicate a medium and borderline significant relationship between the SUM-3 biosignature and the sum of the FIQR, with insignificant correlations for its functional and impact domains. Sum-3 and the symptoms domain showed a large and significant correlation. The relationship between SUM-2 and the sum of the FIQR and its three domains improved significantly. Taken together these results directs to a more meaningful relationship between the metabolites which comprise the biosignature and clinical symptoms related to biochemical perturbations in FMS. This impression is substantiated by the strong and significant relationship between SUM-3 and SUM-2 on the experience of pain (p = 0.004 and 0.016, respectively) and loss of energy (p = 0.006 and 0.001, respectively) in the FMS patients as a group. Notably this relationship is not shared by succinic acid (a metabolite from the Krebs cycle) and taurine (an osmolite), but a good and significant relationship was shown between creatine and the symptoms pain and energy (p = 0.024 and 0.003, respectively). The relationship between the biosignature components to tenderness to touch, the third clinical symptom evaluated, was statistically insignificant (not included in Table 2). All correlation coefficients were positive indicating that patients with high scores on the biosignature will likely also have high FIQR scores.

Discussion

The results of this metabolomics study lead to three main discussion points – whether FMS presents with a unique global metabolic profile which characterizes this disease, whether metabolomics studies contributed to the advancement of an objective clinical diagnosis of FMS in patients so affected and on gut microbial–host metabolic perturbations in FMS.

As the overall health status of individuals is captured in their metabolic state, there exists a prevailing view that metabolomics results embody global biochemical changes in an individual due to a disease and neurological conditions [33], and supported by our results and of two other NMR metabolomics investigations. The first NMR metabolomics study evaluated the diagnostic

Table 3 Relationship between the clinical information of the FIQR and the components of the FMS biosignature

Bivariate components for the correlation analysis	Pearson correlation		Spearman correlation	
	Coeff. (*r*)	*p*-value[b]	Coeff. (*r*)	*p*-value
Correlations of the biosignature (SUM-3)[a] with the FIQR domain categories				
SUM-3 vs Sum of 21 questions of the full FIQR	0.35	0.102	0.42	0.059
SUM-3 vs Sum of 9 questions of the functional domain	0.31	0.134	0.25	0.134
SUM-3 vs Sum of 2 questions of the impact domain	0.15	0.316	0.22	0.241
SUM-3 vs Sum of 10 questions of the symptoms domain	0.41	0.057	0.57	0.011*
Correlations of two components of the biosignature (SUM-2) with the FIQR domain categories				
SUM-2 vs Sum of 21 questions of the full FIQR	0.56	0.016*	0.53	0.021*
SUM-2 *vs*Sum of 9 questions of the functional domain	0.52	0.023*	0.41	0.008**
SUM-2 vs Sum of 2 questions of the impact domain	0.5	0.043*	0.51	0.039*
SUM-2 vs Sum of 10 questions of the symptoms domain	0.59	0.009**	0.57	0.011*
Correlations of components of the biosignature with the symptom of pain[c]				
SUM-3 vs pain experience	0.46	0.037*	0.64	0.004**
SUM-2 vs pain experience	0.52	0.02*	0.54	0.016*
Creatine vs pain experience	0.5	0.025*	0.5	0.024*
Succinic acid vs pain experience	0.08	0.384	0.18	0.249
Taurine vs pain experience	0.39	0.069	0.29	0.135
Correlations of components of the biosignature with the symptom of energy[d]				
SUM-3 vs energy loss	0.32	0.115	0.61	0.006**
SUM-2 vs energy loss	0.68	0.002**	0.72	0.001**
Creatine vs energy loss	0.65	0.003**	0.66	0.003**
Succinic acid vs energy loss	0.15	0.295	0.22	0.221
Taurine vs energy loss	0.22	0.204	0.14	0.307

[a]Biosignature: SUM-3 = creatine + succinic acid + taurine; SUM-2 = creatine + succinic acid
[b]Statistical significance: *significant at $p \leq 0.05$, **significant at $p \leq 0.01$
[c]Pain: No pain = 0; Unbearable pain = 10
[d]Energy: Lots of energy = 0; No energy = 10

accuracy of biomarker profiles in three neurological conditions: idiopathic intracranial hypertension, multiple sclerosis, and cerebrovascular disease relative to controls with either no or combined neurological diseases [34]. It appeared that the metabolomics investigation identified differences in metabolite profiles in patients suffering from these three conditions. A related conclusion was drawn from the second NMR metabolomics study of FMS [14]. Although a relatively small number of patients formed the experimental group, the metabolomics approach was successful in identifying distinct metabolic profiles for FMS patients relative to controls, supporting the concept that the Platelet Activating Factor/Platelet Activating Factor Receptor (PAF/PAFr) system plays a role in modulating pain signalling. Our results furthermore indicated the differentiation of the three control groups used (family members, an age-matched group, and young individuals) and the FMS patients (Additional file 1: Figure S3). Statistical assessment of the outcome of a supervised PLS-DA model confirmed the complete separation between the FMS and young control groups. Good model fit values substantiated some unique differences between the global metabolic profiles of the FMS patients and the healthy young controls. The metabolites principally responsible for the differentiation between our FMS patients and controls included taurine and TMAO which were also reported to be significantly increased ($p < 0.05$) in an FMS patient group in a preliminary targeted NMR study [12]. In addition, we observed perturbed succinic acid suggesting altered energy metabolism in FMS. This result is linked to a study [13] where there was relatively elevated: glucose, the glycolytic intermediate phosphoenolpyruvate, pyruvate and nicotinamide adenine dinucleotide (NAD^+) seen in dried blood spots from FMS patients. This observation was previously reported for patients with chronic widespread pain [35].

A common thread in the metabolomics studies on FMS discussed here is the affirmation of the ability of metabolomics to identify distinct metabolic profiles for FMS patients relative to controls. Some metabolites/biomarkers could therefore contribute to the disease phenotype by having a role in the pathogenesis of FMS. The biomarkers revealed in these metabolomics studies seemed, however, not to be metabolically closely linked, but may be due to the multi-factorial nature of FMS. Noteworthy also are the two main limitations of our own and the other two metabolomics studies: the FMS groups investigated and analytical methods used. Most metabolomics studies are limited by the number of experimental subjects available for investigation, and therefore ultimately call for follow-up validation studies with larger and better-defined experimental groups. Further, given the complexity of the human metabolome and the multi-dimensional nature of biofluids and other biological samples available for metabolomics studies, no single analytical technology can fully disclose and account for the information encapsulated in these samples. Nonetheless, metabolomics retains a promise well beyond the scope of standard clinical chemistry techniques, for affording detailed characterization of metabolic phenotypes and is believed, eventually, to lead to so-called precision medicine in which knowledge of their unique metabolic derangements explains the disease state of individual patients [36]. A third limitation in the present study is the use of the 1990 criteria for FMS (1, 14) as the patient selection was one before publication of the revised criteria in 2011. The use of the revised criteria is now standard practice in our pain clinic.

So, can metabolomics studies contribute to the advancement of objective clinical diagnosis of FMS? The results of the present and the two other metabolomics studies on the disease imply that they can, albeit with qualifications. The analyses of blood spots from FMS patients provided information using IRMS technology that differentiated samples from FMS subjects from those with RA or OA with zero misclassifications (100% accuracy). The accuracy of the metabolomics approach was 75%, but with the advantage of disclosing a prioritized list of metabolites that may underlie the differences identified [9]. The possible role of lysoPCs as biomarkers or as contributors to the FMS phenotype and function in the pathogenesis of this condition suggest they are potential new disease biomarkers and thereby open a new approach for the treatment in FMS [10]. Likewise, the predictive potential of the combination of succinic acid, taurine and creatine proved to be excellent for discriminating between our cases of FMS and controls (AUC = 90%). The combination of creatine and succinic acid also showed a significant correlation with the characteristic symptoms of pain and fatigue in FMS. The inclusion of this predictive information on these three metabolites could in time be considered to form part of the initial evaluation of patients suspected of suffering from the disease, in anticipation of validation of FMS diagnostic markers.

Finally, the involvement of gut microbial–host metabolic perturbations in FMS may prove to contribute significantly in defining the clinical profile in FMS. In health, brain-gut interactions are crucial in the maintaining of homeostasis [37]. It appears that neuroplasticity-related systems and neurotransmitter systems are influenced by the gut–brain axis regulation and perturbed homeostasis may contribute to risk of disease through alterations in gastrointestinal tract, central nervous, autonomic nervous and immune systems [38]. The frequent comorbidity of fibromyalgia with stress related disorders, such as chronic fatigue and irritable bowel syndromes and some CNS related abnormalities, suggests that gut–brain axis regulation may at least be a partial common denominator for these disorders. This view may well be revealed by data from a follow-up targeted metabolomics investigation of high sensitivity, like through mass spectrometric-based technologies.

Conclusions

An untargeted ^{1}H NMR metabolomics analysis of urine samples obtained from a group of clinically well-defined female FMS patients with no psychiatric co-morbidity could be fully differentiated from a group of young healthy women. The presence of metabolic indicators of perturbations in the gut microbiome (hippuric, 2-hydroxyisobutyric and lactic acids) supports the paradigm that regulation of the gut-brain axis becomes affected in stress related disorders, like FMS. Three metabolite markers (taurine, creatine and succinic acid) were important for the differentiation between FMS patients and controls and were significant indicators of the pain and fatigue symptoms in FMS. ROC analysis and odds ratios substantiated the good predictive potential of a combination of these three metabolites for FMS in the present patient group. Follow-up metabolomics research on a larger number of urine samples, including those from individuals at high risk of developing the disease, as well as longitudinal studies on FMS patients during treatment, are needed to validate the findings presented here and to potentially detect effects which would require greater statistical power. These markers may in time provide objective supplementary information together with tender-point measurements and FIQR questionnaires used to confirm FMS.

Abbreviations

^{1}H–NMR: Proton nuclear magnetic resonance; ACR: American College of Rheumatology; AUC: Area under the ROC curve; AUROC: Area under the ROC curve; CF: Group of first-degree relatives of the patients; CN: Group of healthy young subjects; CNS: Central nervous system; CO: Group of age-matched subjects but unrelated to the patients; CV AUROC: Cross-validated AUROC; CWP: Chronic widespread pain; ES: Effect size; FC: Fold change;

FIQR: Fibromyalgia Impact Questionnaire; FM: Fibromyalgia; FMS: Fibromyalgia syndrome; IHCQ: In-house clinical questionnaire; IRMS: Mid-infrared micro-spectroscopy; LC/Q-TOF/MS: liquid chromatography/quadrupole–time of flight/mass spectrometry; LOO CV: Leave-one-out cross-validation; LV: Latent variable; lysoPCs: Lysophosphocholines; MW: Mann–Whitney test; N-acetyl-X: N-acetyl-derivative; NTeMBI: Nuclear Technologies in Medicine and Biosciences Initiative; NWU: North-West University; OA: Osteoarthritis; OR: Odds ratio; PAF/PAFr: Platelet Activating Factor/Platelet Activating Factor Receptor; PC: Principal component; PCA: Principal components analysis; PLS-DA: Partial least squares discriminant analysis; Q^2: Predictive ability parameter; R^2: Goodness-of-fit parameter; RA: Rheumatoid arthritis; ROC: Receiver Operating Characteristic; SN: Substantia nigra; SUM-3: Numerical sum of the concentrations of taurine, creatine and TMAO; TMAO: Trimethylamine-N-oxide; TPs: Tender-points; VIP: Variable important in projection

Acknowledgements
None.

Funding
Research funding for this project was provided by the Technological Innovation Agency (TIA) of the South African Department of Science and Technology (DST) and from the Nuclear Technologies in Medicine and the Biosciences Initiative (NTeMBI) of the Nuclear Energy Corporation of South Africa (NECSA). BM received a post-graduate bursary from the National Research Foundation (NRF) of South Africa and a SAVUSA-SKILL stipend from the Embassy of the Netherlands in Pretoria, enabling her to pursue the NMR analyses at the Radboud University Medical Centre in Nijmegen.

Authors' contributions
This investigation required a multidisciplinary approach and the inputs of all authors were essential to produce the concept and final manuscript. CR and HM defined the aim of the study, developed the experimental design and obtained ethical approval for the study; they are, respectively, the promoter and co-promoter for BM. HM performed the selection and clinical description of the FMS patients and CF and CO control groups and provided the urine samples for these individuals. CR provided it for the CN control group and was responsible for coordination and integration of inputs from the authors. BM conducted all experimental analyses and compiled the clinical information provided by HM. SM and UE gave guidance and assessment on ^{1}H NMR data generation and spectral analyses. RW was responsible for critical evaluation of the analytical aspects of the clinical chemistry data and for their interpretation. MvR performed all the statistical analyses. All authors have given their approval of the version of the manuscript as submitted and agreed to the accountability requirements.

Competing interests
There are no competing interests.

Ethics approval and consent to participate
Informed consent was obtained from all the participants in this study by means of a voluntarily completed consent form. Ethical approval for this study was obtained via the consortium under the Nuclear Technologies in Medicine and Biosciences Initiative (NTeMBI) (ethical approval by Pharma Ethics Pty, Ltd., reference number 11064365). Pharma Ethics confirmed the following: "The study has been accepted as complying to the Ethics Standards for Clinical Research with a new drug in participants based on FDA, ICH GCP and the Declaration of Helsinki guidelines. The Ethics Committee (IRB) granting this approval is in compliance with the Guidelines for Good Practice in the Conduct of Clinical Trials in Human Participants in South Africa (2006), ICH Harmonised Tripartite Guidelines E6: Note: for the Guidance in Good Clinical Practice (CPMP/ICH/135/95) and FDA Code of Federal Regulation Part 50, 56 and 312."

Author details
[1]Centre for Human Metabolomics, Faculty of Natural Sciences, North-West University (Potchefstroom Campus), Private Bag X6001, Potchefstroom, South Africa. [2]Department of Family Medicine, Kalafong Hospital, University of Pretoria, Private Bag X396, Pretoria, South Africa. [3]Translational Metabolic Laboratory, Department of Laboratory Medicine, Radboud University Nijmegen Medical Centre, PO Box 91016500 HB, Nijmegen, The Netherlands.

References

1. Wolfe F, Smythe HA, Yunus MB, Bennett RM, Bombardier C, Goldenberg DL, et al. The American College of Rheumatology 1990 criteria for the classification of fibromyalgia. Arthritis Rheum. 1990;33(2):160–72.
2. Wolfe F, Clauw DJ, Fitzcharles MA, Goldenberg DL, Katz RS, Mease P, et al. The American College of Rheumatology preliminary diagnostic criteria for fibromyalgia and measurement of symptom severity. Arthritis Care Res. 2010;62(5):600–10.
3. Branco JC, Bannwarth B, Failde I, Carbonell JA, Blotman F, Spaeth M, Saraiva F, et al. Prevalence of fibromyalgia: a survey in five European countries. Semin Arthritis Rheum. 2010;39:448–53.
4. Lawrence RC, Felson DT, Helmick CG, Arnold LM, Choi H, Deyo RA, et al. Estimates of the prevalence of arthritis and other rheumatic conditions in the United States: part II. Arthritis Rheum. 2008;58(1):26–35.
5. Russell IJ, Orr MD, Littman B, Vipraio GA, Alboukrek D, Michalek JE, et al. Elevated cerebrospinal fluid levels of substance P in patients with the fibromyalgia syndrome. Arthritis Rheum. 1994;37:1593–601.
6. Yunus MB, Dailey JW, Aldag JC, Masi AT, Jobe PC. Plasma and urinary catecholamines in primary fibromyalgia: a controlled study. J Rheumatol. 1992;19:95–7.
7. Legangneux E, Mora JJ, Spreux-Varoquaux O, Thorin I, Herrou M, Alvado G, et al. Cerebrospinal fluid biogenic amine metabolites, plasma-rich platelet serotonin and [3H]imipramine reuptake in the primary fibromyalgia syndrome. Rheumatol. 2001;40:290–6.
8. Meyer HP. Myofascial pain syndrome and its suggested role in the pathogenesis and treatment of fibromyalgia syndrome. Curr Pain Headache Rep. 2002;6(4):274–83.
9. Levine JS, Burakoff R. Extraintestinal manifestations of inflammatory bowel disease. Gastroenterol Hepatol (NY). 2011;7(4):235–41.
10. Clauw DJ. Fibromyalgia and related conditions. Mayo Clin Proc Elsevier. 2015;90(5):680–92.
11. Dumas M-E, Davidovic L. Metabolic phenotyping and systems biology approaches to understanding neurological disorders. F1000Prime Rep. 2013;5:18.
12. Richards SCM, Bell J, Cheung Y-L, Cleare A, Scott DL. Abstract 382: muscle metabolites detected in urine in fibromyalgia and chronic fatigue syndrome may suggest ongoing muscle damage. 2001.
13. Hackshaw KV, Rodriguez-Saona L, Plans M, Bell LN, Buffington CAT. A bloodspot-based diagnostic test for fibromyalgia syndrome and related disorders. Analyst. 2013;138:4453–62.
14. Caboni P, Liori B, Kumar A, Santoru ML, Asthana S, Pieroni E, et al. Metabolomics analysis and modeling suggest a Lysophosphocholines-PAF receptor interaction in fibromyalgia. PLoS One. 2014;9(9):e107626.
15. Giacomelli C, Sernissi F, Rossi A, Bombardieri S, Bazzichi L. Biomarkers in fibromyalgia: a review. Curr Biomark Find. 2014;4:35–41.
16. Xiao Y, Russell IJ, Liu YG. A brain-derived neurotrophic factor polymorphism Val66Met identifies fibromyalgia syndrome subgroup with higher body mass index and C-reactive protein. Rheumatol Int. 2012;32:2479–85.
17. Bennett RM, Friend R, Jones KD, Ward R, Han BK, Ross RL. The revised fibromyalgia impact questionnaire (FIQR): validation and psychometric properties. Arthritis Res Ther. 2009;11(5):415.
18. Engelke UF, Liebrand-van Sambeek ML, De Jong JG, Leroy JG, Morava É, Smeitink JA, et al. N-acetylated metabolites in urine: proton nuclear magnetic resonance spectroscopic study on patients with inborn errors of metabolism. Clin Chem. 2004;50(1):58–66.
19. Wevers RA, Engelke U, Rotteveel JJ, Heerschap A, De Jong JG, Abeling NG, et al. ^{1}H NMR spectroscopy of body fluids in patients with inborn errors of purine and pyrimidine metabolism. J Inherit Metab Dis. 1997;20(3):345–50.
20. Viant MR, Lyeth BG, Miller MG, Berman RF. An NMR metabolomic investigation of early metabolic disturbances following traumatic brain injury in a mammalian model. NMR Biomed. 2005;18:507–16.
21. Worley B, Powers R. Multivariate analysis in metabolomics. Curr Metabolomics. 2013;1:92–107.

22. Ditre CM, Griffin TD, Murphy GF, Sueki H, Telegan B, Johnson WC, et al. Effects of 2-hydroxy acids on photoaged skin: a pilot clinical, histologic, and ultrastructural study. J Am Acad Dermatol. 1996;34:187–95.
23. Pellerin L, Pellegri G, Bittar PG, Charnay Y, Bouras C, Martin JL, et al. Evidence supporting the existence of an activity-dependent astrocyte-neuron lactate shuttle. Dev Neurosci. 1998;20:291–9.
24. Huxtable RJ. Physiological actions of taurine. Physiol Rev. 1992;72:101–63.
25. Morales I, Dopico JG, Sabate M, Gonzalez-Hernandez T, Rodriguez M. Substantia nigra osmoregulation: taurine and ATP involvement. Am J Physiol Cell Physiol. 2007;292(5):C1934–41.
26. Solanky KS, Bailey NJ, Beckwith-Hall BM, Bingham S, Davis A, et al. Biofluid 1H NMR-based metabonomic techniques in nutrition research - metabolic effects of dietary isoflavones in humans. J Nutr Biochem. 2005;16(4):236–44.
27. Bertini I, Calabro A, De Carli V, Luchinat C, Nepi S, Porfirio B, Tenori L. The metabonomic signature of celiac disease. J Proteome Res. 2008;8(1):170–7.
28. Li M, Wang B, Zhang M, Rantalainen M, Wang S, Zhou H, et al. Symbiotc gut microbes modulate human metabolic phenotypes. Proc Natl Acad Sci U S A. 2008;105:2117–22.
29. Mason S, Reinecke CJ, Kulik W, van Cruchten A, Solomons R, van Furth MT. Cerebrospinal fluid in tuberculous meningitis exhibits only the L-enantiomer of lactic acid. BMC Infect Dis. 2016;16(1):1.
30. Field AP. Discovering statistics using IBM SPSS statistics: and sex and drugs and rock 'n' roll. 3rd ed. London: Sage Publications; 2009.
31. Thompson B. Significance, effect sizes, stepwise methods, and other issues: strong arguments move the field. J Exp Educ. 2001;70:80–93.
32. Cohen J. Statistical power analysis of the behavioural sciences. Revised ed. New York: Academic Press, Inc.; 1988. p. 79–81.
33. Quinones MP, Kaddurah-Daouk R. Metabolomics tools for identifying biomarkers for neuropsychiatric diseases. Neurobiol Dis. 2009;35(2):165–76.
34. Sinclair AJ, Viant MR, Ball AK, Burdon MA, Walker EA, Stewart PM, et al. NMR-based metabolomic analysis of cerebrospinal fluid and serum in neurological diseases- a diagnostic tool? NMR Biomed. 2010;23(2):123–32.
35. Mäntyselkä P, Miettola J, Niskanen L, Kumpusalo E. Glucose regulation and chronic pain at multiple sites. Rheumatology. 2008;47(8):1235–8.
36. Clish CB. Metabolomics: an emerging but powerful tool for precision medicine. Mol Case Stud. 2015;1(1):a000588.
37. Mayer EA, Tillisch K. The brain-gut axis in abdominal pain syndromes. Ann Rev Med. 2011;62
38. Cryan JF, O'Mahony SM. The microbiome-gut-brain axis: from bowel to behavior. Neurogastroenterol Motil. 2011;23(3):187–92.

4

Stability and relative validity of the Neuromuscular Disease Impact Profile (NMDIP)

Isaäc Bos[1*], Jan B.M. Kuks[1], Josué Almansa[2], Hubertus P.H. Kremer[1] and Klaske Wynia[1,2]

Abstract

Background: The aim of this study was to examine the stability and relative validity (RV) of the Neuromuscular Disease Impact Profile (NMDIP) using criterion-related groups. In a previous study the NMDIP-scales showed good internal consistency, convergent and discriminant validity. Known-groups analysis showed that the NMDIP discriminates between categories of extent of limitations.

Methods: A cross-sectional postal survey study was performed on patients diagnosed with a NMD and registered at the Department of Neurology, University Medical Center Groningen, the Netherlands.
Participants were asked to complete the preliminary NMDIP, the Medical Outcome study Short Form Questionnaire (SF-36), the World Health Organization Quality Of Life-abbreviation version (WHOQOL-bref), and two generic domain specific measures: the Groningen Activity Restriction Scale (GARS) and the Impact on Participation and Autonomy Questionnaire (IPAQ). The variables 'Extent of Limitations' and 'Quality of Life' were used to create criterion-related groups. Stability over time was tested using the Wilcoxon Signed Rank Test for paired samples and the intraclass correlation coefficients for repeated measures. RV was examined by comparing the ability of NMDIP with generic multidimensional health impact measures, and domain specific measures in discriminating between criterion-related subgroups using the Kruskal-Wallis H-test.

Results: Response rate was 70% (n = 702). The NMDIP-scales showed sufficient stability over time, and satisfactory or strong RV. In general, the NMDIP scales performed as well as or better than the concurrent measurement instruments.

Conclusions: The NMDIP proved to be a valid and reliable disease-targeted measure with a broad scope on physical, psychological and social functioning.

Keywords: Neuromuscular Disease Impact Profile, Relative validity, Test-retest reliability, Stability, Criterion validity

Background

Neuromuscular Diseases (NMDs) may be caused by an abnormality of the anterior horn cells, sensory ganglion cells (neuronopathy), the peripheral nerves (neuropathy), neuromuscular junctions (myasthenia), or muscle (myopathy). Common symptoms and signs of NMD include muscle weakness, impairment in muscle endurance, involuntary muscle activity (stiffness, myotonia, cramps, and fasciculations), sensory loss, autonomic dysfunction and impairment in control of voluntary movements. Sensations of pain and fatigue are common consequences of muscle and nerve pathology [1, 2]. Easy to apply NMD-specific reliable and validated self-report assessment tools are essential for obtaining insight into the prevalence and severity of the broad range of patient perceived health-related problems in NMDs. This is important for research and for clinical practise as well, in order to narrow the gap between the clinician's and patient's view on the actual health situation and to help to tailor care plans to the patient's need and preferences [3]. We therefore developed the disability-severity Neuromuscular Disease Impact Profile (NMDIP) based on the ICF-Core set for NMDs, a set of categories selected from the International Classification of Functioning, Disability and Health (ICF) [2, 4].

* Correspondence: i.bos@umcg.nl
[1]Department of Neurology, University Medical Center Groningen, University of Groningen, P.O. Box 300019700 RB Groningen, The Netherlands
Full list of author information is available at the end of the article

The NMDIP consists of 36 items that cover all ICF-components and are divided into eight scales and four single items. The NMDIP-scales showed moderate to good Cronbach's alpha and mean inter-item correlation coefficients. Convergent and discriminant validity analysis indicated that the NMDIP measures the impact of neuromuscular disease on physical, psychological and social functioning. The NMDIP discriminates between groups of patients who differ in 'Extent of limitations'. The four single items represent the Environmental Factors component (three items) and one Body Functions item (Seeing function) [4].

The objective of this study was to further examine the psychometric properties of the NMDIP and to build on previous studies on this measurement instrument [2, 4]. We examined its stability over time by assessing the test-retest reliability of the NMDIP-scales. We furthermore compared the ability of the NMDIP scales to discriminate between criterion related subgroups with this ability of four established concurrent measurement instruments, by assessing the Relative Validity (RV) [5, 6]. The RV coefficient indicates how much more or less valid each outcome measure is related to the best outcome measure.

Method

Sample and procedure

A cross sectional study, using a postal survey, was administered to patients diagnosed with a NMD who were registered at the Department of Neurology of the University Medical Center Groningen, University of Groningen, the Netherlands. Inclusion criteria for this study were: diagnosis with a NMD and representing one of Rowland's NMD classification groups: motor-neuron disorders, muscle disorders, junction disorders and peripheral nerve disorders [7]; being aged 18 or older; being able to read and write in Dutch; and being able to give informed consent. No exclusion criteria were formulated.

A total of 1003 eligible patients were selected from the hospital patient records system. To avoid inappropriately sending the questionnaires, we crosschecked for deceased patients using the national population register. Patients received information about the study and were invited to participate.

Respondents completed demographic and disease specific questions, the NMDIP, two criterion variables to measure the 'Extent of Limitations' and 'Quality of Life'. Also, concurrent measures were completed: two generic multidimensional health impact measures (the Medical Outcome study Short Form Questionnaire (SF-36) [8], and the World Health Organization Quality Of Life-abbreviation version (WHOQOL-bref) [9], and two generic domain specific measures the Groningen Activity Restriction Scale (GARS) [10] and the Impact on Participation and Autonomy Questionnaire (IPAQ) [11]. To assess stability over time, the NMDIP was administered on two occasions to patients who agreed to fill in the questionnaire twice. We, arbitrary, selected a time frame from eight to 10 weeks to be sure that patients could not remember their answers on the first questionnaire, and the likelihood of changes in the health situation was minimal.

Measurement instruments

The NMDIP includes 36 items and consists of eight scales and four additional items. The 36 items were divided over the four ICF components. For the Body Functions component items and for the Participation component items scoring options ranged from 0 (no disability) to 4 (complete disability); for the Activities component items scoring options ranged from 0 (no disability) to 3 (complete disability); and for the Environmental Factors component items scoring options ranged from 0 (no support) to 2 (full support) [4]. Item scores were summed into a scale with higher scores indicating more disability. To evaluate the RV, we used the 'Physical Functioning' construct as represented by the 'Activities of Moving around' and 'Self-care and Domestic Activities' scales, the 'Psychological Functioning' construct as represented by the 'Mental Functions and Pain' scale, and the 'Social Functioning' construct as represented by the 'Participation in Life Situations' scale. These scales were selected because items in these scales are closely associated with the scales in the concurrent measures.

The SF-36 was selected as a well-known reliable and valid generic multidimensional health-impact measure used for NMD [12, 13]. The SF-36 [8] comprises 36 items with eight functional dimensions. Three scales were used to examine the RV: 'Physical Functioning', 'Mental Health' and 'Social Functioning'. Item scores were coded, summed and transformed to a score of 0 (worst health) to 100 (best health) for each scale. The overall Cronbach's alpha for these scales was 0.79 in a study of Amyotrophic Lateral Sclerosis patients [14]. In our previous study the Cronbach's alpha for the selected scales ranged from 0.77 to 0.94 [4].

The WHOQOL-bref [9] was selected as a generic measurement instrument for a broad evaluation of quality of life. It consists of 28 items in four constructs and two separate questions. Three scales were used to examine the RV: 'Physical Health and Autonomy', 'Psychological Health', and 'Social Relations'. Item scores from each scale were coded, summed and transformed to a score of 0 (worst health) to 20 (best health). The Cronbach's alpha ranged from 0.63 to 0.81 in a study of Multiple Sclerosis patients [15]. In our previous study the Cronbach's alpha for the selected scales ranged from 0.60 to 0.84 [4].

The GARS [10] is a domain specific generic measurement instrument for assessing disability in 'Activities of daily living' (ADL) and 'Instrumental activities of daily living' (IADL). It consists of eleven ADL items and seven IADL items. A four-category response format was used, and ranged from 1 (no problem in performing without help) to 4 (impossible to perform). The scores were summed for each subscale. The Cronbach's alpha ranged from 0.95 to 0.97 in a study of Multiple Sclerosis patients [15]. In our previous study the Cronbach's alpha ranged from 0.93 to 0.95 [4].

The IPAQ [11, 16] is a domain specific generic measurement instrument for assessing participation. It consists of fifteen items focusing on person-perceived participation and autonomy. The instrument assesses two aspects of participation: perceived participation and the perceived problems with participation. In this study the perceived participation aspect was used since this construct is closely associated with the 'Participation in Life Situations' construct in the NMDIP questionnaire. The sub-domains were 'Autonomy Indoors', 'Family Role', 'Autonomy Outdoors', and 'Social Relations'. The response options ranged from 1 (very good) to 5 (very poor). Scores were summed for each domain. The Cronbach's alpha ranged from 0.86 to 0.94 in a study of Multiple Sclerosis patients [15]. In our previous study the Cronbach's alpha ranged from 0.84 to 0.94 [4].

Criterion variables

Two questions were selected as criterion variables: 'Extent of limitations' and 'Quality of life'.

To evaluate the 'Extent of Limitations' respondents were asked to answer the question: 'To what extent are you limited due to your NMD?' Responses were on a ten-point scale ranging from 1 (not limited at all) to 10 (completely limited). Respondents were classified into one of four groups: Group A with a 'very low extent of limitation' (score 1–2), Group B with a 'moderate extent of limitation' (score 3–5), Group C with a 'high extent of limitation' (score 6–8) and, Group D with a 'very high extent of limitation' (score 9–10).

The second criterion variable for evaluation of quality of life was one of the two single items adapted from the WHOQOL-bref. Respondents were asked: 'How would you rate your quality of life?'. Response options were: 1 = very poor, 2 = poor, 3 = neither poor nor good, 4 = good and 5 = very good. Respondents were classified into three groups: Group A– 'very poor or poor quality of life', Group B– 'neither poor nor good', and Group C– 'good or very good quality of life'.

Analysis

Descriptive statistics were used to characterize the total sample and the test-retest sample. Differences between both samples were examined using the difference in proportions test, the two-sample t-test, and if data are not normally distributed a non-parametric test for independent samples were used.

Test-retest reliability or stability over time was examined using the Wilcoxon Signed Test and the one-way random intraclass correlation coefficients (ICCs) [17].

Relative Validity was examined in several steps. First, the Chi-square was computed for each scale by calculating the Kruskal-Wallis H-test. Second, the RV of each scale was computed by dividing each H-statistic by the H-statistic for the scale with the highest H-statistic, and multiplied by one hundred. The resulting RV-estimate indicates the extent to which a scale or construct is able to discriminate between two groups compared to the measure with the highest H-statistic [18, 19]. Finally, the clinical relevance of the differences between respondent subgroups, and the nonparametric effect size (coefficient r) for unrelated samples, was calculated for statistically significant group differences ($\alpha = 0.05$) with post hoc tests (Bonferroni correction) [20]. Effect sizes where estimated through coefficient r, which was calculated by dividing the z-statistic (obtained from the Mann-Whitney U test) by the root of the sample size (n). To interpret this nonparametric effect sizes (coefficient r), Cohen suggested the following thresholds: an r of <0.10 indicates a trivial effect, an r of ≥ 0.10 to <0.24 a small effect, a r of ≥ 0.24 to <0.37 a moderate effect, and an $r \geq 0.37$ a large effect. A $r \geq 0.10$ reflects a clinically relevant difference between groups [20, 21].

IBM SPSS statistics version 22 was used.

Results

A total of 702 participants (70% response rate) completed the questionnaires. Of the 202 patients who agreed to complete the NMDIP twice 185 participants (92% response rate) actually returned the questionnaire.

The non-respondents from the 1003 eligible patients did not differ from respondents in terms of gender, but non-responders were significantly younger than respondents (p-value < 0.001 not in table).

The total sample (n = 702) and the test-retest sample (n = 185) differed in Age, Years since diagnosis. Participants in the total sample were older and were diagnosed more recently with a NMD compared to the test-retest sample. Also a significant larger proportion of respondents in the total sample was 'Retired due to age' compared to test-retest sample (p-value = 0.007) (Table 1). Finally the NMD category distribution differed significantly between the samples with less patients with Motor-neuron disorders and Muscle disorders and more patients with Peripheral nerve disorders in the total sample compared to the test-retest sample.

Table 1 Patient characteristics of total sample and test-retest sample

Variable	Total sample N = 702	Test-retest sample N = 185	p-value
Gender (%)			
Female	350 (50)	105 (57)	0.095^
Male	352 (50)	80 (43)	0.095^
Age			0.024##
Median (IQR)	61 (21)	57 (18)	
Range	19–92	19–92	
Year since diagnosis			0.003##
Median (IQR)	7 (11)	10 (14)	
Range	0–65	1–64	
Extent of limitations			0.329##
Median (IQR)	5 (4)	6 (4)	
Range	1–10	1–10	
Quality of life (WHOQOL-bref)			0.129##
Median (IQR)	4 (1)	4 (1)	
Range	1–5	1–5	
Relationship status (%)			
Relationship (married/partnership)	515 (73)	135 (76)	0.910^
Single (unmarried/widowed/divorced)	186 (27)	45 (24)	0.549^
Educational level (%)			
Primary school/vocational training	235 (33)	57 (31)	0.492^
Secondary school/vocational training	270 (38)	81 (44)	0.188^
Higher education /vocational training	161 (23)	37 (20)	0.394^
University	28 (4)	8 (4)	0.837^
Employment status (more answers possible) (%)			
Following a training or study	36 (5)	12 (7)	0.468^
Employment (part-time or full time)	173 (25)	43 (23)	0.693^
Voluntary work (part-time or full time)	42 (6)	15 (8)	0.294^
(Partially) retired due to NMD	213 (30)	67 (36)	0.126^
Housewife/househusband	171 (24)	55 (30)	0.136^
Retired due to age	244 (35)	45 (24)	0.007^
NMD category (%)			
Motor neuron disorder (MND)	43 (6)	20 (11)	0.027^
Muscle disorder (MD)	154 (22)	69 (37)	<0.001^
Junction disorder (JD)	234 (33)	66 (36)	0.549^
Peripheral nerve disorder (PND)	271 (39)	30 (16)	<0.001^

^Difference in proportions test, ##Mann-Whitney U test. Interquartile range (IQR) = Q3-Q1

Test-retest reliability

Wilcoxon Signed Rank Test (Table 2) showed no significant score differences between time points for most of the NMDIP scales, indicating stability over time, except for the 'Mental Functions and Pain' scale. However this difference was not clinically relevant (ES 0.18, not shown in table). The ICC of all scales showed sufficient agreement and ranged from 0.79 to 0.97, indicating good stability over time.

Criterion-related relative validity

Median scores of patients with a low 'Extent of limitation' (Table 3) or very poor or poor 'Quality of life' level

Table 2 Test-retest reliability for the NMDIP scales (n = 185)

	Comparison of scores at measurement 0 and 1						Intraclass correlation (one way random)
	Cases (N)	Median (IQR) 0	Cases (N)	Median (IQR) 1	Z-statistic	p-value*	
Muscle Functions	177	4 (2)	179	4 (2)	−2.08	0.037	0.85
Movement Functions	161	2 (3)	153	2 (2)	−.006	0.995	0.88
Excretion and Reproductive Functions	135	2 (3)	144	1 (3)	−1.00	0.318	0.85
Swallowing and Speech Function	172	0 (2)	180	0 (2)	−0.23	0.818	0.91
Mental Functions and Pain	164	4 (4)	162	4 (3)	−3.39	0.001	0.90
Activities of Moving around	185	4 (6)	185	4 (6)	−1.23	0.219	0.96
Self-care and Domestic Activities	185	3 (9)	185	3 (7)	−0.41	0.683	0.97
Participation in Life Situations	180	1 (2)	182	0 (2)	−1.70	0.090	0.79

*Wilcoxon Signed Rank Test, 2-tailed. Interquartile range (IQR) = Q3-Q1

(Table 4) were significantly different in the hypothesized direction when compared to the next higher group mean.

Extent of limitations

About 16% (n = 110) of the respondents reported 'low extent of limitations' (Group A) due to NMD, while 36% (n = 250) reported a 'moderate extent of limitation' (Group B), and 39% (n = 270) reported a 'high extent of limitation' (Group C). About 8% (n = 58) of the respondents reported a 'very high extent of limitations' (Group D).

Comparisons of the RV coefficients, as summarized in Table 3, revealed that the NMDIP 'Activities of Moving around' scale and SF-36 'Physical Functioning' scale were the most valid in discriminating between groups with an increasing extent of limitation.

We then examined the performance of the NMDIP-scales in indicating the differences between extreme groups (A-D) and subgroups (A-B, B-C, C-D) regarding the physical-, psychological- and social functioning constructs, as they relate to similar constructs in the concurrent measurement instruments. Regarding physical functioning, we found that both NMDIP activity scales turned out to be the most sensitive (followed by the 'Muscle Functions' scale) for measuring differences between extreme groups and subgroups. However, the performance of the concurrent SF-36 'Physical functioning' scale and both GARS scales were almost identical. Regarding the psychological functioning construct we found that the NMDIP 'Mental Functions and Pain' scale was the best performing scale compared to the SF-36 'Mental Health' scale and the WHOQOL-bref 'Psychological Health' scale, showing the highest extreme group and subgroup differences. Regarding the social functioning construct the NMDIP 'Participation in Life Situations' scale performed better than the SF-36 'Social Functioning' and the WHOQOL-bref 'Social Relations' scales, and roughly as well as the same as the comparable constructs in the domain-specific IPAQ.

In summary, the NMDIP scales performed sufficient to good in discriminating between (sub) groups with an increasing extent of limitations compared to similar constructs in concurrent measures regarding physical functioning, psychological functioning and social functioning constructs.

Quality of life

Eight percent (n = 53) of the respondents reported poor or very poor quality of life (Group A), while 25% (n = 175) experienced their quality of life as neither poor nor good (Group B) and 67% (n = 474) reported a good or very good quality of life' (Group C).

Comparisons of the RV-coefficients, as summarized in Table 4, revealed that the SF-36 'Psychological Health' scale and IPAQ 'Autonomy outdoors' scales were the most valid in discriminating between groups with differences in quality of life. The 'Mental Functions and Pain' NMDIP scale was the third most valid scale.

When examining the performance of the NMDIP-scales in indicating the differences between extreme and subgroups for quality of life, we found about the same extreme group differences for the physical functioning scales for all concurrent constructs with moderate Effect Sizes (ESs). The same goes for the subgroup differences, although the NMDIP 'Mental Functions and Pain' scale, and the WHOQOL-bref 'Psychological Health' scale performed slightly better than the SF-36 'Mental Health' scale. Finally, when examining the social functioning scales we found that the comparable NMDIP 'Participation in Life Situations' scale performed about as well as the SF-36 'Social Functioning' scale and the IPAQ scales with a moderate to large ESs for extreme group differences. The NMDIP 'Participation in Life Situations' scale also performed better compared to the social functioning construct of the WHOQOL-bref, the 'Social Relations' scale. The same goes for the subgroup differences.

Table 3 Relative validity of the NMDIP, domain specific and generic measurement instruments compared, using subgroups of extent of limitations (n = 702)

	Group A (n = 110) low extent of limitation		Group B (n = 250) moderate extent of limitation		Group C (n = 270) high extent of limitations		Group D (n = 58) very high extent of limitations		Kruskal-Wallis H		Group A-B[a]	Group B-C[a]	Group C-D[a]	Group A-D[a]
	n	Median (IQR)	n	Median (IQR)	n	Median (IQR)	n	Median (IQR)	Chi Square	RV[b]	es	es	es	es
NMDIP														
Muscle Functions	97	2 (2)	231	3 (2)	263	4 (2)	56	6 (3)	221.3	88	0.44	0.30	0.44	0.78
Movement Functions	92	0 (1)	210	2 (2)	232	3 (2)	49	5 (4)	149.3	59	0.34	0.30	0.29	0.72
Excretion and Reproductive Functions	82	0 (1)	182	1 (2)	194	2 (3)	43	3 (3)	47.1	19	0.16	0.18	-	0.51
Swallowing and Speech Function	107	0 (0)	238	0 (1)	258	0 (1)	55	1 (2)	48.6	19	0.17	0.11	0.18	0.50
Mental Functions and Pain	95	2 (2)	205	4 (3)	237	5 (4)	50	6.5 (5)	128.0	51	0.30	0.29	0.21	0.64
Activities of Moving around	110	0 (2)	250	3 (4)	272	6 (7)	58	13 (9)	251.0	99	0.42	0.39	0.39	0.79
Self-care and Domestic Activities	109	0 (1)	250	2 (3)	272	4 (8)	58	16.5 (14)	219.7	87	0.36	0.35	0.37	0.81
Participation in Life Situations	108	0 (0)	249	0 (1)	271	2 (4)	55	4 (4)	168.5	67	0.24	0.33	0.30	0.76
SF-36														
Physical Functioning	109	27 (6)	250	21 (8)	272	16 (7)	58	11 (3)	252.9	100	0.41	0.38	0.43	0.78
Mental Health	110	25 (3)	250	25 (5)	271	24 (6)	58	21.5 (7)	35.2	14	-	0.12	0.14	0.40
Social Functioning	110	10 (1)	250	8 (2)	271	7 (3)	58	5.5 (4)	129.8	51	0.31	0.26	0.22	0.62
WHOQOL-bref														
Physical Health and Autonomy	108	3 (1)	244	3 (0)	271	3 (0)	57	3 (1)	68.0	27	0.21	0.19	-	0.47
Psychological Health	106	4 (0)	246	3.5 (0.5)	271	3.5 (1)	57	3 (0)	68.0	27	0.19	0.14	0.25	0.55
Social Relations	104	4 (1)	238	4 (0)	261	4 (1)	55	4 (1)	30.8	12	-	0.14	-	0.35
GARS														
Activities of Daily Living	110	11 (1)	250	13 (6)	272	17 (10)	58	27 (17)	213.5	84	0.31	0.35	0.39	0.79
Instrumental Activities of Daily Living	109	7 (2)	250	10 (7)	270	15 (9)	58	24 (5)	215.0	85	0.33	0.35	0.39	0.78
IPAQ														
Autonomy Indoors	110	7 (3)	250	13 (6)	272	14 (6)	57	19 (11)	174.3	69	0.37	0.27	0.32	0.75
Family Role	110	8.5 (7)	248	15 (7)	271	18 (7)	58	22 (9)	177.3	70	0.40	0.28	0.22	0.71
Autonomy Outdoors	110	5.5 (4)	249	9 (3)	272	11 (5)	56	14 (4)	238.5	94	0.39	0.40	0.31	0.76
Social Relations	110	9 (6)	250	12 (4)	272	13 (5)	56	13 (4)	87.0	34	0.24	0.23	-	0.52

nmdip, gars, and ipaq: higher scores = more unable to perform activity; sf-36 and WHOQOL-bref scales: higher scores = better quality of life and more able to perform activity. Interquartile range (IQR) = Q3-Q1. - = not statistically significant. Bonferroni correction[a] = 0.0125 (p-value 0.05/4). RV = relative validity,[b] = score indicating the relative validity with score 100 related to the highest H-statistic. ES = effect size

In summary, the NMDIP scales performed well in discriminating between subgroups with differences in quality of life compared to similar constructs in concurrent measures concerning the physical functioning, psychological functioning and social functioning constructs.

Discussion

In this study the NMDIP, that was developed to reflect the prevalence and severity of a broad range of NMD-related disabilities [4], showed stability and performed well in the criterion-related subgroups of NMD-patients who differed in the extent of limitation and quality of life.

The results of the test-retest reliability analysis were sufficient indicating stability in the eight NMDIP scales. Although the results showed a difference for 'Mental Functions and Pain' scale while the effect size was trivial, the intraclass correlation showed sufficient agreement for all NMDIP scales between the two measurement moments.

In general, the NMDIP scales performed well in discriminating between relevant subgroups with increasing extent of limitation. This was the case for constructs evaluating physical, psychological, and social functioning. The NMDIP scales showed satisfactory relative validity and moderate to strong ESs indicating the strength

Table 4 Relative validity of the NMDIP, domain specific and generic measurement instruments compared, using subgroups of Quality of Life (n = 702)

	Group A (n = 53) Very poor or poor QoL		Group B (n = 175) Neither poor nor good QoL		Group C (n = 474) Good or very good QoL		Kruskal-Wallis H Chi Square	RV[b]	Group A-B[a]	Group B-C[a]	Group A-C[a]
	n	Median (IQR)	n	Median (IQR)	n	Median (IQR)			es	es	es
NMDIP											
Muscle Functions	52	5 (2)	167	4 (2)	439	3 (2)	81.4	50	0.34	0.23	0.35
Movement Functions	46	4 (3)	148	3 (2)	400	2 (3)	83.8	51	0.30	0.27	0.35
Excretion and Reproductive Functions	36	3 (5)	129	2 (2)	344	1 (2)	40.6	25	0.21	0.22	0.25
Swallowing and Speech Function	49	2 (3)	162	0 (1)	458	0 (1)	43.6	27	0.26	0.14	0.27
Mental Functions and Pain	45	8 (4)	147	6 (4)	405	3 (4)	147.7	90	0.28	0.42	0.40
Activities of Moving around	53	10 (8)	175	4 (6)	474	3 (5)	75.2	46	0.36	0.19	0.35
Self-care and Domestic Activities	53	10 (13)	175	3 (8)	473	2 (4)	79.9	49	0.32	0.22	0.33
Participation in Life Situations	52	4.5 (5)	175	2 (4)	468	0 (2)	103.7	63	0.32	0.26	0.39
SF-36											
Physical Functioning	53	12 (4)	175	17 (8)	473	21 (10)	85.7	52	0.38	0.23	0.34
Mental Health	53	20 (6)	175	22 (6)	473	25 (4)	132.5	81	0.27	0.35	0.38
Social Functioning	53	5 (3)	175	7 (2)	473	9 (2)	138.3	84	0.31	0.36	0.38
WHOQOL-bref											
Physical Health and Autonomy	53	3 (5)	173	3 (0)	466	3 (0)	117.7	72	0.21	0.41	0.34
Psychological Health	53	3 (0)	173	3 (1)	466	4 (0)	163.8	100	0.31	0.40	0.41
Social Relations	50	3 (1)	170	4 (1)	450	4 (0)	61.3	37	-	0.25	0.25
GARS											
Activities of Daily Living	53	26 (16)	175	17 (10)	474	13 (7)	80.6	49	0.37	0.20	0.35
Instrumental Activities of Daily Living	52	22 (12)	175	15 (9)	472	11 (9)	82.8	51	0.34	0.23	0.33
IPAQ											
Autonomy Indoors	53	19 (9)	175	14 (5)	473	12 (7)	109.6	67	0.32	0.29	0.36
Family Role	53	24 (8)	175	20 (8)	471	15 (8)	127.6	78	0.28	0.34	0.37
Autonomy Outdoors	53	15 (4)	174	11 (5)	471	8 (5)	157.6	96	0.42	0.35	0.43
Social Relations	53	15 (6)	175	13 (3)	472	11 (5)	134.1	82	0.26	0.35	0.37

nmdip, gars, IPAQ scales: higher scores = lower quality of life, sf-36, and WHOQOL-bref scales: higher scores = higher quality of life. Interquartile range (IQR) = Q3-Q1. - = not statistically significant. Bonferroni correction[a] = 0.02 (p-value 0.05/3). *RV* relative validity.[b] = score indicating the relative validity with score 100 related to the highest H-statistic. *ES* effect size

of the differences between subgroups. The NMDIP showed satisfactory performance in discriminating between relevant subgroups with decreasing Quality of Life. This was the case for constructs evaluating physical, psychological and social functioning.

Strength of this study is the inclusion of a large population of patients diagnosed with a NMD. Some potential study limitations should be mentioned. First, RV was examined as criterion-related validity value in this study. Because of the absence of a widely accepted criterion measure we chose to use self-report measures, which turned out to be a useful method. Secondly, the (relatively) small group sizes for 'very high extent of limitations' (Group D) and 'very poor or poor quality of life' (Group A) might have a negative impact on detecting group differences, though the difference between these subgroups and the adjacent groups showed sufficient ESs.

The results in this study permit us to recommend that researchers consider Relative Validity as a useful method to select a valid and 'with caution' a sensitive measure, especially when data from longitudinal studies or intervention studies are lacking. At the same time, we want to stress that RV is not a substitute for the sensitivity-to-change test. The findings in this study cannot be generalized to longitudinal studies. We recommend further research to evaluate the sensitivity to change of the NMDIP scales.

Furthermore generic health measures have some disadvantages against disease-specific health measures in addressing topics of a particular relevance to patients with a specific disease. Therefore it is recommended that the individual items in a scale be examined to estimate the suitability of the scale for a particular patient population [13].

Conclusions

The results in this study confirmed the stability of the NMDIP over time, and showed good relative validity compared to generic QOL and domain-specific measures. In combination with the findings in our previous study [4], the NMDIP proved to be a valid and reliable disease-targeted measure with a broad scope on physical, psychological and social functioning. Further research should examine the responsiveness of the NMDIP scales.

Abbreviations

ADL: Activities of daily living; GARS: Groningen Activity Restriction Scale; IADL: Instrumental activities of daily living; ICC: Intraclass correlation coefficient; IPAQ: Impact on Participation and Autonomy Questionnaire; NMD: Neuromuscular Diseases; NMDIP: Neuromuscular Disease Impact Profile; RV: relative validity; SF-36: Medical Outcome study Short Form Questionnaire; WHOQOL-bref: World Health Organization Quality Of Life-abbreviation version

Acknowledgements

We wish to thank the patients who participated in this study and were so kind to share personal information about the consequences of their disease by taking the time to fill in the questionnaires. We also wish to thank the students who assisted in data collection: Ronald Brans, Kyra van der Beek, Hanna Bosman, Annelies Verschure, Carolien Verschure, and Marieke Verschure.

Funding

Not Applicable.

Authors' contributions

IB contributed to the study design, coordinated the data collection, and drafted the manuscript. JBMK supervised the study and helped drafting the manuscript. JA supervised the statistical analyses and helped drafting the manuscript. HPHK supervised the study and helped drafting the manuscript. KW initiated, coordinated and supervised the study and drafting of the manuscript. All authors read and approved the final manuscript.

Competing interests

The authors declare that they have no competing interests.

Author details

[1]Department of Neurology, University Medical Center Groningen, University of Groningen, P.O. Box 300019700 RB Groningen, The Netherlands.
[2]Department of Health Sciences, Community and Occupational Health, University Medical Center Groningen, University of Groningen, Groningen, the Netherlands.

References

1. Marchettini P, Lacerenza M, Mauri E, Marangoni C. Painful peripheral neuropathies. Curr Neuropharmacol. 2006;4(3):175–81.
2. Bos I, Stallinga HA, Middel B, Kuks JBM, Wynia K. Validation of the ICF core set for neuromuscular diseases. Eur J Phys Rehabil Med. 2013;49(2):179–87.
3. Barry M, Edgman-Levitan S. Shared decision making—the pinnacle of patient-centered care. N Engl J Med. 2012;366:780–1.
4. Bos I, Kuks J, Wynia K. Development and testing psychometric properties of an ICF-based health measure: The Neuromuscular Disease Impact Profile. J Rehabil Med. 2015;47(5):445–53.
5. Ware JE Jr, Kosinski M, Bayliss MS, McHorney CA, Rogers WH, Raczek A. Comparison of methods for the scoring and statistical analysis of SF-36 health profile and summary measures: summary of results from the Medical outcomes study. Med Care. 1995;33(4 Suppl):AS264–79.
6. Fayers PM, Machin D. Developing and testing questionnaires. In: quality of life: assessment, analysis and interpretation. Chichester: John Miley & Sons; 2000. doi:10.1002/9780470024522.
7. Rowland LP, McLeod JG. Classification of neuromuscular disorders. J Neurol Sci. 1994;124(Suppl(0022–510)):109–30.
8. Ware JE Jr, Sherbourne CD. The MOS 36-item short-form health survey (SF-36). I. Conceptual framework and item selection. Med Care. 1992; 30(0025-7079; 0025-7079;6):473–83.
9. The WHOQOL Group. Development of the World Health Organization WHOQOL-bref quality of life assessment. World Health Forum. 1998;28:551–8.
10. Kempen GI, Miedema I, Ormel J, Molenaar W. The assessment of disability with the Groningen activity Restriction scale. Conceptual framework and psychometric properties. Soc Sci Med. 1996;43(0277–9536; 0277–9536; 11): 1601–10.
11. Cardol M, de Haan RJ, de Jong BA, van den Bos GA, de Groot IJ. Psychometric properties of the impact on participation and autonomy questionnaire. Arch Phys Med Rehabil. 2001;82(0003–9993; 0003–9993; 2):210–6.
12. Graham C, Rose M, Grunfeld E, Kyle S, Weinman J. A systematic review of quality of life in adults with muscle disease. J Neurol. 2011;258(9):1581–92.
13. Burns TM, Graham CD, Rose MR, Simmons Z. Quality of life and measures of quality of life in patients with neuromuscular disorders. Muscle Nerve. 2012; 46(1):9–25.
14. Pavan K, Marangoni BEM, Zinezzi M, Schmidt K, Oliveira B, Buainain R, Lianza S. Validation of the amyotrophic lateral Sclerosis assessment questionnaire (ALSAQ-40) scale in the Portuguese language. Arq Neuropsiquiatr. 2010; 68(1):48–51.
15. Wynia K, Middel B, van Dijk JP, De Ruiter H, De Keyser J, Reijneveld SA. The Multiple Sclerosis impact profile (MSIP). Development and testing psychometric properties of an ICF-based health measure. Disabil Rehabil. 2008;30(4):261–74.
16. Cardol M, de Haan RJ, van den Bos GA, de Jong BA, de Groot IJ. The development of a handicap assessment questionnaire: the impact on participation and autonomy (IPA). Clin Rehabil. 1999;13(0269–2155; 0269–2155; 5):411–9.
17. Streiner D, Norman G. Health measurement scales, a practical guide to their development and use. Fourth edition ed. Oxford: Oxford University Press; 2008.
18. McHorney CA, Ware JE, Lu JF, Sherbourne CD. The MOS 36-item short-form health survey (SF-36): III. Tests of data quality, scaling assumptions, and reliability across diverse patient groups. Med Care. 1994;32(1):40–66.
19. Wynia K, Middel B, De Ruiter H, van Dijk JP, De Keyser JHA, Reijneveld SA. Stability and relative validity of the Multiple Sclerosis impact profile (MSIP). Disabil Rehabil. 2008;30(14):1027–38.
20. Andersen M, Johnson U, Lindwall M, Ivarsson A. To adjust or not adjust: nonparametric effect sizes, confidence intervals, and real-world meaning. Psychol Sport Exerc. 2013;14(1):97–102.
21. Cohen J. Statistical power analysis for the behavioural sciences. 2nd ed. Hillsdale: Lawrence Erlbaum Associates; 1988.

5

A possible role of low regulatory T cells in anti-acetylcholine receptor antibody positive myasthenia gravis after bone marrow transplantation

Masahiko Fukatsu[1], Takenobu Murakami[1*], Hiroshi Ohkawara[2], Shunichi Saito[3], Kazuhiko Ikeda[2,3], Suguru Kadowaki[1], Itaru Sasaki[1], Mari Segawa[1], Tomoko Soeda[1], Akihiko Hoshi[1], Hiroshi Takahashi[2], Akiko Shichishima-Nakamura[2], Kazuei Ogawa[2], Yoshihiro Sugiura[1], Hitoshi Ohto[3], Yasuchika Takeishi[4], Takayuki Ikezoe[2] and Yoshikazu Ugawa[1,5]

Abstract

Background: Chronic graft-versus-host disease (GVHD) appears several months following allogenic hematopoietic stem cell transplantation (HSCT) and is clinically analogous to autoimmune disorder. Polymyositis is a common neuromuscular disorder in chronic GVHD, but myasthenia gravis (MG) is extremely rare. Hence, its pathophysiology and treatment have not been elucidated.

Case presentation: A 63-year-old man with a history of chronic GVHD presented with ptosis, dropped head, and dyspnea on exertion, which had worsened over the previous several months. He showed progressive decrement of compound muscle action potential in the deltoid muscle evoked by 3-Hz repetitive nerve stimulation, a positive edrophonium test, and elevated levels of serum anti-acetylcholine receptor antibodies, which suggested a diagnosis of generalized MG. No thymoma was found. Flow cytometric analysis revealed a remarkable depletion of peripheral Tregs ($CD4^+CD25^{high}FOXP3^+$ cells, 0.24% of the total lymphocytes). Administration of prednisolone and tacrolimus was insufficient to alleviate his symptoms; however, the use of rituximab successfully improved his condition.

Conclusions: Myasthenic symptoms appeared in the process of tapering prednisolone for the treatment of chronic GVHD, supporting the diagnosis of MG associated with chronic GVHD. The present case proposes a possibility that reduction of Tregs might contribute to the pathogenesis of MG underlying chronic GVHD. Immunotherapy with rituximab is beneficial for treatment of refractory MG and GVHD.

Keywords: Myasthenia gravis, Hematopoietic cell transplantation, Graft-versus-host disease, Regulatory T cells, Rituximab, Anti-acetylcholine receptor antibody

Background

Myasthenia gravis (MG) is a neuromuscular disorder characterized by muscle weakness and pathological fatigability of skeletal muscles. The pathophysiology of MG is defined as the production of autoantibodies blocking acetylcholine receptors at the neuromuscular junction [1]. Chronic graft-versus-host disease (GVHD) is mediated by the reactivation of donor T cells against recipient tissues and appears several months after allogenic hematopoietic stem cell transplantation (HSCT) in most cases [2]. The major organs involved in GVHD include the skin, gastrointestinal tract, and liver, whereas chronic GVHD features a wide variety of autoimmune disorders, including Sjögren syndrome, scleroderma, bronchiolitis obliterans, and immune cytopenias [3]. Chronic GVHD also affects neuromuscular system. In fact, polymyositis is a common neuromuscular disease present in chronic GVHD; however, MG is extremely rare. Although the 2015

* Correspondence: takebou@fmu.ac.jp
[1]Department of Neurology, Fukushima Medical University, 1 Hikariga-oka, Fukushima, Fukushima 960-1295, Japan
Full list of author information is available at the end of the article

National Institutes of Health Consensus Conference categorized MG under "other features or unclassified entities" of the signs and symptoms for diagnosis and staging of chronic GVHD, there have been a limited number of MG cases following allogeneic HSCT [4], and its pathophysiology and treatment approach have not yet been well established.

We present a case of chronic GVHD developing generalized MG that was successfully treated with advanced immunotherapy. The current case revealed a marked reduction of regulatory T cells (Tregs), suggesting the possible pathogenesis of MG in patients with chronic GVHD.

Case presentation

A 63-year-old man without familial history of MG was diagnosed with secondary acute myeloid leukemia that originated from myelodysplastic/myeloproliferative neoplasms, unclassifiable 2 years prior to the current presentation. He was then treated with intensive chemotherapy, and underwent allogeneic HSCT from a human leukocyte antigen (HLA)-matched unrelated donor in the following year. Prophylaxis against GVHD consisted of tacrolimus and short-term methotrexate. He achieved remission of acute GVHD, and tacrolimus was discontinued on day 86. He then developed mild chronic GVHD of the skin and liver at 7 and 12 months after the transplantation, respectively. Fourteen months after the transplantation, he was admitted to our hospital due to progressive bilateral pleural effusion, which was attributed to pleuritis related to chronic GVHD, and was successfully treated with intravenous methylprednisolone pulse therapy (mPSL) (1 g during the course of 3 days) followed by oral prednisolone (1 mg/kg/day). During the process of tapering oral prednisolone to 7.5 mg/day (20 months after the transplantation), the patient began to complain of bilateral ptosis, dropped head, and dyspnea on exertion, which continued to worsen, and he was admitted to our hospital.

On examination, his general condition was normal, except for the presence of sinus tachycardia (106/min). He had a moon face appearance as well as increased pigmentation and sclerotic changes on the skin. He was alert and had normal cognitive function. The patient had ptosis, dropped head, and mild bilateral weakness involving the craniocervical muscles and deltoid muscles (grade 4 as measured by the Manual Muscle Strength Testing) with fatigability. However, no bulbar symptoms were noted.

Blood sample tests showed an elevated anti-acetylcholine receptor (AChR) antibody (14.0 nmol/L), but negative anti-muscle specific kinase (anti-MuSK) antibody. His HLA genotype consisted of A*24:02-B*52:01-C*12:02-DRB1*12:01 and A*24:02-B*52:01-C*12:02-DRB1*15:02. Although the arterial blood carbon dioxide concentration was within the normal range, a pulmonary function test revealed a substantial reduction of vital capacity (VC) at 1.69 L (45.4% predicted). Polymerase chain reaction analysis of short tandem repeat sequences for peripheral blood showed 100% donor chimerism. Chest computed tomography suggested mild emphysematous changes in the lung field, but thymoma was not found. Intravenous injection of edrophonium remarkably improved the patient's ptosis and dropped head. An electrophysiological study showed 20.0% area decrement of compound muscle action potentials (CMAP) from the right deltoid muscle by 3-Hz repetitive axillary nerve stimulation. These findings confirmed a diagnosis of generalized MG with Myasthenia Gravis Foundation of America clinical classification IIb, quantitative MG score 14 out of 36, and MG-ADL score 8 out of 24.

Flow cytometric analyses were performed by using the patient's peripheral blood because depletion of Tregs after HSCT has been reported to be valuable in predicting chronic GVHD severity [5–7]. The Treg population in the peripheral blood, defined as $CD4^{+}CD25^{high}FOXP3^{+}$ cells, was 0.24% of the total lymphocytes (Fig. 1). This proportion was lower than that of our post-HSCT patients (mean ± SD 0.51 ± 0.15%) and of healthy subjects (0.94 ± 0.19%) [5].

Considering progression to myasthenic crisis, intravenous immunoglobulin was initially administered (0.4 g/kg for 5 days) and the patient showed mild responses for his ptosis and dropped head, but his fatigability and dyspnea on exertion remained unchanged. Subsequent mPSL pulse treatment (1 g for 2 days) exacerbated MG symptoms. We started pyridostigmine 180 mg/day with tacrolimus 3 mg/day, and consequently, his fatigability gradually improved and VC increased to 2.35 L (63.1% predicted) on the 28th hospital day. Follow-up electrophysiological study showed disappearance of significant CMAP decrement (4.5% area decrease). However, these improvements were insufficient for his daily activity. Follow-up anti-AChR antibody was still elevated to 18.0 nmol/L on the 22nd hospital day. The patient was treated with an increased oral prednisolone dose of 50 mg/day and intravenous mPSL pulse (1 g for 3 days), and anti-AChR antibody was decreased to 9.7 nmol/L on the 55th hospital day. Finally, he was administered four courses of weekly rituximab 375 mg/m^2, and his fatigability and weakness continued to improve steadily without pyridostigmine. He was discharged on the 92nd hospital day, receiving tacrolimus 3 mg/day and prednisolone 20 mg/day (Fig. 2). Five months after discharge, minimal manifestations remained, with a VC of 2.95 L (79.2% predicted), and he continued to take oral prednisolone at a dose of 10 mg/day and tacrolimus at 3 mg/day. Titers of anti-AChR antibody were steadily reduced (4.6, 3.7, and 3.2 nmol/L on 3, 6, and 9 months after discharge).

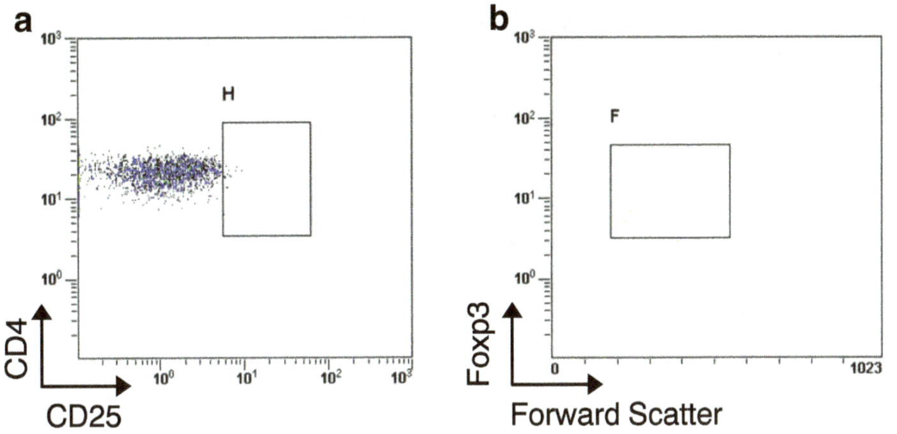

Fig. 1 Decreased CD4$^+$CD25^{high}FOXP3$^+$ cells (Tregs) in peripheral blood mononuclear cells from the patient. **a** Reduced proportion of CD25^{high} cells in gated CD4$^+$ fraction in peripheral blood mononuclear cells (gate H). **b** Most CD4$^+$CD25^{high} cells in gate H (>90%) were positive for Foxp3 (gate F)

Discussion and conclusions

MG is a very rare complication following HSCT, with an occurrence of less than 1%. Myasthenic symptoms typically develop between 22 and 60 months after transplantation [8] and most reported cases are associated with the existence of other symptoms of chronic GVHD, as MG is rarely the sole manifestation [9]. Myasthenic symptoms appear after the discontinuation or tapering of immunosuppressive agents [10], as in the present case. Patients with aplastic anemia as a background would have an increased risk of developing MG after transplantation [11]. Patients with specific HLAs (HLA Cw1, Cw7 or DR2) and a family history of MG are also at an increased risk of developing MG after HSCT [12, 13]. However, none of these risk factors was identified in the present case.

Most patients with MG associated with chronic GVHD test positive for anti-AChR antibodies. Approximately 20% of patients with chronic GVHD show positive anti-AChR antibody without myasthenic symptoms, indicating the existence of higher rates of subclinical MG [14]. In the present case, an elevated titer of anti-AChR antibody supported the diagnosis of MG, and its titer decreased in parallel with the improvement of myasthenic symptoms after immunotherapies. A few reported patients with MG after transplantation revealed

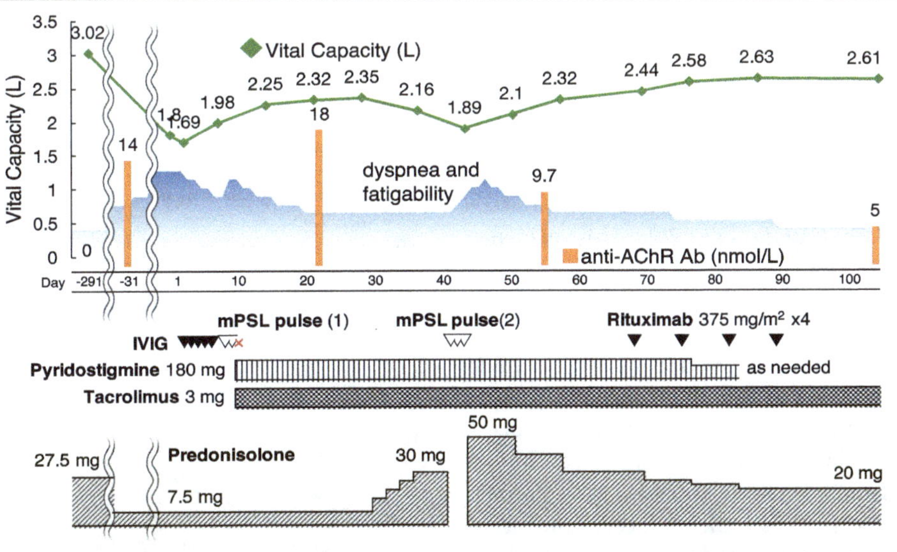

Fig. 2 Clinical courses of the present case. VC (in L) and anti-AChR antibody titer (in nmol/L) are shown in a line chart and a bar graph, respectively. Intravenous immunoglobulin was initially administered (0.4 g/kg for 5 days) with only moderate response. Two courses of mPSL pulse treatment (1 g for 2 to 3 days) rather exacerbated MG symptoms. Meanwhile, he was started on pyridostigmine 180 mg/day and tacrolimus 3 mg/day. Finally, he was administered four courses of weekly rituximab 375 mg/m^2, and his fatigability and weakness continued to improve steadily without pyridostigmine

other antibodies toward non-AChR components of the postsynaptic muscle endplate, e.g. anti-MuSK and anti-striated muscle antibodies [15, 16]. These findings suggest that pathogenic autoantibodies toward the neuromuscular junctions may be produced when discontinuing or tapering immunosuppressive treatments after transplantation.

A unique point in the present case was lower population of Tregs in the peripheral blood. Tregs are a subset of T lymphocytes that modulate the immune system and maintain tolerance to self-antigens [17, 18]. The frequency of Tregs in the peripheral blood has been reported to negatively correlate with GVHD severity [6]. Absence of Tregs coupled with donor-derived T cells leads to development of GVHD [19]. The number of Tregs in the peripheral blood decreases in untreated MG and is normalized by immunotherapy [20]. A functional impairment of thymic Tregs has been reported in the thymus of patients with MG and may play a role in triggering the autoimmune process [21]. Recent studies have reported Treg dysfunction as well as its downstream signal transducer and activator of transcription pathway is associated with immunopathology of MG, and a Treg-based immunotherapeutic approach has been suggested for experimental models of MG [22–24]. We suspect that suppression of Tregs in the present case may have partly contributed to the pathogenesis of MG as a manifestation of chronic GVHD.

Recently, several reports have shown that rituximab, a monoclonal antibody against B cell surface antigen CD20, could be an effective treatment for patients with refractory MG [25, 26]. Rituximab therapy also reduces the incidence of GVHD following allogeneic HSCT and exhibits a beneficial effect on steroid-refractory GVHD [27]. Although rituximab itself directly interacts with B cells, B cell depletion subsequently leads to expansion of Tregs and suppression of autoreactive T cells [28]. Additionally, treatment with rituximab was shown to be successful in two cases of MG associated with chronic GVHD [27, 29]. This evidence supports the utility of rituximab for refractory GVHD and MG against conventional immunotherapies in the present case.

In conclusion, we reported a rare case of chronic GVHD developing systemic MG after allogenic HSCT. Appearance of myasthenic symptoms during the process of tapering prednisolone for the treatment of chronic GVHD is a key feature of MG associated with chronic GVHD. We hypothesize that the reduced number of Tregs might play a possible role in the pathogenesis of MG and chronic GVHD. Immunotherapy with rituximab led to improvements of the patient's myasthenic symptoms, supporting the utility of rituximab for refractory MG and GVHD.

Abbreviations

AChR: Anti-acetylcholine receptor; anti-MuSK: Anti-muscle specific kinase; CMAP: Compound muscle action potentials; GVHD: Graft-versus-host disease; HLA: Human leukocyte antigen; HSCT: Hematopoietic stem cell transplantation; MG: Myasthenia gravis; mPSL: Methylprednisolone; Tregs: Regulatory T cells; VC: Vital capacity

Acknowledgments

Dr. Fukatsu received Young Investigator Award in the 112th Annual Meeting of the Japanese Society of Internal Medicine (2015 Kyoto). The authors wish to thank the Elsevier Language Editing for scientific English editing.

Funding

Dr. Murakami has received research funding from the Research Project Grant-in-aid for Scientific Research from the Ministry of Education, Culture, Sports, Science and Technology No. 15H01563, 16 K09724, the SENSHIN Medical Research Foundation, and the Mitsubishi Tanabe Pharma Corporation. Dr. Hoshi was supported by grants from the Research Project Grant-in-aid for Scientific Research from the Ministry of Education, Culture, Sports, Science and Technology No. 26461314. Dr. Ugawa was supported by grants from the Research Project Grant-in-aid for Scientific Research from the Ministry of Education, Culture, Sports, Science and Technology No. 22390181, 25,293,206, 15H05881, the Research Committee on Degenerative Ataxia from the Ministry of Health and Welfare of Japan, the Uehara Memorial Foundation, and the Novartis Foundation (Japan) for the Promotion of Science.

Authors' contributions

MF, TM, HO: research project conception, organization, execution and writing of the first draft. SS, KI, SK, IS, MS, TS, AH, HT, ASN, KO, YS, HO, and YT: research execution, manuscript review and critique. TI and YU: research project organization and execution, manuscript review and critique. All authors read and approved the final manuscript.

Competing interests

The authors declare that they have no competing interests.

Author details

[1]Department of Neurology, Fukushima Medical University, 1 Hikariga-oka, Fukushima, Fukushima 960-1295, Japan. [2]Department of Hematology, Fukushima Medical University, Fukushima, Japan. [3]Department of Blood Transfusion and Transplantation Immunology, Fukushima Medical University, Fukushima, Japan. [4]Department of Cardiovascular Medicine, Fukushima Medical University, Fukushima, Japan. [5]Fukushima Global Medical Science Center, Advanced Clinical Research Center, Fukushima Medical University, Fukushima, Japan.

References

1. Gilhus NE, Verschuuren JJ. Myasthenia gravis: subgroup classification and therapeutic strategies. Lancet Neurol. 2015;14(10):1023–36.
2. Jamil MO, Mineishi S. State-of-the-art acute and chronic GVHD treatment. Int J Hematol. 2015;101(5):452–66.
3. Vigorito AC, Campregher PV, Storer BE, Carpenter PA, Moravec CK, Kiem HP, Fero ML, Warren EH, Lee SJ, Appelbaum FR, et al. Evaluation of NIH consensus criteria for classification of late acute and chronic GVHD. Blood. 2009;114(3):702–8.
4. Jagasia MH, Greinix HT, Arora M, Williams KM, Wolff D, Cowen EW, Palmer J, Weisdorf D, Treister NS, Cheng GS, et al. National Institutes of Health consensus development project on criteria for clinical trials in chronic graft-versus-host disease: I. The 2014 diagnosis and staging working group report. Biol Blood Marrow Transplant. 2015;21(3):389–401. e381

5. Ngoma AM, Ikeda K, Hashimoto Y, Mochizuki K, Takahashi H, Sano H, Matsumoto H, Noji H, Saito S, Kikuta A, et al. Impaired regulatory T cell reconstitution in patients with acute graft-versus-host disease and cytomegalovirus infection after allogeneic bone marrow transplantation. Int J Hematol. 2012;95(1):86–94.
6. Li Q, Zhai Z, Xu X, Shen Y, Zhang A, Sun Z, Liu H, Geng L, Wang Y. Decrease of CD4(+)CD25(+) regulatory T cells and TGF-beta at early immune reconstitution is associated to the onset and severity of graft-versus-host disease following allogeneic haematogenesis stem cell transplantation. Leuk Res. 2010;34(9):1158–68.
7. Takahashi H, Ikeda K, Ogawa K, Saito S, Ngoma AM, Mashimo Y, Ueda K, Furukawa M, Shichishima-Nakamura A, Ohkawara H, et al. CD4+ T cells in aged or thymectomized recipients of allogeneic stem cell transplantations. Biol Res. 2015;48:41.
8. Grauer O, Wolff D, Bertz H, Greinix H, Kuhl JS, Lawitschka A, Lee SJ, Pavletic SZ, Holler E, Kleiter I. Neurological manifestations of chronic graft-versus-host disease after allogeneic haematopoietic stem cell transplantation: report from the consensus conference on clinical practice in chronic graft-versus-host disease. Brain. 2010;133(10):2852–65.
9. Baron F, Sadzot B, Wang F, Beguin Y. Myasthenia gravis without chronic GVHD after allogeneic bone marrow transplantation. Bone Marrow Transplant. 1998;22(2):197–200.
10. Bolger GB, Sullivan KM, Spence AM, Appelbaum FR, Johnston R, Sanders JE, Deeg HJ, Witherspoon RP, Doney KC, Nims J, et al. Myasthenia gravis after allogeneic bone marrow transplantation: relationship to chronic graft-versus-host disease. Neurology. 1986;36(8):1087–91.
11. Nelson KR, McQuillen MP. Neurologic complications of graft-versus-host disease. Neurol Clin. 1988;6(2):389–403.
12. Dowell JE, Moots PL, Stein RS. Myasthenia gravis after allogeneic bone marrow transplantation for lymphoblastic lymphoma. Bone Marrow Transplant. 1999;24(12):1359–61.
13. Mackey JR, Desai S, Larratt L, Cwik V, Nabholtz JM. Myasthenia gravis in association with allogeneic bone marrow transplantation: clinical observations, therapeutic implications and review of literature. Bone Marrow Transplant. 1997;19(9):939–42.
14. Smith CI, Norberg R, Moller G, Lonnqvist B, Hammarstrom L. Autoantibody formation after bone marrow transplantation. Comparison between acetylcholine receptor antibodies and other autoantibodies and analysis of HLA and gm markers. Eur Neurol. 1989;29(3):128–34.
15. Hon C, Mak W, Kwok AK, Au WY. Immunological and electrophysiological investigations of severe ptosis after bone marrow transplantation. Bone Marrow Transplant. 2004;34(5):455–8.
16. Atassi N, Amato AA. Muscle-specific kinase (MuSK) antibody-associated myasthenia gravis after bone marrow transplantation. Muscle Nerve. 2008; 38(2):1074–5.
17. Vignali DA, Collison LW, Workman CJ. How regulatory T cells work. Nat Rev Immunol. 2008;8(7):523–32.
18. Wing K, Sakaguchi S. Regulatory T cells exert checks and balances on self tolerance and autoimmunity. Nat Immunol. 2010;11(1):7–13.
19. Chen X, Vodanovic-Jankovic S, Johnson B, Keller M, Komorowski R, Drobyski WR. Absence of regulatory T-cell control of TH1 and TH17 cells is responsible for the autoimmune-mediated pathology in chronic graft-versus-host disease. Blood. 2007;110(10):3804–13.
20. Fattorossi A, Battaglia A, Buzzonetti A, Ciaraffa F, Scambia G, Evoli A. Circulating and thymic CD4 CD25 T regulatory cells in myasthenia gravis: effect of immunosuppressive treatment. Immunology. 2005;116(1):134–41.
21. Balandina A, Lecart S, Dartevelle P, Saoudi A, Berrih-Aknin S. Functional defect of regulatory CD4(+)CD25+ T cells in the thymus of patients with autoimmune myasthenia gravis. Blood. 2005;105(2):735–41.
22. Souroujon MC, Aricha R, Feferman T, Mizrachi K, Reuveni D, Fuchs S. Regulatory T cell-based immunotherapies in experimental autoimmune myasthenia gravis. Ann N Y Acad Sci. 2012;1274:120–6.
23. Thiruppathi M, Rowin J, Li Jiang Q, Sheng JR, Prabhakar BS, Meriggioli MN. Functional defect in regulatory T cells in myasthenia gravis. Ann N Y Acad Sci. 2012;1274:68–76.
24. Alahgholi-Hajibehzad M, Oflazer P, Aysal F, Durmus H, Gulsen-Parman Y, Marx A, Deymeer F, Saruhan-Direskeneli G. Regulatory function of CD4 +CD25++ T cells in patients with myasthenia gravis is associated with phenotypic changes and STAT5 signaling: 1,25-Dihydroxyvitamin D3 modulates the suppressor activity. J Neuroimmunol. 2015;281:51–60.
25. Anderson D, Phan C, Johnston WS, Siddiqi ZA. Rituximab in refractory myasthenia gravis: a prospective, open-label study with long-term follow-up. Ann Clin Transl Neurol. 2016;3(7):552–5.
26. Ruzhansky KM, Brannagan TH 3rd. Neuromuscular complications of hematopoietic stem cell transplantation. Muscle Nerve. 2015;52(4):480–7.
27. Zaja F, Bacigalupo A, Patriarca F, Stanzani M, Van Lint MT, Fili C, Scime R, Milone G, Falda M, Vener C, et al. Treatment of refractory chronic GVHD with rituximab: a GITMO study. Bone Marrow Transplant. 2007;40(3):273–7.
28. Lund FE, Randall TD. Effector and regulatory B cells: modulators of CD4+ T cell immunity. Nat Rev Immunol. 2010;10(4):236–47.
29. Unal S, Sag E, Kuskonmaz B, Kesici S, Bayrakci B, Ayvaz DC, Tezcan I, Yalnizoglu D, Uckan D. Successful treatment of severe myasthenia gravis developed after allogeneic hematopoietic stem cell transplantation with plasma exchange and rituximab. Pediatr Blood Cancer. 2014;61(5):928–30.

6

Case report: a novel frameshift mutation in the *mitochondrial cytochrome c oxidase II* gene causing mitochondrial disorder

Laura Kytövuori[1,2,3*], Mikko Kärppä[1,2,3], Hannu Tuominen[4], Johanna Uusimaa[2,5,6,7], Markku Saari[8], Reetta Hinttala[2,5,6,7] and Kari Majamaa[1,2,3]

Abstract

Background: *Mitochondrial cytochrome c oxidase 2, MT-CO2*, encodes one of the three subunits, which form the catalytic core of cytochrome c oxidase (COX), complex IV. Mutations in *MT-CO2* are rare and the associated phenotypes are variable including nonsyndromic and syndromic forms of mitochondrial diseases.

Case presentation: We describe a 30-year-old man with cognitive decline, epilepsy, psychosis, exercise intolerance, sensorineural hearing impairment, retinitis pigmentosa, cataract and lactic acidosis. COX-deficient fibers and ragged red fibers were abundant in the muscle. Sequencing of mitochondrial DNA (mtDNA) revealed a novel frameshift mutation m.8156delG that was predicted to cause altered C-terminal amino acid sequence and to lead to truncation of the COX subunit 2. The deletion was heteroplasmic being present in 26% of the mtDNA in blood, 33% in buccal mucosa and 95% in muscle. Deletion heteroplasmy correlated with COX-deficiency in muscle histochemistry. The mother and the siblings of the proband did not harbor the deletion.

Conclusions: The clinical features and muscle histology of the proband suggested a mitochondrial disorder. The m. 8156delG deletion is a new addition to the short list of pathogenic mutations in the mtDNA-encoded subunits of COX. This case illustrates the importance of mtDNA sequence analysis in patients with an evident mitochondrial disorder.

Keywords: Neuromuscular disorders, Mitochondrial diseases, Cytochrome c oxidase deficiency, Case report

Background

Complex IV (CIV) in the mitochondrial respiratory chain is composed of 13 subunits, three of which are encoded by genes in mitochondrial DNA (mtDNA). *Cytochrome c oxidase II, MT-CO2*, codes for structural subunit 2, which participates in the formation of the catalytic core of CIV. Rare mutations have been described in *MT-CO2* in patients with various phenotypes, such as severe lactic acidosis [1], MELAS (mitochondrial encephalomyopathy, lactic acidosis, and stroke-like episodes) [2], encephalomyopathy [3], or rhabdomyolysis [4]. The 10 nuclear genes encoding the remaining subunits are even more rarely mutated than the mitochondrial ones and only a handful of mutations have been described to date [5–10]. Most of the cases with complex IV deficiency harbor causative mutation in the genes encoding non-structural factors [11, 12].

We describe a male patient with heteroplasmic de novo deletion, m.8156delG, in *MT-CO2* leading to truncation of subunit 2 in cytochrome c oxidase (COX). The patient had a clinically apparent mitochondrial disorder with prominent findings in muscle histology.

Case presentation

The patient is a 30-year-old man with negative family history of neuromuscular disorders. Early childhood development was normal. Sensorineural hearing impairment with tinnitus and mild memory deficit were the first symptoms, which were noticed at the age of 12 years. Neuropsychological examination revealed a moderate cognitive decline at the age of 24 years.

* Correspondence: laura.kytovuori@oulu.fi
[1]Research Unit of Clinical Neuroscience, University of Oulu, P.O. Box 5000, FI-90014 Oulu, Finland
[2]Medical Research Center Oulu, Oulu University Hospital and University of Oulu, Oulu, Finland
Full list of author information is available at the end of the article

Retinitis pigmentosa was diagnosed at the age of 25 years and premature cataract at the age of 29 years. The bilateral cataracts were operated soon after the diagnosis. Generalized epilepsy and psychosis were diagnosed at the age of 29 years, but because of poor tolerance and compliance he does not use medications. Moreover, he has exercise intolerance and mild balance disorder. He lives alone with supervision.

Neurological examination at the age of 29 years revealed cognitive decline, clumsy movements, abnormal balance tests and impaired visual acuity. Hearing was impaired and he had hearing aid in both ears. Ophthalmoplegia was not found. Walking and muscle strength were normal. His height is 170 cm and weight 57 kg.

Blood lactate was first measured at the age of 23 years and was 3.06 mmol/l (laboratory reference, 0.33–1.33 mmol/l). Muscle histology at the age of 23 years revealed a substantial number of COX-deficient fibers and ragged red fibers (Fig. 1). Muscle ultrastructural analysis revealed large intramitochondrial inclusions. In brain MRI ventricular enlargement, moderate cerebellopontine atrophy and hyperintense signals in both basal ganglia were found. Cardiac examination and electrophysiological studies of the muscle and nerve were normal.

Molecular methods and cell culture

DNA extraction from blood, buccal swab and myoblasts was done by using QIAamp DNA Blood Mini Kit (QIAGEN, Hilden, Germany). From muscle biopsy, the purification was done with Wizard® Genomic DNA purification kit (Promega Corporation, Madison, WI). The mitochondrial DNA was amplified and sequenced in 12 overlapping fragments.

Mutation heteroplasmy in tissues from the patient, his mother and the four siblings was determined by cloning as described previously [13]. One hundred colonies per cloned sample were screened for the mutation with the conformation sensitive gel electrophoresis.

A muscle sample was obtained from *vastus lateralis* and myoblast culture was established as described previously [14]. Cells were immunostained with myoblast-specific antibody for desmin (BioGenex, Fremont, CA, U.S.A.).

Laser-capture microdissection of COX-SDH stained frozen sections was done using Zeiss P.A.L.M. microscope (Microlaser Technologies GmbH, Bernried, Germany) in Turku Centre for Biotechnology. Ten COX-negative, COX-positive and COX-deficient fibers were collected in tubes with adhesive caps (Carl Zeiss MicroImaging GmbH, Munich, Germany). DNA was released from the ten pooled fibers of each COX phenotype using lysis buffer (200 mM KOH, 50 mM DTT) and 30 min incubation at 65 °C. The lysis reaction was then neutralized with Tris-HCl (900 mM, pH 8.3) and 4 μl of the solution was used for PCR. PCR was carried out using Phusion High-Fidelity DNA polymerase (Thermo Fisher Scientific, Waltham, MA, U.S.A.) in a 50 μl reaction that was established according to the provided protocol. The reaction conditions are available on request. The heteroplasmy was determined by cloning.

Novel mutation in MT-CO2

Sequencing of mtDNA revealed a novel frameshift mutation m.8156delG in the *MT-CO2* gene of the proband (Fig. 2). The mutation was heteroplasmic and the proportion of the mutant genome was 26% in blood, 33% in epithelial cells from buccal swab and 95% in the skeletal muscle. The deletion was not detected in the blood or buccal mucosa from the mother or in the blood from the siblings of the patient suggesting de novo mutation. Single-fiber analysis showed that the proportion of the mutation required to cause a biochemical defect was high. Pooled blue COX-negative fibers contained 98% of mutant DNA. The proportion was 96% in COX-deficient

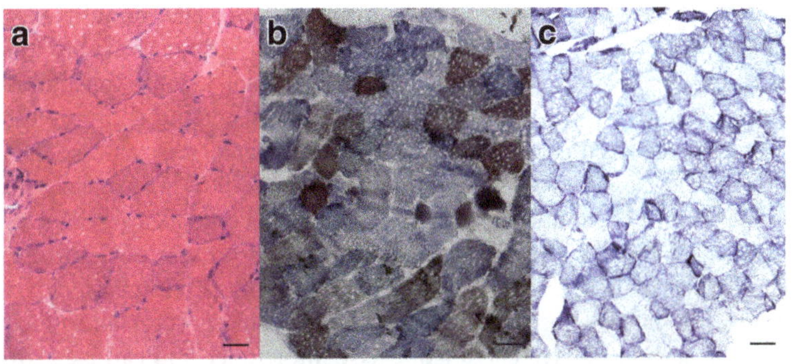

Fig. 1 Histology of *vastus lateralis* muscle from the patient harboring the m.8156delG mutation. **a** Hematoxylin and eosin stainings show ragged *red fibers*. Bar = 50 μm (**b**) SDH-COX staining shows that COX-deficient fibers encompass more than half of the fibers. Bar = 50 μm (**c**) NADH staining shows mitochondrial proliferation. Bar = 100 μm

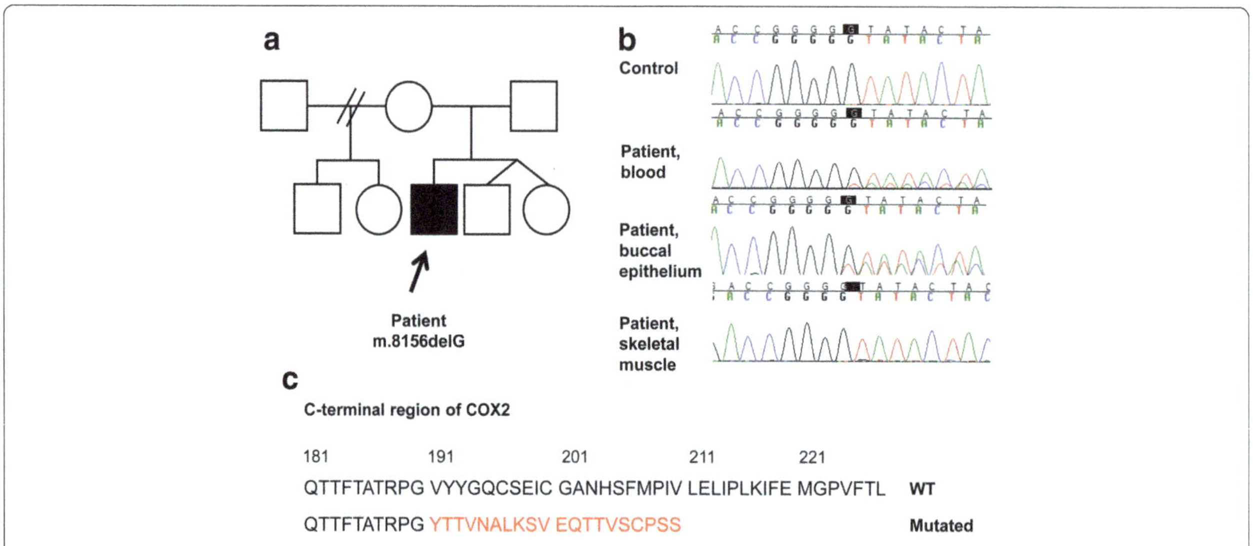

Fig. 2 Novel frameshift mutation in *MT-CO2* alters and truncates the C-terminus of COX2. **a** The deletion m.8156delG was found in the proband, but not in the asymptomatic mother or siblings, suggesting that the mutation had arisen de novo. **b** The deletion was found in three tissues of the proband. **c** The mutation alters the amino acid sequence of the C-terminus of COX2 beyond amino acid 190 and creates a stop codon at position 211

fibers with intermediate color and 88% in biochemically normal fibers.

The mutation is predicted to lead to an altered amino acid sequence from position 191 and extending towards the C-terminus of the COX2 subunit. The mutation creates a termination codon resulting in premature truncation of the protein at amino acid 210, while the wild type protein consists of 227 amino acids. Three suggested copper binding sites are located in the affected region. The mtDNA belonged to haplogroup U8a1a1.

Four cell cultures were established from two muscle biopsies obtained on separate occasions. The first two cell cultures turned out to be fibroblasts with less than 20% of the mutant mtDNA. The other two cell cultures were desmin-positive verifying their muscular identity. Surprisingly, the mutation could not be detected in any of the subcultures.

Discussion

We found a novel mutation m.8156delG that is suggested to result in an altered protein sequence and truncation of subunit COX2 in a patient with mitochondrial disorder. Previously, five mutations that are predicted to lead to truncated COX2 have been reported in patients with phenotypes of variable severity. In addition, six missense mutations in *MT-CO2* have been reported in patients with variable phenotypes in MITOMAP database [15]. Furthermore, nine variants have been reported with disease associations, but later studies have classified them as polymorphisms.

A frameshift deletion m.8042_8043delTA is one of the truncating mutations destroying one third of the COX2 and resulting in severe lactic acidosis and death at the age of few days [1]. The mutation load was 20% in the skeletal muscle and complex IV activity was decreased to half of the normal. The presence of the truncated form of COX2 was not verified in tissues, however. In contrast, the m.7630delT deletion has been found in a patient with MELAS syndrome that was fatal only at the age of 23 years [2]. The predicted length of COX2 was 16 amino acids, mutation heteroplasmy was 93%, and residual activity of CIV was only a few percent of the normal. Moreover, the protein level of COX2 was substantially reduced, but mRNAs of CIV subunits including that of mutant COX2 were significantly increased. The presence of the mutant protein was not investigated. Furthermore, a m.7896G > A nonsense mutation with a heteroplasmy of 60–80% has been reported to result in a 104-amino-acid protein, to lead to 13% activity of complex IV and to cause a severe early-onset multisystem disorder [16]. The amount of wild type COX2 was reported to be decreased, but the truncated protein was not detected. Finally, the mutation p.Glu129* has been found in a patient with adolescence-onset hearing impairment and psychiatric disorder. Mutation heteroplasmy was 90% in skeletal muscle and the remaining activity of complex IV was 12% [3]. Again, the mutant form of the protein was not investigated. At age 25 years he had developed bilateral cataract and within few years, the syndrome progressed to include gait instability, exercise intolerance and cardiac arrhythmia. The patient died from cardiac arrest at the age of 35 years.

These four cases show that in the presence of a truncating mutation the activity of CIV is decreased.

Interestingly, there is a lack of correlation between decreased activity and clinical severity suggesting that the truncated proteins may interfere with respiratory chain or other cellular processes by gaining an abnormal function. Unfortunately, the studies have failed to show the presence of truncated COX2 or the existence has not been investigated.

The G stretch spanning between the nucleotides m.8152–8156 in *MT-CO2* has previously been found to be mutated in an adult patient with exercise-induced myoglobinuria and rhabdomyolysis [17]. This mutation was a heteroplasmic duplication m.8156dupG with a 56% mutation load in skeletal muscle causing decreased activity of CIV. In our patient, the predicted truncation of C-terminal sequence resulted in a mitochondrial disorder with various classical features of mitochondrial dysfunction. However, similar to the previous reports with frameshift mutations in *MT-CO2*, the presence of the truncated protein could not be verified.

The m.8156delG mutation was undetectable already in the first passages of the myoblast cultures despite of the high mutation load in the skeletal muscle showing that the mutation was present in highly differentiated myotubes. It is possible that the healthy cells benefitted from the culture conditions optimized for myoblasts leading to the disappearance of the mutant containing cells. Similar findings have previously been reported in a patient with m.9789 T > C in the *MT-CO3* with a heteroplasmy of 50% [3] and in a patient with m.9952G > A with a heteroplasmy of 57% [18]. Furthermore, m.7671 T > A in *MT-CO2* has been reported to be absent in myoblasts despite the very high heteroplasmy of 90% in the muscle [19]. In contrast, the m.6930G > A mutation in *MT-CO1* has been found at 33% heteroplasmy in myoblasts, while the mutation heteroplasmy was 75% in muscle [20]. Furthermore, heteroplasmic disease-causing deletions have been found to be present only in a minority of myoblast subcultures, even though the proportion of the deletion in the satellite cells was shown to be similar to that in the skeletal muscle [21]. In that study, the heteroplasmy decreased during further culturing and differentiation to myotubes. The authors suggested that there might be two periods of selection against the mutated mtDNA, the first occurring during satellite cell activation and second in the replication phase [21].

Conclusions

Frameshift mutations in *MT-CO2* are rare and clinically variable. We presented here a patient with a progressive mitochondrial syndrome and a novel frameshift mutation m.8156delG in *MT-CO2* as a cause. This case illustrates the importance of mtDNA sequence analysis in patients with a suspected mitochondrial disorder.

Abbreviations

mtDNA: mitochondrial DNA; *MT-CO2: mitochondrial cytochrome c oxidase 2;* COX: cytochrome c oxidase; MELAS: mitochondrial encephalomyopathy, lactic acidosis, and stroke-like episodes

Acknowledgements

The authors gratefully acknowledge the expert technical assistance of Ms. Anja Heikkinen and Ms. Pirjo Keränen. Laser capture microdissection was performed at the Cell Imaging Core, Turku Centre for Biotechnology, University of Turku and Åbo Akademi University.

Funding

The study was supported by grants from the Sigrid Juselius Foundation, Medical Research Center, University of Oulu and Oulu University Hospital, State research funding from Oulu University Hospital, and the Academy of Finland (R.H., decision numbers 266,498 and 273,790).

Authors' contributions

L.K. carried out molecular analyses and wrote the first draft of the manuscript. M.K. performed clinical examinations. H.T. analyzed muscle histology. M.S. designed and conducted the LCM protocol. J.U. participated in designing of the study. R.H. participated in designing and conduction of the study. K.M. participated in designing the project, and all investigations occurred under his supervision. All authors have revised the manuscript and approved the manuscript for submission.

Competing interests

The authors declare that they have no competing interests.

Author details

[1]Research Unit of Clinical Neuroscience, University of Oulu, P.O. Box 5000, FI-90014 Oulu, Finland. [2]Medical Research Center Oulu, Oulu University Hospital and University of Oulu, Oulu, Finland. [3]Department of Neurology, Oulu University Hospital, P.O. Box 20OYS, FI-90029 Oulu, Finland. [4]Department of Pathology, Cancer and Translational Medicine Research Unit, University of Oulu and Department of Pathology, Oulu University Hospital, Oulu, Finland. [5]PEDEGO Research Unit, University of Oulu, P.O. Box 5000FI-90014 Oulu, Finland. [6]Department of Children and Adolescents, Division of Pediatric Neurology, Oulu University Hospital, Oulu, Finland. [7]Biocenter Oulu, University of Oulu, P.O. Box 5000FI-90014 Oulu, Finland. [8]Turku Centre for Biotechnology, Cell Imaging Core, University of Turku, FI-20520 Turku, Finland.

References

1. Wong LJ, Dai P, Tan D, Lipson M, Grix A, Sifry-Platt M, et al. Severe lactic acidosis caused by a novel frame-shift mutation in mitochondrial-encoded cytochrome c oxidase subunit II. Am J Med Genet. 2001;102:95–9.
2. Rossmanith W, Freilinger M, Roka J, Raffelsberger T, Moser-Their K, Prayer D, et al. Isolated cytochrome c oxidase deficiency as a cause of MELAS. J Med Genet. 2008;45:117–21.
3. Horváth R, Schoser BG, Müller-Höcker J, Volpel M, Jaksch M, Lochmüller H. Mutations in mtDNA-encoded cytochrome c oxidase subunit genes causing isolated myopathy or severe encephalomyopathy. Neuromuscul Disord. 2005;15:851–7.
4. McFarland R, Taylor RW, Chinnery PF, Howell N, Turnbull DM. A novel sporadic mutation in cytochrome c oxidase subunit II as a cause of rhabdomyolysis. Neuromuscul Disord. 2004;14:162–6.
5. Massa V, Fernandez-Vizarra E, Alshahwan S, Bakhsh E, Goffrini P, Ferrero I, et al. Severe infantile encephalomyopathy caused by a mutation in COX6B1, a nucleus-encoded subunit of cytochrome c oxidase. Am J Hum Genet. 2008;82:1281–9.
6. Shteyer E, Saada A, Shaag A, Al-Hijawi FA, Kidess R, Revel-Vilk S, et al. Exocrine pancreatic insufficiency, dyserythropoietic anemia, and calvarial hyperostosis are caused by a mutation in the COX4I2 gene. Am J Hum Genet. 2009;84:412–7.

7. Indrieri A, van Rahden VA, Tiranti V, Morleo M, Iaconis D, Tammaro R, et al. Mutations in COX7B cause microphthalmia with linear skin lesions, an unconventional mitochondrial disease. Am J Hum Genet. 2012;91:942–9.
8. Abdulhag UN, Soiferman D, Schueler-Furman O, Miller C, Shaag A, Elpeleg O, et al. Mitochondrial complex IV deficiency, caused by mutated COX6B1, is associated with encephalomyopathy, hydrocephalus and cardiomyopathy. Eur J Hum Genet. 2015;23:159–64.
9. Tamiya G, Makino S, Hayashi M, Abe A, Numakura C, Ueki M, et al. A mutation of COX6A1 causes a recessive axonal or mixed form of charcot-marie-tooth disease. Am J Hum Genet. 2014;95:294–300.
10. Hallmann K, Kudin AP, Zsurka G, Kornblum C, Reimann J, Stüve B, et al. Loss of the smallest subunit of cytochrome c oxidase, COX8A, causes leigh-like syndrome and epilepsy. Brain. 2016;139:338–45.
11. Zhu Z, Yao J, Johns T, Fu K, De Bie I, Macmillan C, et al. SURF1, encoding a factor involved in the biogenesis of cytochrome c oxidase, is mutated in leigh syndrome. Nat Genet. 1998;20:337–43.
12. Leary SC, Antonicka H, Sasarman F, Weraarpachai W, Cobine PA, Pan M, et al. Novel mutations in SCO1 as a cause of fatal infantile encephalopathy and lactic acidosis. Hum Mutat. 2013;34:1366–70.
13. Martikainen MH, Kytövuori L, Majamaa K. Juvenile parkinsonism, hypogonadism and leigh-like MRI changes in a patient with m.4296G>a mutation in mitochondrial DNA. Mitochondrion. 2013;13:83–6.
14. Shoubridge EA, Johns T, Boulet L. Use of myoblast cultures to study mitochondrial myopathies. Methods Enzymol. 1996;264:465–75.
15. MITOMAP: A Human Mitochondrial Genome Database. http://www.mitomap.org, accessed 10 Sept 2016.
16. Campos Y, Garcia-Redondo A, Fernandez-Moreno MA, Martínez-Pardo M, Goda G, Rubio JC, et al. Early-onset multisystem mitochondrial disorder caused by a nonsense mutation in the mitochondrial DNA cytochrome C oxidase II gene. Ann Neurol. 2001;50:409–13.
17. Vissing CR, Duno M, Olesen JH, Rafiq J, Risom L, Christensen E, et al. Recurrent myoglobinuria and deranged acylcarnitines due to a mutation in the mtDNA MT-CO2 gene. Neurology. 2013;80:1908–10.
18. Hanna MG, Nelson IP, Rahman S, Lane RJ, Land J, Heales S, et al. Cytochrome c oxidase deficiency associated with the first stop-codon point mutation in human mtDNA. Am J Hum Genet. 1998;63:29–36.
19. Rahman S, Taanman JW, Cooper JM, Nelson I, Hargreaves I, Meunier B, et al. A missense mutation of cytochrome oxidase subunit II causes defective assembly and myopathy. Am J Hum Genet. 1999;65:1030–9.
20. Bruno C, Martinuzzi A, Tang Y, Andreu AL, Pallotti F, Bonilla E, et al. A stop-codon mutation in the human mtDNA cytochrome c oxidase I gene disrupts the functional structure of complex IV. Am J Hum Genet. 1999;65:611–20.
21. Spendiff S, Reza M, Murphy JL, Gorman G, Blakely EL, Taylor RW, et al. Mitochondrial DNA deletions in muscle satellite cells: implications for therapies. Hum Mol Genet. 2013;22:4739–47.

7

Single-fiber electromyography in the orbicularis oculi muscle in patients with ocular myasthenia gravis symptoms: does abnormal jitter predict response to treatment?

Goran Rakocevic[1*], Mark Moster[2] and Mary Kay Floeter[3]

Abstract

Background: Seronegative ocular myasthenia gravis (OMG) is diagnosed by ocular symptoms with supporting SFEMG, typically of frontalis or extensor digitorum muscles. We aimed to determine the sensitivity and specificity of orbicularis oculi SFEMG to diagnose and exclude myasthenia gravis and predict response to therapy.

Methods: Orbicularis oculi SFEMG studies were conducted in 142 consecutive patients with symptoms and/or findings of OMG and negative AChR antibody during the period of 5 years. Retrospective chart review was conducted 2 years after the SFEMG to determine whether treatments were given and responses to treatment.

Results: Orbicularis oculi SFEMG was abnormal in 31 patients and normal in 111 patients. Twenty-nine patients with abnormal SFEMG were treated, and 25 had a good response. Twenty-four patients with normal SFEMG received treatment; none responded to treatment or developed generalized myasthenia.

Conclusion: An abnormal orbicularis oculi SFEMG in patients with seronegative OMG has a high predictive value for response to therapy. Our study findings may affect the treatment decisions in practice and aid better management of myasthenic patients.

Keywords: Ptosis, Diplopia, Single-fiber EMG, Neuromuscular jitter, Acetylcholine receptor antibody

Background

SFEMG is the most sensitive diagnostic test for diagnosis of seronegative myasthenia gravis [1–3]. Frontalis, orbicularis oculi and extensor digitorum communis (EDC) are commonly tested muscles in the electrophysiological exam. There are no current guidelines to apply when deciding what and how many muscles to evaluate in order to increase the yield of diagnostic sensitivity and specificity. Based on several studies comparing SFEMG of frontalis and or EDC muscles with repetitive nerve stimulation (RNS) [4–6], SFEMG is established as more sensitive test for diagnosing NMJ disorder than RNS. More recent studies investigated the utility of SFEMG in orbicularis oculi muscles in diagnosing MG. These studies, carried out on a mixed population of patients with focal or generalized myasthenic symptoms, found that SFEMG of the orbicularis oculi was reliable for diagnosis of MG [7] and had prognostic value for predicting the severity of patients' clinical course [8]. We postulated that SFEMG in orbicularis oculi muscle would be particularly relevant for diagnosis and predicting response to therapy in a cohort of seronegative patients with typical visual symptoms of ocular myasthenia.

* Correspondence: goran.rakocevic@jefferson.edu
[1]Department of Neurology, Thomas Jefferson University, 901 Walnut Street, Room 408, Philadelphia, PA 19107, USA
Full list of author information is available at the end of the article

Methods

Eighty-six women and fifty-six men with negative AChR antibody and fluctuating ocular symptoms (double vision in 79, ptosis in 37, and both in 51 patients) were referred for evaluation of ocular myasthenia gravis. The clinical diagnosis of ocular myasthenia (OMG) was based on the presence of at least one of cardinal visual symptom (diplopia) and/or findings on exam (variable extraocular muscle weakness and ptosis) by two examiners: a referring neuro-ophthalmologist and examining neurologist. All patients had ocular symptoms and/or findings for at least one month prior to SFEMG. Three patients were adolescents of 15, 16 and 17 years of age. A complete neuro-ophthalmologic evaluation including an MRI of brain with orbital protocol was performed in all patients to exclude other neurological disorders. All patients had laboratory testing for serum AchR and six were tested for anti-MuSK antibody. No patients had undergone genetic testing for other possible causes of external ophthalmoplegia prior to SFEMG, and during the follow up period after electrophysiological study.

SFEMG in orbicularis oculi muscle was intended as the measured variable, while the clinical criterion used as the gold standard was objective eyelid and/ or orbicularis oculi and extraocular muscle weakness on exam with fluctuating symptoms and findings.

SFEMG was performed on both orbicularis oculi muscles in all patients by the same examining neurologist in a single center (GR), using a SFEMG needle with standard techniques. A minimum of twenty pairs of muscle fibers were recorded from right and left orbicularis oculi muscle from all patients. The SFEMG study was considered abnormal: 1) if the mean jitter (MCD) in twenty pairs exceeded normal values for the orbicularis oculi and the patient's age [7, 9]; or 2) if >10% of all studied pairs had jitter above the maximum allowed for a single pair using values adjusted for age.

Following the SFEMG study, treatment decisions were determined by referring physicians. Two-year follow up information for all patients was acquired by chart review, phone contact and office examination. The determination of generalized MG was based on development of symptomatic bulbar and/ or limb weakness confirmed by clinical examination by referring or treating neurologist. The medical charts were reviewed and patients' symptoms and response to therapy, if any, were documented during a 2-year follow-up period. The determination about a therapeutic response and whether generalized myasthenia (GMG) developed were based on the examinations by neuro-ophthalmologists and treating neurologists in the clinic and documented in the medical records or by a telephone interview.

T-tests were used to compare demographic data of patients with normal SFEMG to those with abnormal SFEMG, with $p < 0.05$ as threshold for significance. A positive response to therapy was defined as objective improvement of symptoms and findings on exam. The relationship between a positive response and an abnormal SFEMG was calculated using Fisher's exact test. The sensitivity and specificity of orbicularis oculi muscle SFEMG to predict treatment-responsive OMG and development of generalized MG were also calculated. Statistics were carried out in Prism 6 (www.graphpad.com).

Results

One hundred and eleven patients had normal jitter and thirty-one had abnormal jitter. There was no significant difference in the mean age or disease duration of the two groups. Gender was equal in the group with abnormal jitter. Women made up 63% of the patients in the group with normal jitter.

Twenty-nine of 31 patients with abnormal jitter received treatment: pyridostigmine first, and if favorable but suboptimal response, by adding prednisone until resolution of symptoms. Two were not treated and 1 patient's follow-up information was missing.

Twenty-five patients had a positive response to treatment as defined by improvement of ocular symptoms and signs, and based on objective neurologic or ophthalmologic exam (Table 1). In the group of patients with normal jitter, 24 patients were treated and 87 patients were not treated. Pyridostigmine alone and/or combined with oral steroids did not provide benefit in non-responders regardless of an underlying etiology, which was not conclusively established for each non-responder. More women than men with normal jitter were treated. This difference in treatment by gender was significant. None of the treated patients with normal jitter had a positive response to treatment. Thus, abnormal jitter was significantly associated with a beneficial response to treatment (Fisher exact test $p < 0.001$). Abnormal jitter had 100% sensitivity and 85.7% specificity for response to therapy. The positive predictive value was 86.2% and negative predictive value was 100% for response to treatment.

Four patients with negative MuSK antibody were given pyridostigmine trial with no benefit. Another patient was later found to have MuSK antibodies after a normal SFEMG, but did not receive any myasthenic therapy due to intercurrent cancer. A single patient who presented with ocular symptoms and had an abnormal SFEMG eventually developed generalized myasthenia.

Table 1 Response to MG therapy and SFEMG findings in patients with fluctuating ocular symptoms

Data analyzed	No response	Responded	Total
Group with abnormal jitter	4	25	29
Group with normal jitter	24	0	24
Total	28	25	53

Discussion

This study confirms usefulness of SFEMG for detecting a NMJ disorder in patients with fluctuating extraocular muscle weakness and negative antibodies by recording SFEMG from orbicularis oculi muscles. Additionally, we have shown that abnormal jitter in orbicularis oculi muscles in patients presenting with a clinical picture of ocular myasthenia correlated with response to myasthenic therapies. The sensitivity and specificity of SFEMG was studied in this patient cohort retrospectively and correlated with their response to myasthenic therapy, if administered by referring physicians. An abnormal SFEMG was not predictive of subsequent development of generalized MG as only one of 29 patients with an abnormal SFEMG subsequently developed generalized MG. No patient with normal SFEMG responded to treatment or developed generalized MG. Our findings are in concordance with Rostedt et all retrospective study in EDC [10] and Padua's prospective study [7] demonstrating SFEMG in orbicularis oculi muscle as the test of highest value in diagnosing ocular and generalized myasthenia.

Conclusion

A high diagnostic sensitivity of SFEMG in orbicularis oculi muscle in identifying patients who are unlikely to respond to myasthenic therapies is the most objective diagnostic tool available to clinicians managing patients with fluctuating ocular symptoms and negative NMJ antibodies. The relevance of our study highlights importance of SFEMG in the treatment decisions and management of patients with ocular myasthenia.

Abbreviations

AchR: Acetylcholine Receptor; CT: Computerized tomography; EDC: Extensor digitorum communis; GMG: General myasthenia gravis; MCD: Mean consecutive discharge; MRI: Magnetic resonance imaging; MuSK: Muscle-specific kinase; NMJ: Neuromuscular junction; OMG: Ocular myasthenia gravis; RNS: Repetitive stimulation study; SFEMG: Single fiber EMG

Acknowledgements

Not applicable.

Funding

Dr. Floeter is supported by the Intramural Research Program of the National Institutes of Health, NINDS.

Authors' contributions

Research project conception and execution: GR and MKF. Statistical analysis: GR and MKF. Manuscript preparation and critical revision: GR, MKF and MM. All authors read and approved the final manuscript.

Competing interests

The authors declare that they have no competing interests.

Author details

[1]Department of Neurology, Thomas Jefferson University, 901 Walnut Street, Room 408, Philadelphia, PA 19107, USA. [2]Wills Eye Hospital, Thomas Jefferson University, Philadelphia, PA, USA. [3]EMG Section, National Institute of Neurological Disorders and Stroke, National Institutes of Health, Bethesda, MD, USA.

References

1. Stalberg E, Trontelj JV, Schwartz MS. Single-muscle-fiber recording of the jitter phenomenon in patients with myasthenia gravis and in members of their families. Ann N Y Acad Sci. 1976;274:189–202.
2. Sanders DB, Howard JF Jr, Johns TR. Single-fiber electromyography in myasthenia gravis. Neurology. 1979;29:68–76.
3. Weinberg DH, Rizzo JH III, Hayes MT, Kneeland MD, Kelly JJ. Ocular myasthenia gravis: predictive value of single-fiber electromyography. Muscle Nerve. 1999;22:1222–7.
4. Cui LY, Guan YZ, Wang H, Tang XF. Single fiber electromyography in the diagnosis of ocular myasthenia gravis: report of 90 cases. Chin Med J. 2004; 117(6):848–51.
5. Katzberg HD, Bril V. A comparison of electrodiagnostic tests in ocular myasthenia gravis. J Clin Neuromuscular Dis. 2005;6:109–13.
6. Gomez-Fernandez L, Vega-Treto H, Lestayo-Ofarril Z. Single fiber electromyography in the diagnosis of myasthenia gravis. Rev Neurol. 2000;30(7):609–13.
7. Padua L, Caliandro P, Di Iasi G, Pazzaglia C, Ciaraffa F, Evoli A. Reliability of SFEMG in diagnosing myasthenia gravis: sensitivity and specificity calculated on 100 prospective cases. Clin Neurophysiol. 2014;125(6):1270–3.
8. Baruca M, Leonardis L, Podnar S, Hojs-Fabjan T, Grad A, Jerin A, et al. Single fiber emg as a prognostic tool in myasthenia gravis. Muscle Nerve. 2016; 54(6):1034–40.
9. Stalberg E, Trontelj JV. Single Fiber EMG. Studies in Healthy and Diseased Muscle. 2nd ed. New York: Raven Press; 1994. p. 254.
10. Rostedt A, Saders LL, Edards LJ, Massey JM, Sanders DB, Stalberg EV. Predictive value of single-fiber electromyography in the extensor digitorum communis muscle of patients with ocular myasthenia gravis: a retrospective study. J Clin Neuromuscul Dis. 2000;2(1):6–9.

8

Characteristic differences in the mini-mental state examination used in Asian countries

Yong S. Shim[1,6*], Dong Won Yang[2], Hee-Jin Kim[3], Young Ho Park[4] and SangYun Kim[4,5*]

Abstract

Background: The mini-mental state examination (MMSE) was adapted by individual countries according to their languages and cultures, though it has not been systematically compared. The objective of this study was to compare the linguistic and cultural variations of the MMSE used in various Asian countries. With this, we can analyze the strengths and weaknesses of the MMSE and consider using a common version in future international clinical studies in Asia.

Methods: We collected the MMSEs used in 11 Asian nations. After translating those into English, we compared them to understand the differences in the questionnaires with regard to cultural aspects.

Results: Many items may be applicable or comparable with a little modification, for Asian countries. However, attention and calculation and repetition may be incomparable. There were some differences in the contents and the ways to administer.

Conclusions: The lack of consideration of the cultural differences and their influences on the interpretation of the same cognitive test makes cross-cultural studies difficult. Some items of MMSE tasks need readjusting for, if any, multi-national studies. This study might serve as a first step in the development of a standardized cross-cultural cognitive instrument, especially in Asia.

Keywords: Mini-mental state examination, Culture, Asia, Multi-national studies, Cognitive screening test

Background

The Mini–Mental State Examination (MMSE) was originally developed by Folstein et al. in 1975, to differentiate organic from functional psychiatric patients [1], and the standard MMSE form is currently used with minor subsequent modifications by the authors, based on its original conceptualization. The MMSE requires no specialized equipment or training for administration, and has both validity and reliability for the diagnosis and longitudinal assessment of Alzheimer's disease (AD) [1, 2]. Although there are some reported disadvantages including that it is affected by demographic factors such as age and education, and it has problematic items to administer in other languages with the lack of standardization [2–4], the MMSE is still used extensively in clinical and research settings to measure cognitive impairment or to screen for dementia. It is also used to estimate the severity and progression of cognitive impairment and to follow the course of cognitive changes in an individual over time.

With the increase in the aged population, dementia, which can cause disability in older adults, is gradually increasing the great economic burden in many countries [5]. In particular, the Asian population in 2009 was estimated at 4 billion, comprising 59% of the total global population of 6.8 billion [6]. In 2005, a study using the Delphi method reported that 60% of all dementia patients live in developing countries, and China, India, Japan, and Indonesia are among the top 7 countries with the largest number of dementia patients [7]. Therefore, many researchers have proposed clinical trials aimed at reducing the burden of dementia in Asia, and many

* Correspondence: ysshim@catholic.ac.kr; neuroksy@snu.ac.kr
[1]Department of Neurology, Bucheon St. Mary's Hospital, College of Medicine, The Catholic University of Korea, Seoul, Republic of Korea
[4]Department of Neurology, Seoul National University College of Medicine & Clinical Neuroscience Center, Seoul National University Bundang Hospital, Seoul, Republic of Korea
Full list of author information is available at the end of the article

collaborative studies are currently being planned and conducted in Asian societies [8].

Multi-national studies have to consider cultural variations and cross-cultural comparisons [9, 10]. Collaborative cross-cultural research is especially difficult in Asia due to the drastically different languages, ethnicities, and customs. One cross-cultural study, which was "a multi-national study to identify treatment discontinuation rate in de novo patients with Alzheimer's disease who have been newly prescribed with donepezil in Asia" (https://clinicaltrials.gov/ct2/show/NCT02262975), assessed 41 centers from 11 countries with a feasibility questionnaire screening for dementia. All of the centers (41 centers, 100%) used the MMSE [1], which is a commonly used, brief screening test for dementia. However, disadvantages of the MMSE include the need to adjust scores for age, education, and ethnicity [2–4]. In multi-national clinical trials, patients with the different severities of dementia can be recruited in the different countries by the same MMSE. Notably, the MMSEs were adapted by individual countries taking into account their languages and cultures, though the different versions of the MMSEs were not systematically compared.

The primary objective of this study was to compare the linguistic and cultural variations of the MMSE used in various Asian countries. With this, we can analyze the strengths and weaknesses of the MMSE and consider using a common version in future international clinical studies in Asia. This can be the first step for the Asian version of MMSE if needed.

Methods

We collected the different versions of MMSE used in 11 Asian nations. Further information on the MMSEs was available by searching databases including MEDLINE (PubMed), SCOPUS, PsycINFO, EBSCO, or GOOGLE. The MMSEs were available from China (Chinese) [11], Hong Kong (Chinese & English) [12], India (Hindi) [13], Indonesia (Indonesian) [14], Japan (Japanese) [15], Korea (Korean) [16], Malaysia (Malay) [17], the Philippines (English with a few Tagalog words) [18], Singapore (English with Chinese and Malay phases) [19], Taiwan (Chinese) [20], and Thailand (Thai) [21]. The MMSE questionnaires were written using a given country's domestic languages. We translated all 11 versions of the MMSE back into English and compared them to understand the differences in the questionnaires with regard to cultural aspects in Asian countries.

First, we compared the contents in 5 domains (orientation to time and orientation, registration and recall, attention and calculation, and language and visuospatial function) across the 11 versions of MMSE, and then summarized the modifications (Table 1). The difference in the ways of administering the tests was also compared.

Results

Comparison of content across the 11 versions of the MMSE used in Asia

The MMSE test includes items assessing orientation, word recall and registration, attention and calculation, and language and visuospatial abilities [1]. All 11 versions included all these domains.

Orientation to time (5 points)

The traditional MMSE inquires about time by asking the respondent about the date (month, day, and year) and the season. Contrary to the habitual use of the Western calendar, some Asian nations use 24 seasonal divisions according to the lunar calendar. In addition, some nations in Southeast Asia have no seasonal changes. Thus, changes were made to the questionnaire as needed. In Taiwan, respondents could report the recent or upcoming feasts from the lunar calendar. Furthermore, when the season was not relevant, questions probed respondents as to whether it was morning, noon, afternoon, or evening. In Malaysia, the question about the season was replaced with time, and Singapore replaced it with the knowledge of an upcoming festival. In India, the question regarding the year was replaced with whether it was morning, afternoon, or evening.

Orientation to place (5 points)

Orientation to place requires familiarity with the Western style addresses in the traditional MMSE [3]. Some questions were changed to reflect the geographical/political nomenclature of the study location; that is, rather than a direct translation for "state, province, or city," the names of the administrative districts in the individual countries were used.

It seems it was difficult to generate 5 distinct questions about the place orientation in small countries. In Singapore, which is a city-country, the only correct answer to the question about the city was Singapore, which is also the country name, so some questions were replaced with knowledge of a nearby landmark instead of a city and with the district instead of the province. China, Hong Kong, India, Japan, Taiwan, and Thailand did not ask the name of the country, because the name of the country would be a test of common knowledge, not of place orientation. Especially, Taiwan presented a more generous set of questions, where the examiner could choose the 5 most appropriate questions out of 8 total questions according to where the test was performed (at home or clinic). The Taiwanese questions were: 1) What do you do in this place?; 2) Which department?; 3) What floor?; 4) Name of the building; 5) Location of the hospital; 6) District; 7) Town; and 8) Street. In addition, Thailand had two kinds of versions depending on where the test took place. At the hospital, the

Table 1 Comparison of individual items in 11 versions of the MMSE used in Asia

	China	Hong Kong	India	Indonesia	Japan	Korea	Malaysia	The Philippines	Singapore	Taiwan	Thailand
Time orientation (5)[a]											
Year			M, A, E[b]								
Month											
Day											
Date											
Season							Time		Festival	Alternatives[c]	
Place orientation (5)[d]											
Country	Department	Place nature	Post office		Prefecture						
Province		Region	District		Region			Street (barangay)	District		
City		District	Village			Place nature			Landmark		
Hospital		Building	Block (zip code)			Place name	Building	Place name			
Floor			Place name								
Registration (3) and Recall (3)	Rubber ball	Apple	Mango	Apple	any three[e]	Plane	any three[e]	Mango	Pen	any three[e]	Flower
	National flag	Newspaper	Chair	Table		Pencil		Table	Apple		River
	Tree	Train	Coin	Coin		Pine tree		Money	Cat		Train (tree, ocean, car)[f]
Attention and Calculation (5)	Serial 7's	Serial 7's or		Serial 7's or	Serial 7's or	Serial 7's	Serial 7's or		Serial 7's or	Serial 7's	Serial 7's or
					Serial 5's or		Serial 3's from 20 or				
		Digit span	Name,	Spell	Spell		Spell	Spell	Spell		Spell
		backwards	Date	"WAHYU"	"Fujinoyama"		"WORLD"	"KARNE"	"WORLD"		"MANĀW"
			backwards	backwards (means revelation)	backwards		backwards	backwards (means meat)	backwards		backwards (means lemon)
Language and Visuospatial function (9)											
Naming (2)			*touch*[g]								
Pencil	Pen		Pen			Ballpoint pen				any two[h]	
Watch				Book							

Table 1 Comparison of individual items in 11 versions of the MMSE used in Asia *(Continued)*

Repeat (1)											
	"Si shi si zhi shi zi"	"Yi fu mai yu chang"	"Na tō yaha na hī vaha"	"Namun, tanpa, bila"	"Min'na de, ryokuo awasete tsunao hikimasu"	"Baek mun e bul yeo il geoun"	"Tak mungkin dan cukup mustahil"	"Minikaniko ni monikaang makina"	"Marah, merah, murah"	Random[k]	"Cry- cry – kai- ggai – kai"
(meaning)	(It is forty-four stone lions.)	(Uncle is buying fish guts.)[i]	(neither this nor that: *proverb*)	(However, without, if)	(Everyone, pull the rope to fit the power.)	(Seeing is believing.)	(No, it is impossible.)	unknown *(tongue-twister)*	(angry, red, cheap)[j]		(who, desire, chicken, egg)
Command (3)											
Take a paper in your right hand,	in your right hand			in your hand		Turn the paper		with your non-dominant hand		in your left hand	
fold it in half, and											
put it on the floor (table).	on your thigh	on your lap	give it to me	on the floor	on the desk	give it to me	put it on the floor	on your lap		give it to me	
Reading (1)			*follow*[l]								
Writing (1)			(no score)[m]								
Inter-locking pentagons (1)			3 points[m]								

[a]Order of items asked could be changed
[b]Instead of the year, a question about the time of day is asked, i.e., morning (M), afternoon (A), or evening (E)
[c]Alternatives are lunar feasts, current time, and morning, noon, afternoon, or evening, etc
[d]Order of items asked could be changed
[e]Any three unrelated words could be used
[f]If the questionnaire was administered to the same respondent a second time within 2 months
[g]Respondents could touch objects
[h]Any two objects were selected
[i]In Hong Kong, the English version used "No ifs, ands, or buts"
[j]In Singapore, the English version used "No ifs, ands, or buts" and the Chinese version used "Si shi si zhi shi shi zi"
[k]Any random sentence could be used
[l]Respondents followed the researcher's speech
[m]In India, there was no score for the writing item. Instead, the drawing item consisted of a diamond within a square and was scored out of 3 points

questions included, 1) What is the name of this place and what do you do in this place?; 2) What floor?; 3) District, province; 4) Town; and 5) Which part? At the patient's home, 1) Area/address; 2) Town, street, and district; 3) Province; 4) Rural, and 5) Which part?

Registration (3 points) & recall (3 points)

The "3 objects" used in the registration/recall test were different across many versions of the MMSE. The original English version also does not specify the 3 objects to be used for the test. Each country had different standardized appointed objects except Japan, Malaysia, and Taiwan, where the examiner chose any 3 unrelated objects. All countries used concrete nouns but not abstract words such as love, cold, sweet, and beauty. In the instructions, examiners choose what a subject has experienced or used in everyday life and avoid unrealistic words. Things within the field of the test environment were excluded, as far as possible, which eliminate the clues that the subjects can remember. It is recommended to use the specific objects with different types (e.g. nose, car, sun). However, it is not recommended that objects that are too similar or too closely related such as "nose, eye, mouth", "train, car, ship" or "star, moon, sun", are not used. Since the test is performed based on listening, homonymous words such as "flower" or "flour" and "ant" or "aunt" are not used to cause confusion. In Thailand, a different set of objects was used if the patient was administered the test a second time within 2 months (e.g., flower, river, and train the first time and tree, ocean, and car the second time).

Attention and calculation (5 points)

Although either spelling the word "WORLD" backwards or serial sevens were originally used [22, 23], serial sevens have been suggested to be more appropriate to a non-native English population [24]. Accordingly, serial sevens were most often used in the Asian MMSEs. China, Korea, and Taiwan performed only serial sevens, though some countries used serial sevens or spelling backwards; Indonesia used "WAHYA" meaning revelation, Japan used "Fujinoyama" meaning Fuji Mountain, Thailand used "MANǍW" meaning lemon, and Singapore and Malaysia used "WORLD". Instead of serial sevens, serial fives (Japan), serial threes from 20 (Malaysia), or digit span backwards from 42,731 (Hong Kong) were used. In the Philippines, only spelling "KARNE," meaning meat in Filipino language, backwards was used, and in India, respondents had to name the date backwards.

Language and visuospatial function (9 points)

There are 6 components in this domain: naming, reading, writing, repetition, motor skill, and visuospatial function.

Naming a pencil and a watch (2 points)

This was almost the same in all versions of the MMSE. However, in Taiwan, the examiner let the respondent name any two objects that the subject seemed to have previously experienced and, in India, naming after touching the objects with the hand was also accepted. Pencil and watch were used in general, although some countries used other objects. Instead of a pencil, a ballpoint pen was used in Korea, a fountain pen was used in China, and a pen was used in India. A book instead of a watch was used in Indonesia.

Repetition, speaking back a phrase: "no ifs, ands, or buts" (1 point)

"No ifs, ands, or buts" is not an easily translated phrase. When translated into other languages, its articulation complexity can be lost. Furthermore, the phrase may be unfamiliar in many countries as it is linguistically irregular [25, 26]. Instead of a direct translation of "No ifs, ands, or buts," each country used a non-familiar phrase or a sentence with a different meaning and pronunciation, as appropriate. India and Korea used a type of proverb, and China, the Philippines, and Thailand used a type of a tongue-twister. In Taiwan, the examiner chose any sentence that came to his or her mind during the test. However, using other phrases may assess a different cognitive domain, and the validity of this item is questioned.

Completing a three-stage command (3 points)

In the original command, respondents are required to take a paper with their right hand. The standardized version provides more specific instructions, i.e., to take the paper with the non-dominant hand (if right-handed, the respondent is asked to use the left hand, and vice versa) [22].

Many countries let the respondent take the paper with the right hand. However, in the Philippines, the examiner asked the respondent to take it with the non-dominant hand, Taiwan with the left hand, and the Indonesian version did not specify which hand; China, Hong Kong, and the Philippines instructed the respondent to place the paper on the lap, instead of the floor or the table. In India, Korea, and Taiwan, the respondent was asked to give the paper back to the examiner, not to place it on the table. In Korea, respondents were asked to turn the paper over instead of taking the paper.

Reading (1 point)

This section was almost the same for all versions of the MMSE. In the traditional version, the patient is asked to read and obey a written command on a paper stating, "Close your eyes." However, in India, the respondent was asked to imitate the examiner's facial expression, not follow a written command.

Writing (1 point)

The patient is asked to write a sentence with at least a subject and a verb, and this section was also almost always the same. However, this test was not included in the total score in India.

Copying interlocking pentagons (1 point)

This was almost the same in all versions of the MMSE. However, in India, a diamond within a square was used with 3 points. Having no points for writing, the total score in India was 31 points instead of 30 points (2 additional points for drawing and 1 less point for writing).

Summary of the modifications

A summary of the modifications is shown below with possible reasons/justifications.

1) Regarding orientation to time, the traditional MMSE inquires about the season; however, there are no astronomical seasons in some countries. Thus, the question on seasons was replaced with questions such as the current time of day or cognizance of an upcoming festival. Taiwan used knowledge of recent or upcoming feasts on the lunar calendar.

2) Because of the different administrative districts used, the individual name of the administrative district of their country was used. Some countries did not ask the name of the country, because the name of the country could be a test of common knowledge, not for place orientation. In Taiwan and Thailand, the examiner selected appropriate questions according to the place the test was administered, at hospital or home.

3) For registration and recall, each country used unrelated, specified objects according to the words or syllables of their language. In Thailand, a different set of objects was appointed if the patient repeated the test a second time within 2 months.

4) Regarding attention and calculation, the traditional MMSE asked respondents to spell the word "WORLD" backwards or perform serial sevens. However, spelling "WORLD" backwards may be inappropriate where English is not the first language. Instead, countries used another word, phrase, or sentence with 5 syllables. Serial sevens may be less relevant to other cultural groups [27]; hence, it was eliminated in some versions.

5) Among items of the language and related functions, first, for repetition, instead of the original phrase, "No ifs, ands, or buts," many other language versions used a phrase or a sentence with a different meaning and pronunciation. Second, many people in Asia tend to think it is polite to take with both two hands in when they receive something from a stranger. Korean version requires the respondent to turn the paper, instead of taking it with the right hand. Next, the Hindi MMSE awarded no points for writing and 3 instead of 1 point for drawing, so the total score in India was 31 points instead of 30 points.

6) On the whole, scores of time and place orientation, registration and recall, and visuospatial and related functions excluding repeat may be applicable for many Asian countries. Other items are also be comparable with a little modification, if needed. However, attention and calculation (5 points) and repeat (1 point) may be incomparable and need readjusting for, if any, multinational studies in Asia.

Discussion

It is difficult to compare older adults with different cultural backgrounds using the same cognitive measures. In addition, diverse language and culture cannot be overcome through a simple, direct translation of the instrument. Direct literal translations may have different meanings or syllables from the original instrument. Thus, many countries developed their MMSE versions according to their cultures and languages. In general, scores of time and place orientation, registration and recall, and visuospatial and related functions excluding repeat may be applicable and alike for many Asian countries. Others can also be comparable with a little modification, if needed. However, attention and calculation (5 points) and repeat (1 point) may be incomparable and need readjusting for, if any, multi-national studies in Asia.

There are many different countries, languages, ethnicities, and cultural differences in Asia. Asia also includes countries with no written language and one nation with many languages. Many Asian nations developed their MMSEs by translating the original English MMSE and modifying it according to their languages and cultures. In addition, there are sometimes different versions of the MMSE within the same country. For example, China and other countries have various versions of the MMSE [28–31]. Moreover, in Korea, different versions of the MMSE were developed by different groups [16, 32, 33]. Furthermore, as time goes by, revised and modified versions of the MMSE are derived [34–37, 40]. This study is limited in that we selected only one version of the MMSE per country for comparison.

In addition to the cultural and language differences, demographic factors such as age and education also should be considered. Previous studies have reported that the MMSE total score was affected by age and education, and normative data were provided for age and education [2, 38–40]. In a Korean version of the MMSE (MMSE-K) [34], 4 additional points were given to illiterate patients. Other versions of the Korean MMSE used the mean scores according to age and education level [16, 35, 36]. Other Asian versions have used different cut-off scores with mean scores adjusted for education, age, or sex. In the Chinese version [11] included in this study, cut-off scores for illiterate was ≤19; for elementary level ≤ 22; for high educational level ≤ 26. The sensitivity was 90.7% in the urban area; 97.1% in the rural area. At the cut-off score of 19/20 of the Cantonese MMSE of Hong Kong, sensitivity was 97.5% and specificity was 97.3% [12]. Illiterates were included 46.3% and mean education period was 3.5 ± 7.9 years. In the Hindi MMSE, a subject is classified as impaired if he/she scores 19 or less on the test, and/or obtains scores at or below the 10th percentile on a memory test and at least one other test [41]. In a study on 100 illiterate elderly subjects, the Hindi MMSE was 94% sensitive and 98% specific [42]. Cut-off score used in the Indonesian MMSE was 24 [43]. MMSE score at or below 24 was classified as cognitive dysfunction/dementia. This showed sensitivity 88% and specificity 96%. Cut-off score was 18 for 0–6 years of education and 25 for >6 years of education. The Japanese MMSE used in this study [44], score less than 23 was classified as cognitive impairment. In a current study, MMSE had an excellent sensitivity (97%) and good specificity (89%) for screening AD at the cut-off point of 28/29, but it had poor specificity (58%) for screening MCI at the cut-off point of 29/30) [45]. In Malaysia, cut-off score was 22 with sensitivity 88.5% and specificity 75.3% [17]. In the Philippines [46], the subjects were identified to have dementia if they scored 23 or less on the MMSE. To adjust for education bias, a cut-off score of 17 or less was used for those who attained primary level of education. The Singapore MMSE [19] compared in this study was validated in 1092 community living Asians from Singapore. There were significant ethnic differences in the total score between Chinese, Malays and Indians in the non-educated participants. At a cut-off score of 23/24, sensitivity was 97.5% and specificity was 75.6%. Specificity decreased with lower education levels. In Taiwan [20], Normal cognition results were defined as a score > 24 in literate elders and >13 in illiterate elders. The MMSE-Thai 2002 [21] of Thai MMSEs was compared in this study, and the suggested cut-off score was ≤14 for illiterates, ≤ 17 for elementary school, and ≤22 for over elementary school.

Instruments are often considered different from the original version once after they have been culturally and linguistically adapted [39]. For example, in the Hindi Mental State Exam (HMSE) [13], 16 of the original items were changed to adapt for rural older adults in India, who have little or no education. Another 3 Korean versions of the MMSE (not included in this analysis) measured judgment instead of reading and writing with 2 questions [34–36], "Why do you clean your clothes?" and "How do you give back another's belongings when you get them by chance?" or a Korean proverb, "What does it mean that many a little make a mickle [a large amount]?".

Some new tests without cultural bias have also been attempted [3, 47]. These culture-free tests could enable older adults to demonstrate their cognitive abilities fully regardless of language, education, and so on. However, these new culture-free tests require further validations, especially in Asia, which has various languages, religions, and ethnicities, even in the same country. Currently, the lack of understanding of the differences of various cultures and how these differences may affect the interpretation of the same cognitive test, such as MMSE, makes multinational, cross-cultural studies difficult. Any international version of the MMSE that accounts for differences in cultures may be needed for an optimal cross-cultural study. This study serves to help understand how individual cultures adapt one cognitive test to best suit their needs. It serves as a first step in the development of a standardized cross-culturally sensitive cognitive instrument, especially in Asia.

Conclusions

The MMSEs used in Asian countries showed many differences in the contents and the ways to administer, although many items may be applicable or comparable with a little modification. Some items of MMSE tasks need readjusting for, if any, multi-national studies. No consideration of the cultural differences and their influences on the interpretation of the same cognitive test makes cross-cultural studies difficult. This study might serve as a first step in the development of a standardized cross-cultural cognitive instrument, especially in Asia.

Abbreviations

HMSE: Hindi mental state exam; MMSE: Mini-mental state examination; MMSE-K: Korean version of the MMSE

Acknowledgements

Not applicable.

Funding

This research did not receive any specific grant from funding agencies in the public, commercial, or not-for-profit sectors.

Authors' contributions

Study design: YSS and SYK; Data acquisition: YSS, DWY, HJK, and YHP; Analysis and interpretation: YSS, HJK, and SYK; Manuscript drafting: YSS and SYK; Final approval: YSS, DWY, HJK, YHP, and SYK; Agreement to be accountable: YSS, DWY, HJK, YHP, and SYK.

Competing interests

The authors declare that they have no competing interests.

Author details
[1]Department of Neurology, Bucheon St. Mary's Hospital, College of Medicine, The Catholic University of Korea, Seoul, Republic of Korea. [2]Department of Neurology, Seoul St. Mary's Hospital, College of Medicine, The Catholic University of Korea, Seoul, Republic of Korea. [3]Department of Neurology, College of Medicine, Hanyang University, Seoul, Republic of Korea. [4]Department of Neurology, Seoul National University College of Medicine & Clinical Neuroscience Center, Seoul National University Bundang Hospital, Seoul, Republic of Korea. [5]82, Gumi-ro 173 beon-gil, Bundang-gu, Seongnam-si, Gyeonggi-do 13620, South Korea. [6]327 Sosa-ro, Wonmi-gu, Bucheon-si, Gyeonggi-do 14647, South Korea.

References

1. Folstein MF, Folstein SE, McHugh PR. "mini-mental state." a practical method for grading the cognitive state of patients for the clinician. J Psychiatr Res. 1975;12:189–98.
2. Crum RM, Anthony JC, Bassett SS, Folstein MF. Population-based norms for the mini-mental state examination by age and educational level. JAMA. 1993;269:2386–91.
3. Parker C, Philp I. Screening for cognitive impairment among older people in black and minority ethnic groups. Age Ageing. 2004;33:447–52.
4. Espino DV, Lichtenstein MJ, Palmer RF, Hazuda HP. Ethnic differences in mini-mental state examination (MMSE) scores: where you live makes a difference. J Am Geriatr Soc. 2001;49:538–48.
5. WHO. Dementia: a public health priority. Geneva: World Health Organization; 2012.
6. Bremner J, Haub C, Lee M, Mather M, Zuehlke E. [document on the internet] World population highlights: key findings from PRB's 2009 world population data sheet. Population BulletinWashington: Population Reference Bureau; 2009. [cited October 6, 2009]. Available from http://www.prb.org/.
7. Ferri CP, Prince M, Brayne C, Brodaty H, Fratiglioni L, Ganguli M, et al. Global prevalence of dementia: a Delphi consensus study. Lancet. 2005;366:2112–7.
8. Asian Society Against Dementia (ASAD): http://www.asiandementia.org/.
9. Salmon DP, Riekkinen PJ, Katzman R, Zhang M, Jin H, Yu E. Cross-cultural studies of dementia. A comparison of mini-mental state examination performance in Finland and China. Arch Neurol. 1989;46:769–72.
10. Baiyewu O, Bella AF, Jegede RO. The effect of demographic and health variables on a modified form of mini-mental state examination scores in Nigerian elderly community residents. Int J Geriatr Psychiatry. 1993;8:503–10.
11. Zhang Z, Hong X, Li H. The mini-mental state examination in the Chinese residents population aged 55 years and over in the urban and rural areas of Beijing. Chin J Neurol. 1999;3:149–53.
12. Chiu HF, Lee HC, Chung WS, Kwong PK. Reliability and validity of the Cantonese version of mini-mental state examination—a preliminary study. J Hong Kong Col Psychiatrists. 1994;4:25–8.
13. Ganguli M, Ratcliff G, Chandra V, Sharma S, Gilby J, Pandav R, et al. A Hindi version of the MMSE: the development of a cognitive screening instrument for a largely illiterate rural elderly population in India. Int J Geriatr Psychiatry. 1995;10:367–77.
14. Sjahrir H, Ritarwan K, Tarigan S, Rambe AS, Lubis ID, Bhakti I. The mini mental state examination in healthy individuals in Medan, Indonesia by age and education level. Neurol J Southeast Asia. 2001;6:19–22.
15. Kitamura T. Mini-Mental State (MMSE). In: Ootsuka T, Honma A, editors. Assessment manual of intellectual function for the demented elderly. Tokyo: World Planning; 1991. p. 35–8. (in Japanese).
16. Kang Y, Na DL, Hahn S. A validity study on the Korean mini-mental state examination (K-MMSE) in dementia patients. J Korean Neurol Assoc. 1997;15: 300–8.
17. Ibrahim NM, Shohaimi S, Chong HT, Rahman AH, Razali R, Esther E, et al. Validation study of the mini-mental state examination in a Malay-speaking elderly population in Malaysia. Dement Geriatr Cogn Disord. 2009;27:247–53.
18. Ligsay AD. Validation of the mini-mental state examination among the Filipino elderly. Manila: M.Sc. Thesis, University of the Philippines; 2004.
19. Ng TP, Niti M, Chiam PC, Kua EH. Ethnic and educational differences in cognitive test performance on mini-mental state examination in Asians. Am J Geriatr Psychiatry. 2007;15:130–9.
20. Shyu YI, Yip PK. Factor structure and explanatory variables of the mini-mental state examination (MMSE) for elderly persons in Taiwan. J Formos Med Assoc. 2001;100:676–83.
21. Thai Cognitive Test Development Committee 1999. Mini-mental state examination-Thai 2002. Bangkok: Institute of Geriatric Medicine, Department of Medical Services, Ministry of Public Health, Thailand; 2002.
22. Ganguli M, Ratcliff G, Huff FJ, Belle S, Kancel MJ, Fischer L, et al. Serial sevens versus world backwards: a comparison of the two measures of attention from the MMSE. J Geriatr Psychiatry Neurol. 1990;3:203–7.
23. Molloy DW, Alemayehu E, Roberts R. Reliability of a standardized mini-mental state examination compared with the traditional mini-mental state examination. Am J Psychiatry. 1991;148:102–5.
24. Espino DV, Lichtenstein MJ, Palmer RF, Hazuda HP. Evaluation of the mini-mental state examination's internal consistency in a community-based sample of Mexican-American and European-American elders: results from the San Antonio longitudinal study of aging. J Am Geriatr Soc. 2004;52:822–7.
25. Folstein MF. Mini-mental and son. Int J Geriatr Psychiatry. 1998;13:290–4.
26. Werner P, Heinik J, Lin R, Bleich A. 'yes' ifs, ands or buts: examining performance and correlates of the repetition task in the mini-mental state examination. Int J Geriatr Psychiatry. 1999;14:719–25.
27. Katzman R, Zhang MY, Ouang-Ya-Qu WZY, Liu WT, Yu E, et al. A Chinese version of the mini-mental state examination: impact of illiteracy in a shanghai dementia survey. J Clin Epidemiol. 1988;41:971–8.
28. Steis MR, Schrauf RW. A review of translations and adaptations of the min-state examination in languages other than English and Spanish. Res Gerontol Nurs. 2009;2:214–24.
29. Rowland J, Conforti D, Basic D, Vrantsidis F, Hill K, LoGiudice D, et al. A study to evaluate the Rowland universal dementia assessment scale (RUDAS) in two populations outside the Sydney south west area health service: south west area health service and the National Ageing Research Institute, report for the Australian Government Department of Health and ageing; 2007.
30. Xu G, Meyer JS, Huang Y, Du F, Chowdhury M, Quach M. Adapting mini-mental state examination for dementia screening among illiterate or minimally educated elderly Chinese. Int J Geriatr Psychiatry. 2003;18:609–16.
31. Zhang MY, Katzman R, Salmon D, Jin H, Cai GJ, Wang ZY, et al. The prevalence of dementia and Alzheimer's disease in shanghai, China: impact of age, gender and education. Ann Neurol. 1990;27:428–37.
32. Sahadevan S, Lim PPJ, Tan NJL, Chan SP. Diagnostic performance of two mental status tests in the older Chinese: influence of education and age on cut-off values. Int J Geriatr Psychiatry. 2000;15:234–41.
33. Lee SM, Lin X, Haralambous B, Dow B, Vrantsidis F, Tinney J, Blackberry I, Lautenschlager NT, LoGiudice D. Factors impacting on early detection of dementia in older people of Asian background in primary healthcare. Asia Pac Psychiatry. 2011;3:120–7.
34. Park JH, Kwon YC. Modification of the mini-mental state examination for use in the elderly in a non-western society. Part 1. Development of Korean version of mini-mental state examination. Int J Geriatr Psychiatry. 1990;5: 381–7.
35. Lee DY, Lee KU, Lee JH, Kim KW, Jhoo JH, Youn JC, et al. A normative study of the mini-mental state examination in the Korean elderly. J Korean Neuropsychiatr Assoc. 2002;41:508–5.
36. Kim TH, Jhoo JH, Park JH, Kim JL, Ryu SH, Moon SW, et al. Korean version of mini mental status examination for dementia screening and its' short form. Psychiatry Investig. 2010;7:102–8.
37. Feng L, Chong MS, Lim WS, Ng TP. The modified mini-mental state examination test: normative data for Singapore Chinese older adults and its performance in detecting early cognitive impairment. Singapore Med J. 2012;53:458–62.
38. Tombaugh TN, McIntyre NJ. The mini-mental state examination: a comprehensive review. J Am Geriatr Soc. 1992;40:922–35.
39. Tombaugh TN, McDowell I, Kristjansson B, Hubley AM. Mini-mental state examination (MMSE) and the modified MMSE (3MS): a psychometric comparison and normative data. Psychol Assess. 1996;8:48–59.
40. Ideno Y, Takayama M, Hayashi K, Takagi H, Sugai Y. Evaluation of a Japanese version of the mini-mental state examination in elderly persons. Geriatr Gerontol Int. 2012;12:310–6.
41. Ganguly M, Chandra V, Gilby JE, Ratcliff G, Sharma SD, Pandav R, et al. Cognitive test performance in a community-based nondemented elderly sample in rural India: the indo-US cross-national dementia epidemiology study. Int Psychogeriatr. 1996;8:507–24.

42. Tsolaki M, Iakovidou V, Navrozidou H, Aminta M, Pantazi T, Kazis A. Hindi mental state examination (HMSE) as a screening test for illiterate demented patients. Int J Geriatr Psychiatry. 2000;15:662–4.
43. Ismail RI, Mansyur M, Fidiansjah, Maharani P, Rahardjo TB. Module detection cognitive status. 1st ed. Ismail RI, ed. Jakarta: Center for Ageing Studies UI; 2010:6.
44. Fujiwara Y, Watanabe S, Kumagai S, Yoshida Y, Takabayashi K, Morita M, et al. Prevalence and characteristics of older community residents with mild cognitive decline. Geriatr Gerontol Int. 2002;2:57–67.
45. Fujiwara Y, Suzuki H, Yasunaga M, Sugiyama M, Ijuin M, Sakuma N, et al. Brief screening tool for mild cognitive impairment in older Japanese: validation of the Japanese version of the Montreal cognitive assessment. Geriatr Gerontol Int. 2010;10:225–32.
46. Abat MEM, Reyes FA, Ramos MA Jr. Mini-mental status examination profile of the elderly Filipino hemodialysis patient. Phil J Intern Med. 2009;47:161–73.
47. Chiu HF, Lam LC. Relevance of outcome measures in different cultural groups - does one size fit all? Int Psychogeriatr. 2007;19:457–66.

9

Phenotypic expressions of hereditary Transthyretin Ala97Ser related Amyloidosis (ATTR) in Taiwanese

Hui-Ching Hsu[2], Ming-Feng Liao[1], Jung-Lung Hsu[1], Ai-Lun Lo[1], Hung-Chou Kuo[1], Rong-Kuo Lyu[1], Victor Chien-Chia Wu[3], Chih-Wei Wang[4] and Long-Sun Ro[1*]

Abstract

Background: The disease course and early signs specific to ATTR Ala97Ser, the most common endemic mutation in Taiwan, have not been well described. Since new medications can slow down the rate of disease progression, the early diagnosis of this heterogeneous and fatal disease becomes critical.

Methods: We retrospectively reviewed the characteristics of genetically confirmed ATTR Ala97Ser patients at a tertiary referral medical center.

Results: Eight patients from 7 different families were enrolled (61.7 ± 5.5 years). Gastrointestinal symptoms, dyspnea or chest tightness, rather than sensory symptoms, were the initial symptoms in two patients (2/7 = 29%). Body weight loss (3/7 = 43%), muscle wasting (4/7 = 57%), or dysphagia (3/7 = 43%) were the consecutive symptoms. Orthostatic symptoms including orthostatic hypotension (7/7 = 100%), dizziness (6/7 = 86%) and syncope (5/7 = 71%) tended to develop in the late phase of the disease. Autonomic dysfunction was conspicuous. Cardiographic findings included a combination of ventricular wall thickening and pericardial effusion (7/7 = 100%), a granular sparkling appearance of the ventricular myocardium (4/7 = 57%), or conduction abnormalities (5/7 = 71%).

Conclusions: This study broadens the recognition of the initial signs and symptoms, including cardiographic findings and longitudinal manifestations in Taiwanese individuals with ATTR Ala97Ser mutation. These manifestations should prompt doctors to perform further studies and make an early diagnosis.

Keywords: Familial amyloid polyneuropathy, Transthyretin-related amyloidosis, Ala97Ser Mutation

Background

Hereditary transthyretin-related amyloidosis (ATTR) is the most common form of familial systemic amyloidosis and is caused by dominantly inherited transthyretin (TTR) mutations [1–3]. ATTR is a rare but widely distributed disease with a clinical picture that varies in persons from different geographic, ethnic or genetic backgrounds, even among those with the same mutation or within the same family [4, 5]. Ala97Ser, the most common endemic mutation in Taiwan, is much less prevalent in the rest of the world. Only three articles (fewer than 60 cases in Taiwan) have been reported thus far [6–8]. The various clinical presentations of ATTR were available in the existing literature. Nevertheless, the early signs/symptoms specific to ATTR Ala97Ser and the progression of ATTR Ala97Ser over time have not been described previously.

Transthyretin mutations result in the deposition of amyloid fibrils in the peripheral and autonomic nerves, gastrointestinal tract and myocardium, typically presenting with an axonal predominant, length-dependent sensorimotor polyneuropathy (thus, the disorder is also termed familial amyloid polyneuropathy, FAP [2]) that frequently coexists with autonomic dysfunction, cardiac involvement and weight loss [9].

In addition, because emerging data suggest that the TTR-stabilizers can be more beneficial when treatment

* Correspondence: cgrols@adm.cgmh.org.tw
[1]Department of Neurology, Chang Gung Memorial Hospital Linkou Medical Center and Chang Gung University College of Medicine, No.199, Tung Hwa N. Rd., Songshan Dist, Taipei City 105, Taiwan, Republic of China
Full list of author information is available at the end of the article

begins earlier [10, 11], there is an increasing necessity to identify the early signs and symptoms of this progressive and fatal disease so that early diagnosis can be made and treatment can be initiated earlier.

Methods

Clinical data

This research was carried out in accordance with the guidelines and regulations approved by the Institutional Review Board of Chang Gung Memorial Hospital and University (License no. 100-4470A3 and 104-2462A3). Informed consents were obtained from all patients. We enrolled patients with diagnoses of TTR Ala97Ser FAP based on a genetic analysis from 2010 to 2013 (see Additional file 1: Figure S1). We retrospectively reviewed the entire medical records in our hospital until October 2016 and compared clinical manifestations among subjects. We evaluated the onset age of the signs and symptoms and compared the sequential presentations among individuals. We reviewed other data, including the chief complaints, family history, clinics visited before the neurology referral, biopsy studies if available, reports of electrophysiological tests, electrocardiography (ECG), echocardiography findings, and major events including the placement of a permanent pacemaker and cardiopulmonary-cerebral resuscitation (CPCR). Positive ratios of the clinical data reported in two published articles of Ala97Ser in Taiwan were also compared with the results of the present study.

Genetic analyses of mutations

Genomic DNA was isolated from the peripheral blood samples. The intronic primers applied to expand the promoter region, and all exons of the TTR gene were chosen according to previous research [12]. Polymerase chain reaction (PCR) used Tag 'T' DNA polymerase. Amplification proceeded for 29 cycles with denaturation at 94 °C for 30 s, annealing at 51 °C for 30 s, and extension at 72 °C for 45 s. There was a 10-min post-elongation at 72 °C. All PCR products were alkali denatured and submitted to electrophoresis in a 1× TBE buffer. Electrophoresis was performed at room temperature. The PCR products were directly sequenced by an autosequencing machine (DNA Engine, Platier Thermal Cycler, Hercules, CA, USA).

Histopathology

Patients received colonoscopic or salivary gland biopsies if amyloidosis was suspected. The slides of hematoxylin and eosin stain were examined. Congo red staining was then performed and the slides were viewed under a polarized microscope light. (LEITZ LABORLUX S, Solmes, Germany).

Table 1 Clinical course of patients with ATTR Ala97Ser mutation

																						Cardiographic findings					Major events				
Patient No.	Gender	Age at first symptoms onset	Family members with similar symptoms	Body weight loss	Dyspnea on exertion	Chest tightness	Pain	Lower limb sensory	Upper limb sensory	Muscle atrophy / wasting	Frequent dysphagia	Gastrointestinal symptoms	Lower limb motor	Upper limb motor	Orthostatic hypotension	Impaired walking capacity	Dizziness	Syncope	Clinics visited before the neurology referral	Neurology consultation & NCV study	PND disease staging at neurology consultation	First degree AV block	Wall thickening	Pericardial effusion + ventricular wall thickening	Bundle-branch block	Elevated BNP	Permanent pacemaker	CPCR / TCP	Death	Latest follow-up	Tissue biopsy
1	M	60	V	–	1	1	F	F	F	1	–	1	F	F	2	2	3	3	2 (CV)	2	IV	2	2	2	2[b]	3	2	–	4	4	(-) rectal
2[a]	F	–	V	–	–	–	–	–	–	–	–	–	–	–	–	–	–	–	–	–	–	–	–	–	–	ND	–	–	–	Loss	ND
3	F	68	V	–	F	F	–	F	F	–	2	4	F	F	2	–	3	4	F (CV) 2 (GI)	3	–	F	3	4	7	ND	–	4,7	7	7	ND
4	M	66	V	–	–	–	–	F	1	1	–	F	1	–	1	1	1	–	–	1	II	–	1	1	–	ND	–	–	–	Loss	(-) rectal
5	F	69	–	–	–	–	3	F	F	–	–	3	F	–	3	2	4	3	1 (ort)	3	III	3[b]	3	4	3	4	5	–	–	6	(-) salivary
6	M	55	V	7	–	7	F	F	8	–	7	–	[8]	10	7	9	7	7	7 (NS)	10	II	–	10	10	–	ND	[9]	–	–	Loss	(+) rectal
7	M	59	V	6	–	F	–	8	–	[9]	[–]	8	[8]	–	9	9	5	7	F(CV) 5(NS) 7(chest) 8(OH-) 9(GI, CV) 10(ort)	10	III	9[b]	9	9	9[b]	11	11	11	–	14	(+) rectal
8	M	55	–	2	2	–	1	1	1	1	3	F	–	–	5	–	–	–	2(GI) 3(CV) 4(psych, rheuma, hema)	5	–	5	3	5	3	ND	–	–	–	Loss	ND

For the sake of simplicity, an "F" stands for the year of the first symptoms or findings for each subject, and the ordinal number in each row stands for the interval (years) between the onset of the first and consecutive symptoms or events. The progressions in individuals are illustrated in rows

[a]Patient 2 is the daughter of patient 1, and patient 2 was excluded from the age analysis because she had normal NCV study findings

[b]The patients had developed higher degree AV block or complete BBB during the observation period. Please see the Results section

CPCR/TCP: cardiopulmonary-cerebral resuscitation or transcutaneous cardiac pacing use

CV Cardiology, *GI* Gastrology, *ort* Orthopedics, *NS* Neurosurgeon, *chest* chest, OH-: negative results after survey at other hospital, psych: psychiatrist, rheuma: rheumatology, hema: hematology

Values that are enclosed indicate patient who reported similar symptoms/events in their family members

PND disease staging [5]: polyneuropathy disability staging, Stage 0: no impairment, Stage I: sensory disturbances but preserved walking capability, Stage II: impaired walking capability but ability to walk without a stick or crutches, Stage IIIA: walking only with the help of one stick or crutch, Stage IIIB: walking with the help of two sticks or crutches, Stage IV: confined to a wheelchair or bedridden

ND: not done

Results

Clinical manifestations and progression of ATTR Ala97Ser

All patients gradually developed peripheral neuropathy, including progressive tingling, occasional throbbing/ shooting pain, or paresthesia/dysesthesia in the feet. Symptoms started in the distal parts of the lower limbs and then progressed to the upper limbs, with resultant walking difficulty (5/7, 71%) and/or functional impairment of the hands (3/7, 43%) in variable time intervals (see Table 1).

Gastrointestinal (GI) symptoms (6/7, 86%), dyspnea on exertion (3/7, 43%), or chest tightness (4/7, 57%), rather than sensory symptoms, were the initial symptoms in patients 7 and 8 (Table 1). GI symptoms were common and included chronic constipation, diarrhea or constipation alternating with diarrhea [5, 7]. Chest tightness occurred particularly at night (with orthopnea). Patient 7 complained of chest tightness over the substernal area with cold sweating for up to 2 h. Cardiac involvement was common and could lead to symptoms of heart failure. Patients 1, 5 and 7 presented with elevated brain natriuretic peptide (BNP) [5] at levels up to 200, 108, and 232 pg/ml at 3, 4, and 11 years after the initial symptom onset, respectively (Table 1).

The progression of the disease was accompanied by the occurrence of body weight loss (BWL), muscle wasting, or dysphagia. Persistent BWL of up to 20 kg were found within a duration of 3 ~ 20 years. Patients may have suffered from GI symptoms or unexplained BWL before typical neurological symptoms presented. Muscle atrophy/wasting (4/7, 57%) bilaterally affected the hands, thighs, or shoulder girdles. Frequent choking or progressive dysphagia were not related to stroke (normal brain MRIs). A negative panendoscope and PET scan results in patient 6 excluded the presence of an esophageal tumor. Esophagography revealed probable esophageal dysmotility in patient 3 [3]. Patient 7 did not develop dysphagia, but his brother did. Family members with similar symptoms were observed in six patients (6/8, 75%; Table 1).

Orthostatic hypotension, dizziness and recurrent syncope usually occurred in the late phase of the disease. Exertional syncope usually lasted for seconds and occurred during defecation, after voiding [13], after deep breathing, standing from a sitting position, or while driving. Cold sweat and decreased blood pressure (systolic blood pressure 70 ~ 80 mmHg) often accompanied frequent falls [13].

The unfavorable events (syncope/cardiac arrest/CPCR) occurred approximately 4 years after the appearance of the initial neurological symptoms (Fig. 1). CPCR or temporary transcutaneous cardiac pacing (TCP) implantation were observed in three episodes. Patient 3 was implanted with a TCP device at our emergency department at the

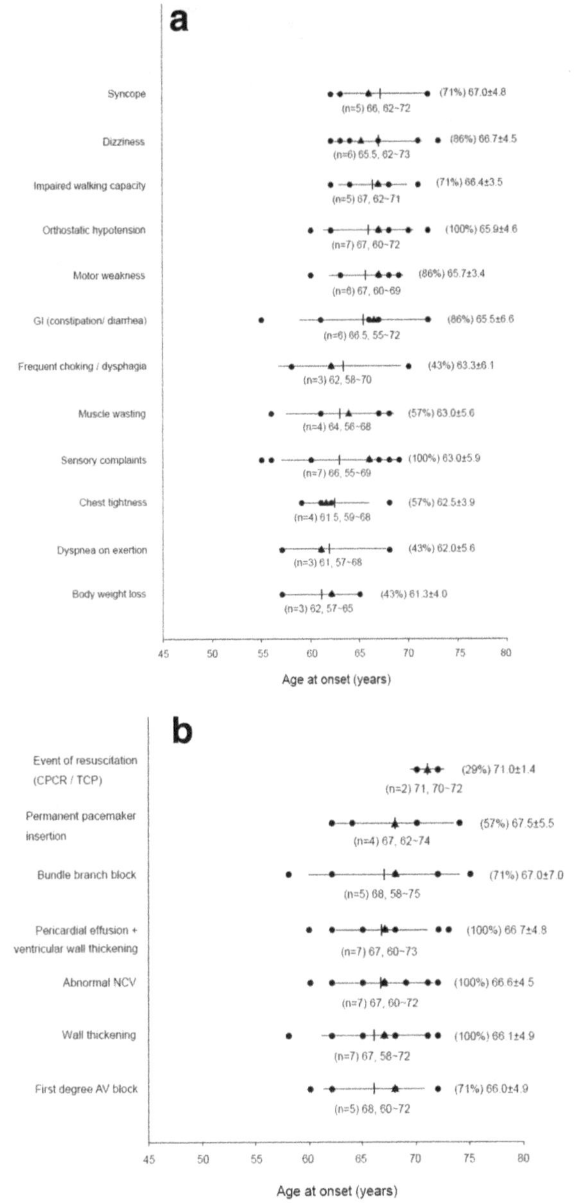

Fig. 1 The onset age of warning symptoms (**a**) and signs (**b**) in patients with ATTR Ala97Ser mutation. Data are presented as (patient number), median, range below the bars and (%), mean ± standard deviation on the right side of the bars. Circles: age at onset of each subject; ▲symbols: median; bars with vertical line: mean ± standard deviation

age of 72 because of a sudden sinus arrest (a slow junctional escape rhythm with shock status), which was suspected to result from an amiodarone-related side effect. Patient 7 was revived with CPCR after sudden cardiac arrest. Ventricular tachyarrhythmia and high degree atrioventricular (AV) block were detected in this patient.

Patients 5 and 7 were alive as the present study ended and returned to clinics for regular follow-up appointments. Patients 1 and 3 died from severe sepsis.

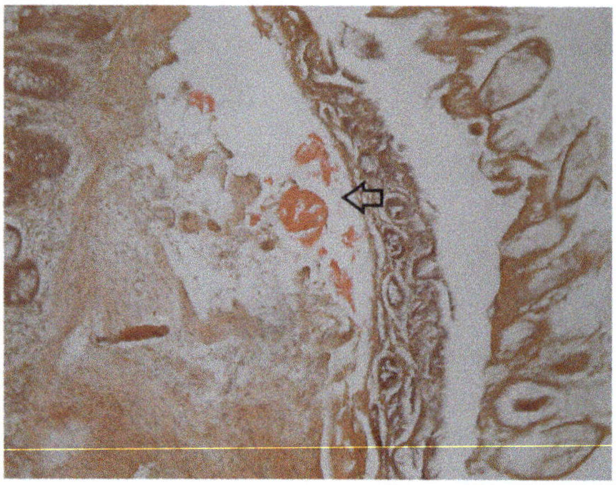

Fig. 2 A representative colonic biopsy of patient 6 showed a portion of amyloid deposits in the submucosa; the deposits stained positive for Congo red stain (arrow, 100X)

Paraclinical and histopathological findings

Electrophysiological tests

The most common finding on nerve conduction studies was an axonal predominant, length-dependent sensorimotor polyneuropathy (7/7, 100%). Bilateral carpal tunnel syndromes were detected in patients 4, 6 and 8. In contrast, patient 2 had a normal nerve conduction study at the age of 37. Current perception threshold testing (CPT) of 4 patients revealed the dysfunction of both large and small sensory nerves in 3 patients (3/4, 75%) and the dysfunction of A beta-fibers of both feet in one patient (1/4, 25%). A sympathetic skin response (SSR) was absent in the palms and soles of five patients (5/6, 83%) and in the soles alone of one patient (1/6, 17%), among the 6 patients who were evaluated for SSR.

Histopathology

Colonic tissue biopsies were positive for Congo red staining in patients 6 and 7 (Fig. 2). Amyloid fibrils were not found on Congo red stained sections of the other three patients.

Electrocardiography and echocardiography

In our study, the most common ECG and echocardiography findings, including pericardial effusion associated with progressive ventricular wall thickening (7/7, 100%; Fig. 3 and Fig. 4) [2], AV block (5/7, 71%), and bundle-branch block (BBB; 5/7, 71%; Table 1).

All patients exhibited progressive left ventricular (LV) wall thickening on echocardiography, but none had electrocardiographic signs of LV hypertrophy. Only two patients had low voltage QRS in the limb leads and the precordial leads, respectively [2]. Echocardiogram a granular sparkling appearance of the ventricular myocardium in four patients (57%; Fig. 3) [2, 4, 14]. Concentric LV hypertrophy was noted in patients 3, 4, 5 and 7 [2]. Except for patient 3, none had systemic hypertension that could explain ventricular hypertrophy [2].

Patients 1 and 7 developed complete left BBB. Patient 8 had left anterior fascicular block. Patients 3 and 5 had right BBB. Patients 5 and 7 developed second- and third-degree AV block at 3 and 11 years after the initial symptom onset, respectively [15]. Pan-conduction system disease was also identified in patient 1. Other findings included left atrial enlargement (patients 1, 4, 6 and 7; Fig. 3) [15], atrial fibrillation (patients 1 and 7) [2], and left axis deviation (patients 5 and 8) [15].

Search for a constellation of progressive manifestations as warning symptoms

Table 1 lists common manifestations and warning symptoms and reveals a rapid progression of autonomic dysfunction and cardiac involvement along with progressive polyneuropathy. Core features of clinical and laboratory manifestations were summarized in Table 2.

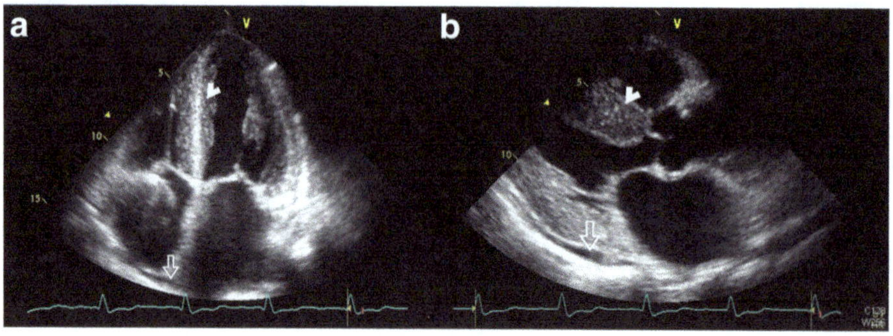

Fig. 3 a In an apical 4-chamber view, biventricular wall thickening, granular sparkling (arrowhead), thickening of the mitral and tricuspid valves, and a trivial amount of pericardial effusion next to the right atrium are visible in the systolic phase (arrow) (patient 6, age 65). **b** In a parasternal long-axis view, a left atrium dilatation and a very thick granular myocardium (arrowhead) with some pericardial effusion (arrow) at the baso-posterior wall are evident (patient 6, age 65)

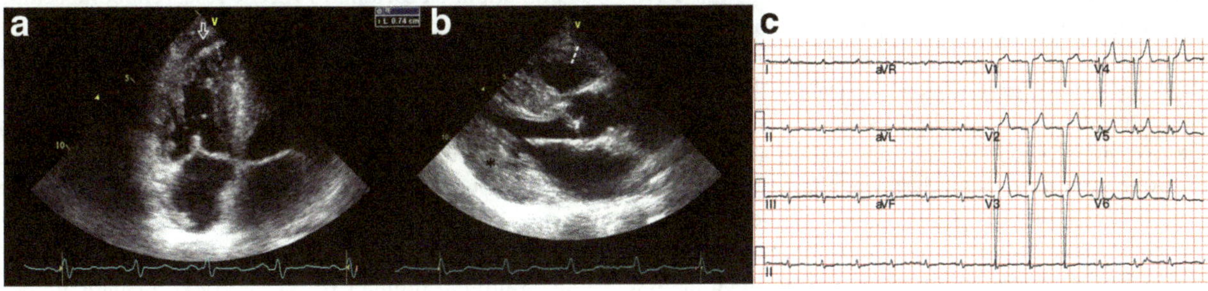

Fig. 4 a In a right ventricle-centered view, a thickened right ventricular wall and a small amount of pericardial effusion next to the right ventricular apex (arrow) are apparent (patient 7, age 68). Among the serial echocardiographic studies this patient received, this is the earliest echo image in which the combination of ventricular wall thickening and pericardial effusion can be identified. **b** In this parasternal long-axis view, a thickening of the right ventricular free wall at 0.74 cm (dashed line) and very thick left ventricular walls (asterisk) are apparent (patient 7, age 69). **c** The ECG of this patient shows a normal sinus rhythm and a complete left bundle branch block (age 69)

Discussion

In this study, we aimed to describe a constellation of easily recognized manifestations that could alert physicians to diagnose ATTR Ala97Ser in Taiwan. Patients initially presented with warning symptoms that might be easily overlooked (including GI symptoms, dyspnea, chest tightness, body weight loss, muscle wasting, or dysphagia). A rapid progressive course was conspicuous and included autonomic disturbances, severe axonal predominant, length-dependent sensorimotor polyneuropathy, and abnormal cardiographic findings [16]. The presence of these manifestations in patients 50–60 years old, as well as similar symptoms among family members, should prompt clinicians to consider the probability of a diagnosis of ATTR.

An intriguing observation was that most patients visited different clinics before receiving a final diagnosis at a neurology department of a referral hospital (Table 1). Cardiologists and gastrologists were most frequently consulted because of chief concerns, the warning symptoms, including chest tightness, dyspnea, dizziness, BWL, constipation (or diarrhea), or frequent choking. These findings revealed a serious issue: patients did not consult a neurologist for their sensory complaints until neurologic symptoms became apparent. Subspecialists did not connect the patients' chief concerns with ATTR, and thus did not vigilantly investigate sensory deficits, family history or other manifestations listed in Table 1. However, the diagnosis of ATTR is particularly challenging

Table 2 Core features of the clinical and laboratory manifestations of patients with ATTR Ala97Ser mutation

	(n = number of patients, males: females)	This study (*n* = 8, 5:3)	Liu et al., 2008 (*n* = 5, 3:2)	Chao et al., 2015 (*n* = 28, 25:3)
Core features	1. Late onset age (years, mean ± SD, median, range)	61.7 ± 5.5, 60, 55–69	50.4 ± 5.6, 49, 46–60	59.9 ± 6.0, 59, 48–71
	2. Progressive polyneuropathy[a]	7/7 (100.0%)	5/5 (100.0%)	28/28 (100.0%)
	3. Progressive autonomic dysfunction[b]	7/7 (100.0%)	5/5 (100.0%)	22/28 (78.6%)
	4. Family members with similar symptoms or documented ATTR	6/8 (75.0%)	5/5 (100.0%)	NA
Supportive laboratory findings	1. Progressive axonal predominant, length-dependent, sensorimotor polyneuropathy on electrophysiology	7/7 (100.0%)	5/5 (100.0%)	28/28 (100.0%)
	2. Ventricular wall thickening in association with pericardial effusion on echocardiography	7/7 (100.0%)	NA	NA
	3. LVH in association with low to normal QRS voltage on electrocardiography	7/7 (100.0%)	NA	NA
	4. Granular sparkling appearance of the ventricular myocardium on echocardiography	4/7 (57.1%)	NA	NA
	5. Hypertrophic cardiomyopathy in the absence of other causes[c]	7/7 (100.0%)	3/5 (60.0%)	NA
	6. Conduction abnormalities on ECG	5/7 (71.4%)	3/5 (60.0%)	NA
	7. Amyloid deposition on tissue biopsy	2/5 (40.0%)	3/5 (60.0%)	> 1/3 (> 33.3%)

[a]Data are presented as ratio. The denominators differ according to the availability of the data. NA: not available

[b]Autonomic dysfunction including gastrointestinal (constipation, diarrhea, or nausea/vomiting), orthostatic (hypotension, dizziness, syncope) and genitourinary symptoms (sexual dysfunction, urinary incontinence, urinary retention)

[c]Increased thickness of the ventricular wall, atrial septum, interventricular septum, or atrioventricular valve

in patients without overt neurological symptoms [2]. TTR-FAP can present as non-familial particularly in late-onset cases [1, 17].

Newly observed presentations or events that had not been reported regarding ATTR Ala97Ser in Taiwan include occasional shooting pain or tingling accompanied with lower limb numbness, dyspnea, chest tightness, frequent choking or dysphagia, dizziness, frequent episodes of syncope, abnormal cardiographic findings (Table 2), and CPCR. Other presentations or events documented in this study as well as by Liu's study [7] are corroborated and worth our attention; these include muscle atrophy resulting from denervation [1, 18], BWL, permanent pacemaker placement, and a preceding carpal tunnel syndrome [5].

Syncope is predisposed by induction of a Valsalva maneuver and is a risk factor for sudden cardiac death [13, 19, 20]. The high ratio of autonomic dysfunction (Table 2) and the exacerbations of orthostatic symptoms suggest that autonomic dysfunction in ATTR Ala97Ser may not be as mild as other types of late-onset FAP [1, 7].

The serial ECGs and/or echocardiography that are often the initial work-ups in these patients play an important role in providing supportive clues since late-onset TTR-related amyloidosis often has cardiac involvement [16, 18, 21]. An ECG or echocardiography finding alone is relatively nonspecific, but the combination of clinical presentations can be more suggestive of ATTR Ala97Ser. Possible sampling errors, the uneven distribution of amyloid fibrils, and the predominant non-fibrillar amyloid precursor material in late-onset specimens may lead to a false negative finding and the low positive ratio of tissue biopsies in this study [5, 17, 18]. Therefore, DNA testing, the most reliable test for TTR-FAP, should be performed without being misled by a negative biopsy in patients with clinical suspicion of TTR-FAP [1, 17].

ATTR Ala97Ser appears to be a late-onset disorder [18, 22, 23]. Nonetheless, there are some differences between ATTR Ala97Ser and other amyloidoses. Left BBB was not as rare as other TTR variants [2]. Unlike light-chain (AL) amyloidosis and early-onset TTR Met 30 FAP [23], renal impairment was less frequent in our subjects. Unlike other TTR variants [1], ocular manifestations were also rare; only patient 5 had glaucoma [24].

There are some limitations in this study. First, the data were collected from a single referral medical center. Second, as this was a retrospective chart review, clinical information and measures were not uniform. Repeated neuropathy impairment score (NIS) and modified body mass index (mBMI) that can reflect disease progression were incomplete [25]. Laboratory studies were not performed early or serially. Three subjects refused biopsy due to personal reasons. No one received a postmortem examination. According to recent research, bone scintigraphy for detection of ATTR cardiac amyloidosis should be performed in the future, because it may replace the traditional requirement for histological confirmation [26]. Third, we were unable to collect complete longitudinal data on patients who were followed up at other hospitals because of personal preference or convenience.

Conclusion

Only a limited number of ATTR Ala97Ser patients have been reported to date in Taiwan. Although rare, careful clinical characterization can facilitate early diagnosis and intervention, which can improve the prognosis of patients with ATTR Ala97Ser. Thus, a further nationwide, prospective enrollment and data collection is warranted.

Abbreviations

ATTR: Hereditary transthyretin related amyloidosis; AV: Atrioventricular; BBB: Bundle-branch block; BNP: brain natriuretic peptide; BWL: Body weight loss; CPCR: Cardiopulmonary-cerebral resuscitation; CPT: Current perception threshold testing; ECG: Electrocardiography; FAP: Familial amyloid polyneuropathy; GI: Gastrointestinal; LV: Left ventricular; mBMI: Modified body mass index; NIS: Neuropathy impairment score; SSR: Sympathetic skin response; TCP: Temporary transcutaneous cardiac pacing; TTR: Transthyretin

Acknowledgements

We wish to thank Miss Shin-Fun Wu for her help in the preparation of the figures.

Funding

This study was supported by a grant from the Chang Gung Medical Research Program (CMRPG3C0371, CMRPG3C0372, CMRPG3C0373) and IRB 100-4470A3, 104-2462A3, Taiwan, ROC.

Authors' contributions

HCH contributed to analysis and interpretation of data, preparation of the manuscript. MFL contributed to patient data acquisition and review of the manuscript. JLH contributed to analysis and interpretation of data and review of the manuscript. ALL contributed to patient data acquisition of the manuscript. HCK contributed to analysis and interpretation of data. RKL contributed to review of the manuscript. VCCW contributed to analysis of the cardio-graphic findings. CWW contributed to interpretation of the pathological findings. RSL contributed to analysis of data, and review of the manuscript. All the authors have read and approved the final version of the manuscript.

Competing interests

The authors have no conflicts of interest to declare.

Author details

[1]Department of Neurology, Chang Gung Memorial Hospital Linkou Medical Center and Chang Gung University College of Medicine, No.199, Tung Hwa N. Rd., Songshan Dist, Taipei City 105, Taiwan, Republic of China. [2]Department of Traditional Chinese Medicine, Division of Chinese Acupuncture and Traumatology, Chang Gung Memorial Hospital Linkou Medical Center and Chang Gung University College of Medicine, No.5, Fuxing St., Guishan Dist, Taoyuan City 333, Taiwan, Republic of China. [3]Department of Cardiology, Chang Gung Memorial Hospital Linkou Medical Center and Chang Gung University College of Medicine, No.5, Fuxing St., Guishan Dist, Taoyuan City 333, Taiwan, Republic of China. [4]Department of Anatomic Pathology, Chang Gung Memorial Hospital Linkou Medical Center and Chang Gung University College of Medicine, No.5, Fuxing St., Guishan Dist, Taoyuan City 333, Taiwan, Republic of China.

References

1. Planté-Bordeneuve V, Said G. Familial amyloid polyneuropathy. Lancet Neurol. 2011;10(12):1086–97.
2. Rapezzi C, Quarta CC, Riva L, Longhi S, Gallelli I, Lorenzini M, Ciliberti P, Biagini E, Salvi F, Branzi A. Transthyretin-related amyloidoses and the heart: a clinical overview. Nat Rev Cardiol. 2010;7(7):398–408.
3. Sattianayagam PT, Hawkins PN, Gillmore JD. Systemic amyloidosis and the gastrointestinal tract. Nat Rev Gastroenterol Hepatol. 2009;6(10):608–17.
4. Ikeda S, Nakazato M, Ando Y, Sobue G. Familial transthyretin-type amyloid polyneuropathy in Japan: clinical and genetic heterogeneity. Neurology. 2002;58(7):1001–7.
5. Ando Y, Coelho T, Berk JL, Cruz MW, Ericzon BG, Ikeda SI, Lewis WD, Obici L, Planté-Bordeneuve V, Rapezzi C, et al. Guideline of transthyretin-related hereditary amyloidosis for clinicians. Orphanet J Rare Dis. 2013; doi:10.1186/1750-1172-8-31.1.
6. Yang NC, Lee MJ, Chao CC, Chuang YT, Lin WM, Chang MF, Hsieh PC, Kan HW, Lin YH, Yang CC, et al. Clinical presentations and skin denervation in amyloid neuropathy due to transthyretin Ala97Ser. Neurology. 2010;75(6):532–8.
7. Liu YT, Lee YC, Yang CC, Chen ML, Lin KP. Transthyretin Ala97Ser in Chinese-Taiwanese patients with familial amyloid polyneuropathy: genetic studies and phenotype expression. J Neuro Sci. 2008;267(1–2):91–9.
8. Chao CC, Huang CM, Chiang HH, Luo KR, Kan HW, Yang NCC, Chiang H, Lin WM, Lai SM, Lee MJ, et al. Sudomotor innervation in transthyretin amyloid neuropathy: pathology and functional correlates. Ann Neurol. 2015;78(2):272–83.
9. Mead S, Reilly MM. A new prion disease: relationship with central and peripheral amyloidoses. Nat Rev Neurol. 2015;11(2):90–7.
10. Coelho T, Maia LF, Da Silva AM, Cruz MW, Planté-Bordeneuve V, Suhr OB, Conceiçao I, Schmidt HHJ, Trigo P, Kelly JW, et al. Long-term effects of tafamidis for the treatment of transthyretin familial amyloid polyneuropathy. J Neurol. 2013;260(11):2802–14.
11. Coelho T, Maia LF, Da Silva AM, Cruz MW, Planté-Bordeneuve V, Lozeron P, Suhr OB, Campistol JM, Conceição IM, Schmidt HHJ, et al. Tafamidis for transthyretin familial amyloid polyneuropathy: a randomized, controlled trial. Neurology. 2012;79(8):785–92.
12. Patrosso MC, Salvi F, De Grandis D, Vezzoni P, Jacobson DR, Ferlini A. Novel transthyretin missense mutation (Thr34) in an Italian family with hereditary amyloidosis. Am J Med Genet. 1998;77(2):135–8.
13. Mathias CJ. Autonomic diseases: clinical features and laboratory evaluation. J Neurol Neurosurg Psychiatry. 2003;74(suppl 3):iii31–41.
14. Rapezzi C, Merlini G, Quarta CC, Riva L, Longhi S, Leone O, Salvi F, Ciliberti P, Pastorelli F, Biagini E, et al. Systemic cardiac Amyloidoses. Circulation. 2009;120(13):1203–12.
15. Cacciapuoti F. The role of echocardiography in the non-invasive diagnosis of cardiac amyloidosis. J Echocardiogr. 2015;13(3):84–9.
16. Rapezzi C, Quarta CC, Obici L, Perfetto F, Longhi S, Salvi F, Biagini E, Lorenzini M, Grigioni F, Leone O, et al. Disease profile and differential diagnosis of hereditary transthyretin-related amyloidosis with exclusively cardiac phenotype: an Italian perspective. Eur Heart J. 2013;34(7):520–8.
17. Plante-Bordeneuve V, Ferreira A, Lalu T, Zaros C, Lacroix C, Adams D, Said G. Diagnostic pitfalls in sporadic transthyretin familial amyloid polyneuropathy (TTR-FAP). Neurology. 2007;69(7):693–8.
18. Dohrn MF, Röcken C, De Bleecker JL, Martin JJ, Vorgerd M, Van Den Bergh PY, Ferbert A, Hinderhofer K, Schröder JM, Weis J, et al. Diagnostic hallmarks and pitfalls in late-onset progressive transthyretin-related amyloid-neuropathy. J Neurol. 2013;260(12):3093–108.
19. Sayed RH, Rogers D, Khan F, Wechalekar AD, Lachmann HJ, Fontana M, Mahmood S, Sachchithanantham S, Patel K, Hawkins PN, et al. A study of implanted cardiac rhythm recorders in advanced cardiac AL amyloidosis. Eur Heart J. 2015;36(18):1098–105.
20. Chamarthi B, Dubrey SW, Cha K, Skinner M, Falk RH. Features and prognosis of exertional syncope in light-chain associated AL cardiac amyloidosis. Am J Cardiol. 1997;80(9):1242–5.
21. Sato C, Takaya T, Mori S, Hasegawa K, Soga F, Tanaka H, Watanabe Y, Nishii T, Kono AK, Morinaga Y, et al. An isolated case of late-onset amyloidogenic transthyretin type familial amyloid polyneuropathy associated with a mutant transthyretin substituting methionine for valine at position 30 showing latent progressive cardiac involvement confirmed by serial annual electrocardiograms. Intern Med. 2017;56(2):163–8.
22. Takahashi K, Sakashita N, Ando Y, Suga M, Ando M. Late onset type I familial amyloidotic polyneuropathy: presentation of three autopsy cases in comparison with 19 autopsy cases of the ordinary type. Pathol Int. 1997;47(6):353–9.
23. Koike H, Misu K, Sugiura M, Iijima M, Mori K, Yamamoto M, Hattori N, Mukai E, Ando Y, Ikeda S, et al. Pathology of early- vs late-onset TTR Met30 familial amyloid polyneuropathy. Neurology. 2004;63(1):129–38.
24. Ishida K, Nishida T, Niimi Y, Suemori S, Mochizuki K, Kawakami H, Kimura A, Hirayama T. Elderly onset vitreous opacities as the initial manifestation in hereditary transthyretin (ATTR Val30Met) carries. Ophthalmic Genet. 2017; doi:10.1080/13816810.2016.1232413.1-5.
25. Coelho T, Vinik A, Vinik EJ, Tripp T, Packman J, Grogan DR. Clinical measures in transthyretin familial amyloid polyneuropathy. Muscle Nerve. 2016; doi:10.1002/mus.25257.
26. Gillmore JD, Maurer MS, Falk RH, Merlini G, Damy T, Dispenzieri A, Wechalekar AD, Berk JL, Quarta CC, Grogan M, et al. Nonbiopsy diagnosis of cardiac Transthyretin Amyloidosis. Circulation. 2016;133(24):2404–12.

10

Electrocardiographic assessments and cardiac events after fingolimod first dose

Volker Limmroth[1†], Tjalf Ziemssen[2†], Michael Lang[3], Stephan Richter[4], Bert Wagner[4], Judith Haas[5], Stephan Schmidt[6], Kathrin Gerbershagen[1], Christoph Lassek[7], Luisa Klotz[8], Olaf Hoffmann[9], Christian Albert[9], Katrin Schuh[10], Monika Baier-Ebert[10], Guillaume Wendt[10], Heinke Schieb[10], Susanne Hoyer[10], Ralf Dechend[11†] and Wilhelm Haverkamp[12*†]

Abstract

Background: First dose observation for cardiac effects is required for fingolimod, but recommendations on the extent vary. This study aims to assess cardiac safety of fingolimod first dose. Individual bradyarrhythmic episodes were evaluated to assess the relevance of continuous electrocardiogram (ECG) monitoring.

Methods: START is an ongoing open-label, multi-center study. At the time of analysis 3951 patients were enrolled. The primary endpoints are the incidence of bradycardia (heart rate < 45 bpm) and second-/third-degree AV blocks during treatment initiation. The relevance of Holter was assessed by matching ECG findings with the occurrence of clinical symptoms as well as by rigorous analysis of AV blocks with regard to the duration of pauses and the minimal heart rate recorded during AV block.

Results: Thirty-one patients (0.8%) developed bradycardia (<45 bpm), 62 patients (1.6%) had second-degree Mobitz I and/or 2:1 AV blocks with a lowest reading (i.e. mean of ten consecutive beats) of 35 bpm and the longest pause lasting for 2.6 s. No Mobitz II or third-degree AV blocks were observed. Only one patient complained about mild chest discomfort and fatigue. After 1 week, there was no second-/third-degree AV block.

Conclusions: Continuous Holter ECG monitoring in this large real-life cohort revealed that bradycardia and AV conduction abnormalities were rare, transient and benign. No further unexpected abnormalities were detected. The data presented here give an indication that continuous Holter ECG monitoring does not add clinically relevant value to patients' safety.

Keywords: Fingolimod, First dose, Electrocardiogram, Cardiac effects, Bradycardia, Atrioventricular conduction

Background

Fingolimod (FTY720, brand name Gilenya®) has been approved for the treatment of relapsing remitting multiple sclerosis (RRMS). It exerts its therapeutic effects via modulation of sphingosine-1-phosphate (S1P-) receptors on lymphocytes, which results in the retention of circulating lymphocytes in the lymph nodes [1–4]. As a result, peripheral blood lymphocyte counts are reversibly reduced to approximately 30%, which is postulated to reduce recirculation of autoreactive lymphocytes and to prevent infiltration into the central nervous system [5, 6].

Receptors of this class, predominantly S1P1, are also expressed on atrial myocytes [7]. Fingolimod binding to S1P1 mediates a decrease in heart rate and prolongation of atrioventricular (AV) conduction. These effects are transient as fingolimod also induces internalization of these receptors, causing functional antagonism. Consequently,

* Correspondence: wilhelm.haverkamp@charite.de
†Equal contributors
[12]Charité Universitaetsmedizin Berlin, Campus Virchow Klinikum, Augustenburger Platz 1, Berlin 13353, Germany
Full list of author information is available at the end of the article

the negative chronotropic effects are limited to treatment initiation [6, 8–10].

A first-dose observation procedure is recommended. The exact procedure is defined by local product labels and differs between countries. It is generally required to observe patients for bradycardia by hourly measurements of pulse and blood pressure for at least six hours and to obtain an electrocardiogram (ECG) prior to dosing and at the end of the observation period. In contrast to the United States (US) and the Australian labels, the European Union (EU) label additionally recommends a continuous Holter ECG for six hours. In Japan, continuous ECG and observation of heart rate and blood pressure for 24 hours are recommended.

START is a prospective study designed to assess the cardiac safety of fingolimod first dose in detail and in a much larger cohort compared to previous studies. Patients and study sites were selected to closely resemble the broad range of fingolimod patients and treatment circumstances in daily practice. The study follows the EU label recommendations by obtaining a Holter ECG for six hours in addition to clinical monitoring and pre-/post first dose ECG. Therefore, START is the first interventional study that investigates in a large cohort whether continuous ECG monitoring detects clinically meaningful findings beyond pre-/post first dose ECG. The results might facilitate guidance on the degree of observation that is necessary to ensure patient safety.

Methods

Study design

START (NCT01585298) is an ongoing open-label, multicenter study in Germany in patients with RRMS receiving fingolimod at a daily dose of 0.5 mg. Its purpose is (a) to assess cardiac safety of fingolimod first dose with a special focus on bradycardia and AV conduction abnormalities, and (b) to analyze individual arrhythmic episodes more extensively in order to evaluate the clinical relevance of continuous ECG monitoring. Up to 7000 patients are planned to be enrolled based on a two-sided 95% confidence interval with a precision of 0.23%. Sample size calculation was based on the observed incidence of 0.963% of second-degree or higher AV blocks in the first 1000 patients enrolled. Annual interim analyses are planned per protocol to review whether the sample size needs to be adjusted. The results of the 2015 interim analysis are reported here. At the time of the interim analysis, the number of patients included has largely exceeded the sample size of previous studies, thereby adding significantly to the state of knowledge on the cardiac effects of fingolimod.

Endpoints

The primary endpoints are the incidence of bradycardia, defined as heart rate < 45 bpm, and the incidence of second- and third-degree AV blocks during the six-hour monitoring period. For this analysis, three types of second-degree blocks were distinguished: Mobitz type I (progressive prolongation of the PR interval with the subsequent occurrence of a single non-conducted P wave, i.e. atrial impulse that creates a pause), 2:1 (second-degree block with a fixed 2:1 ratio of conducted and non-conducted P waves, that can be the result of either Mobitz I or Mobitz II type blocks) or Mobitz type II (constant PR interval followed by a non-conducted P wave, such that either an occasional dropped P wave or a regular conduction pattern of 2:1, 3:1, and so on is observed). Secondary endpoints include the incidence of other conduction abnormalities such as first-degree AV block (PR-interval prolongation), and QTc prolongation. The latter is defined as QTc > 450 ms in males and > 470 ms in females. Additionally, QTc prolongations > 500 ms are identified as these patients required overnight monitoring as specified by the EU label.

To analyze the incidence of bradycardia, pulse palpation by study personnel was used. In detail, study personnel were advised to measure the heart rate for at least 15 s. Second- and third-degree AV blocks were identified from continuous Holter ECG recordings. The remaining variables, i.e. PR- and QT-interval, were taken from 12-lead ECG data. Fridericia formula was used for correction of the QT intervals.

Safety assessments

The incidence of adverse events (AE) and serious adverse events (SAE) was determined applying the definitions and standards of the ICH guideline on clinical safety data management. Further, the incidence of AE suggestive for cardiac events was determined using the following MedDRA preferred terms: Angina pectoris, chest discomfort, dizziness, dyspnoea, exertional dyspnoea, fatigue, palpitations, syncope, vertigo, positional vertigo, and blurred vision.

The incidence of overnight hospitalization was defined as the number of patients who experienced a cardiac AE (any AE out of the system organ class "cardiac disorders") starting on the day of the first fingolimod intake and who were hospitalized for this event.

Clinical relevance of continuous ECG monitoring

To assess the relevance of continuous ECG monitoring, the identified second-degree AV blocks were assessed for clinical relevance, i.e. the occurrence of any cardiac symptoms in these patients. Furthermore, continuous ECG recordings of patients with AV blocks were evaluated rigorously. The duration of pauses (RR intervals) and the minimal heart rate during second-degree AV blocks were determined post hoc by the cardiologist. The minimal heart rate during AV blocks was defined as the mean heart rate of 10 beats during an AV block to detect short lasting changes in heart rate. Holter ECG data of patients with cardiac symptoms were assessed for any abnormalities that might have predicted the symptoms. Alignment of evaluations of bradycardia as assessed by study nurse and the Holter ECG were also evaluated post hoc. No statistical comparison between Holter ECG and 12-lead ECG plus pulse palpation assessment with respect to the incidence of cardiac events was performed.

Results of START were analyzed descriptively. Where indicated, statistical tests were performed based on Student's *t*-test unless otherwise noted.

Approval and participants

The study protocol was approved by the respective state and institutional ethical standards committees at all participating sites (Competent ethics committee: Ethikkommission der Ärztekammer Nordrhein; EUDRACT No. 2012-000653-32-DE). Patients have to give written informed consent. The inclusion and exclusion criteria were defined to select patients with RRMS who were eligible for treatment with fingolimod (Gilenya®) according to the EU label. Patients were excluded if they received class Ia or III antiarrythmic drugs or beta blockers, heart-rate-lowering calcium channel blockers or other substances which may decrease heart rate (e.g. digoxin, anticholinesteratic agents or pilocarpine). Furthermore, patients were excluded if they have a history of second-degree Mobitz Type II or higher-degree AV block, Sick-sinus syndrome, Sino-atrial heart block, significant QT prolongation, symptomatic bradycardia or recurrent syncope, known ischemic heart disease, cerebrovascular disease, myocardial infarction, hypokalemia, congestive heart failure, cardiac arrest, uncontrolled hypertension, or severe sleep apnea.

Study procedures

Patients' eligibility was determined during a 4-week screening phase (visit 1). At the first-dose visit (visit 2), patients underwent baseline assessments of basic demographic and relevant clinical characteristics including MS status, concomitant medication, vital signs, blood count and blood chemistry. A 12-lead ECG prior to the first dose of fingolimod was recorded. After the first intake of the study drug, patients were monitored for six hours by continuous Holter ECG recording, while heart rate and blood pressure were measured simultaneously, every hour. Afterwards, a second 12-lead ECG was recorded. The 6-hour monitoring period reflects the current EU label and was considered sufficient as the nadir of the heart rate decrease usually occurs four hours post-dose [9]. At visit 3, i.e. 1 week after study drug initiation, a third 12-lead ECG is recorded and vital signs, blood count and blood chemistry were assessed (Fig. 1). Adverse events were recorded at all visits.

If the patient's heart rate at the end of the 6-hour period is the lowest following first dose administration, the monitoring had to be extended by at least two hours and until the heart rate rises. In those patients with evidence of clinically important cardiac events (e.g. persistent new-onset second-degree or third-degree AV block, heart rate < 45 bpm at six hours after first dose, QTc interval ≥ 500 msec), monitoring had to be extended until full resolution of symptoms, including overnight monitoring. If a patient required pharmacologic intervention during the first dose observation, the first dose monitoring strategy had to be repeated after the second dose of fingolimod. Study medication had to be interrupted or discontinued in cases of atypical neurological deterioration, lymphopenia < 200/µl, and a more than 5-fold elevation of liver function tests. In other cases the decision on continuation of study drug was at the discretion of the physician and the patient.

Each study site was equipped with the ECG-device CardioMem® CM3000-12, a 12-lead-continuous-ECG-digital recorder. The ECG recordings were pseudonymized and immediately transmitted via internet to the cardiology reading center for evaluation. The results of ECG analysis were available to the treating physician within less than 40 min. To identify AV blocks all Holter ECG recordings were assessed according to the same automated analysis process. Subsequently, two independent cardiologists manually reviewed every second- or third-degree AV block episode to determine the exact AV block subtype per episode, the number of episodes, the duration of the longest pause and the minimal heart rate (mean of ten consecutive beats).

Twice a year, an external and independent Data Safety Monitoring Board (DSMB), consisting of two neurologists and a cardiologist, reviewed safety-related issues. The DSMB was entitled to recommend changes in study conduct.

Results

Study patients and conduct

The present analysis is based on 3951 patients recruited between June 2012 and January 2015. The majority of the patients were seen by office-based neurologists. Baseline demographics and MS history are presented in Tables 1 and 2. A Holter ECG was recorded at visit 2 in 3906 out of 3951 patients who received fingolimod (Fig. 1). 25 patients had discontinued medication after the first or second dose, and another 25 patients had discontinued the study drug further on (Table 3). In 38 patients (0.96%) adverse events were the primary reason for discontinuation. In the remaining 12 patients abnormal laboratory values or other reasons prompted to stop the study drug. 13 patients out of those who discontinued study drug did not show up for visit 3 (Fig. 2). These patients were followed-up separately confirming that they were alive and did not suffer from cardiac sequelae.

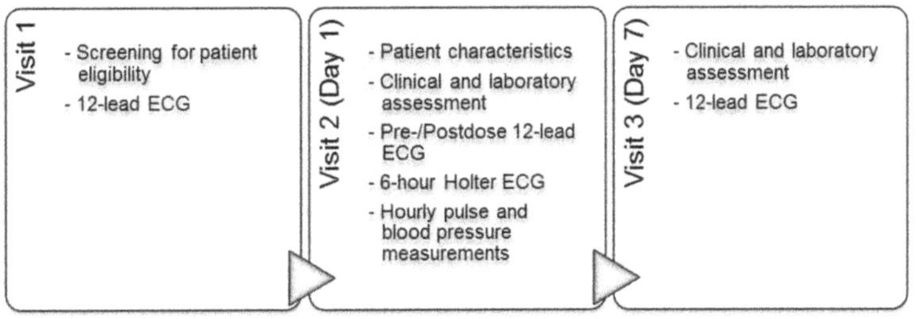

Fig. 1 Visit schedule

Changes in heart rate

Patients receiving the first dose of fingolimod experienced on average a slight and transient decline in heart rate. 87.4% of the patients reached the nadir before the end of the 6-hour post-dose observation period. In 31 patients (0.8%) the heart rate dropped below 45 bpm. Holter ECG confirmed 23 of the 31 cases with a heart rate below 45 as measured by study personnel. For three patients no Holter was available und two other patients had an insufficient Holter ECG reading. Table 4 presents the heart beat dynamics of patients by subgroup, i.e. by time of the lowest heart rate measurement, by presence of bradycardia and by presence of AV blocks.

AV conduction abnormalities

First-degree AV blocks (PR-interval > 200 ms in the ECG assessments) occurred in 2.7% of the patients before and in 5.8% of the patients after the first dose of fingolimod. In 62 patients (1.6%) a second-degree AV block was observed. Type 2:1 AV blocks were identified for 18 patients (Table 5). In 16 patients the 2:1 blocks emerged from Mobitz I blocks.

Table 1 Patient demographics and relevant baseline characteristics

	Fingolimod 0.5 mg ($N = 3951$)
Age groups in years, n (%)	
18–30	880 (22.3)
> 30–40	1222 (30.9)
> 40–55	1622 (41.1)
> 55–65	208 (5.3)
> 65	18 (0.5)
Sex	
Female, n (%)	2779 (70.3)
Duration of MS since first symptoms in years, mean ± SD	10.0 ± 7.6
Number of relapses in previous year, mean ± SD	1.6 ± 1.2
EDSS, mean ± SD	2.8 ± 1.6
DMT treatment within the last 6 months, n (%)	
No	827 (20.9)
Yes	3124 (79.1)

In the two patients with 2:1 block not emerging from Mobitz I, the event was limited to a single episode. No Mobitz II second-degree AV blocks or third-degree AV blocks occurred (Table 5). On average the first second-degree AV blocks occurred 3.62 h after drug intake (SD 1.26, range 0.62 to 5.87). The mean minimal heart rate during second-degree AV block as assessed by Holter ECG (mean of ten consecutive beats) was 51.5 bpm (range 35 to 80 bpm) with no significant difference between the two types of second-degree AV blocks, Mobitz type I and 2:1 ($p = 0.235$). The longest pause observed in association with second-degree AV blocks was 2.6 s. The mean value was 1.9 s (SD 0.3), with no difference between 2:1 and Wenckebach-type AV blocks ($p = 0.887$). Heart rate dynamics of patients with second-degree AV blocks as measured by study personnel are shown in Fig. 3 and Table 4.

Effects on repolarisation

The mean QTc interval in the overall population was 413.8 ms (range 352 to 470 ms) before and 417.7 ms (range 239 to 479 ms) after first dose. Applying > 450 ms in men and > 470 ms in women as a conservative threshold, only two men and four women had QTc intervals above their respective thresholds after fingolimod intake. None of these patients had symptoms suggestive of cardiac events and none required additional medication during first dose monitoring. All of these patients were continued on study medication. No patient had a QTc interval exceeding 500 ms, which would have warranted overnight monitoring as defined in the current EU label.

Adverse events and cardiac symptoms

AEs were observed in 1350 patients (34.2%) and 117 patients (2.96%) experienced SAEs (Table 6). The most frequent types of AEs causing discontinuation of medication were cardiac, gastrointestinal, and nervous system disorders (Table 7). Symptoms reported as AE during the 6-hour monitoring suggestive of cardiac events occurred in 120 patients (3.04%, Table 6). Holter ECG revealed no rhythm abnormalities in these patients, as confirmed by the cardiologist. Only one case of symptomatic second-degree AV block (0.03%) and one case of symptomatic bradycardia

Table 2 Patient characteristics with potential relevance for cardiac events and frequency of symptoms by subgroup

	Overall population	Patients with bradycardia	Patients with second-degree AV block	Patients with AE	Patients with symptoms suggestive of cardiac events at visit 2	Patients who discontinued study drug due to AE
	N = 3951	*N* = 31	*N* = 62[a]	*N* = 1350	*N* = 120	*N* = 38
Demographics						
Age (years), mean ± SD	39.3 ± 10.4	42.1 ± 10.9	40.4 ± 11.7	39.3 ± 10.4	39.6 ± 10.4	42.3 ± 12.4
Female, n (%)	2779 (70.3)	14 (45.2)	57 (91.9)	1023 (75.8)	96 (80.0)	29 (76.3)
Concomitant medication known to prolong QT interval:						
SSRI n (%)	339 (10.1)	1 (3.2)	4 (6.5)	152 (11.3)	17 (14.2)	6 (15.8)
TCA n (%)	92 (2.3)	0	0	38 (2.8)	2 (1.7)	1 (2.6)
Amantadin n (%)	42 (1.1)	0	0	18 (1.3)	2 (1.7)	0
Carbamazepin n (%)	29 (0.7)	0	1 (1.6)	14 (1.0)	3 (2.5)	1 (2.6)
Fampridine n (%)	299 (7.6)	3 (9.7)	5 (8.1)	81 (6.0)	8 (6.7)	1 (2.6)
Heart rate at visit 2 pre-dose						
Heart rate (bpm), mean ± SD	73.9 ± 10.4	59.5 ± 8.0	75.0 ± 8.5	73.4 ± 10.4	73.3 ± 11.6	75.8 ± 10.6
Blood pressure at visit 2 pre-dose						
Systolic (mmHg), mean ± SD	121.8 ± 14.0	125.7 ± 20.3	117.5 ± 13.7	122.0 ± 14.1	123.9 ± 14.5	120.4 ± 15.4
Diastolic (mmHg), mean ± SD	78.5 ± 9.7	78.1 ± 13.1	75.7 ± 9.0	78.7 ± 9.8	79.9 ± 10.0	76.1 ± 11.1
Potassium levels at visit 2						
< 3.5 mmol/L	13 (0.3)	0	0	5 (0.4)	0	0
≥ 3.5–5.5 mmol/L	3853 (98.3)	31 (100)	61 (98.4)	1320 (98.5)	119 (99.2)	38 (100.0)
> 5.5 mmol/L	54 (1.4)	0	1 (1.6)	15 (1.1)	1 (0.8)	0
Symptoms suggestive of cardiac events[b] during 6 h first-dose observation						
Patients with symptoms, n (%)	120 (3.0)	1 (3.2)[c]	1 (1.6)[d]	120 (8.9)	120 (100.0)	1 (2.6)

[a]One of the patients had both, bradycardia and second-degree AV block and is therefore included in both groups
[b]Cardiac symptoms are defined as the following MedDRA preferred terms: Angina pectoris, chest discomfort, dizziness, dyspnoea, dyspnoe exertional, fatigue, palpitations, syncope, vertigo, vertigo positional, blurred vision
[c]Fatigue and chest discomfort
[d]Palpitations

(0.03%) were observed (Table 2). Neither syncope nor dyspnoea were observed in these patients. No patient required medical treatment for bradycardia or AV block. The patient with the lowest heart rate measured (31 bpm) was asymptomatic. In total, 42 patients (1.06%) were hospitalized overnight due to any cardiac adverse event that started during day 1 after first dose administration. Patient characteristics potentially increasing the risk for cardiac events by subgroup are presented in Table 2.

Table 3 Doses of study drug intake prior to discontinuation of study drug

	Fingolimod 0.5 mg *N* = 50
Number of capsules taken	n (%)
1	17 (34.0)
2	8 (16.0)
3–7	21 (42.0)
> 7	3 (6.0)
Missing	1 (2.0)

Follow up

At visit 3, first-degree AV blocks were found in 2.8% of patients. 12-lead ECG did not reveal any second- or third-degree AV blocks. However, since no continuous ECG was recorded at visit 3, accidental second- or third-degree AV blocks might have been missed. Bradycardia was present in only two patients with heart rates of 44 bpm (51 bpm at baseline) and 43 bpm (55 bpm at baseline). No symptoms were associated. Only two men and one woman had QTc intervals above the relevant thresholds (>450 and > 470 ms, respectively). None of the patients developed clinically relevant QTc interval prolongation (i.e. arrhythmias).

Discussion

The data presented here demonstrate that 0.8% patients had bradycardia and 0.03% had symptomatic bradycardia with mild self-limiting symptoms. Transient second-

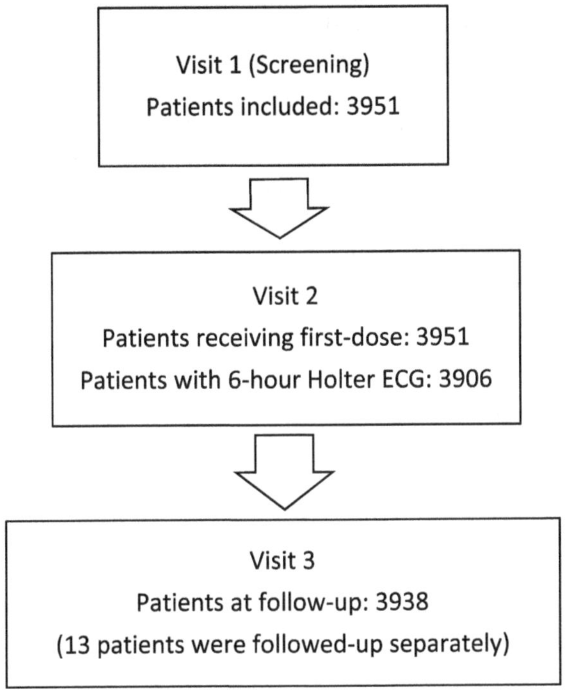

Fig. 2 Patient disposition

degree AV blocks (Mobitz Type I and 2:1) were detected in 1.6% of patients. Bradycardia and AV block did not result in pre-syncope or syncope, demonstrating the benign and self-limiting nature of these cardiac effects. Despite the large size of the cohort and the transient occurrence of second-degree AV blocks Type I and 2:1, no Mobitz II or third degree AV blocks were observed. At visit 3, no patient had second- or third-degree AV blocks and the lowest heart rate was 43 bpm. The decrease in heart rate of patients with second-degree AV-blocks did not significantly differ from that in patients without such an event. Interestingly, the baseline mean heart rate of patients who developed bradycardia during first dosing was below 60, whereas in all other groups the mean baseline heart rate was above 70. This could be an indication that a patient with a low heart rate at onset may be at risk to develop substantial bradycardia.

Drug-related effects on myocardial repolarization (QT interval >450/470 ms) were observed in five patients, however, without a need for intervention. No patient required overnight monitoring due to QT interval prolongation > 500 ms, as warranted by the EU label. Although single reports on spontaneous arrhythmias have been published [11–16], no such events were observed in this large cohort.

The results of START are consistent with previous studies. Incidence of bradycardia and second-degree AV blocks in previous studies were 1.3 to 1.4% (bradycardia), 1.3 to 2.6% (Mobitz type I second-degree AV block, Wenckebach) and 0.5 to 1.4% (2:1 second-degree AV block) [7–10]. In a cohort of 625 healthy volunteers, transient type I second-degree AV blocks (Wenckebach) were observed in 14 (2.2%) individuals during nighttime.

Table 4 Heart rate dynamics by subgroup within 6 h post-dose

	Number of patients	Pre-dose heart rate[a] (bpm)	Lowest post-dose heart rate[a] (bpm)	Maximum decline in heart rate[a] (bpm)
	n (%)	Mean (range)	Mean (range)	Mean (SD)
	Fingolimod, $N = 3951$			
Overall population				
Overall population	3951 (100.0)	73.9 (45–132)	62.1 (31–101)	11.8 (8.47)
By time of lowest heart rate				
Patients with lowest heart rate at < 6 h	3455 (87.4)	73.8 (45–132)	61.9 (31–101)	11.9 (8.42)
Patients with lowest heart rate at 6 h	496 (12.6)	74.6 (48–114)	63.5 (38–90)	11.1 (8.76)
p-value[b]				0.0394
By presence of bradycardia				
Patients with bradycardia	31 (0.8)	59.5 (46–80)	41.6 (31–44)	17.9 (8.30)
Patients without bradycardia	3920 (99.2)	74.0 (45–132)	62.2 (45–101)	11.7 (8.45)
p-value[b]				0.0001
By presence of second-degree AV block				
Patients with second-degree AV block	62 (1.6)	75.0 (56–95)	62.7 (42–83)	12.2 (8.12)
Patients without second-degree AV block	3889 (98.4)	73.8 (45–132)	62.1 (31–101)	11.8 (8.48)
p-value[b]				0.691

[a]as measured by on-site study personnel
[b]Students *t*-test

Table 5 Second- and third-degree AV blocks during treatment initiation

	Fingolimod 0.5 mg $N = 3951$
Patients with 12-lead ECG recording, n	$N = 3951$
Patients with first-degree AV block, n (%)	280 (7.1)
Pre-dose	96 (2.7)
Post-dose	206 (5.8)
Patients with Holter ECG recording, n	$N = 3906$
Patients with second-degree AV block, n (%)	62 (1.6)
Mobitz Type I (Wenckebach)	60 (1.5)[a]
2:1	18 (0.5)[a]
Mobitz Type II (Mobitz)	0
Patients with third-degree AV block, n (%)	0

[a]A patient might experience both Mobitz type I and 2:1 AV blocks during the six-hour monitoring

In three cases, AV blocks were also observed during daytime [17]. The occurrence of AV blocks beyond the 6-hour observation interval including nocturnal events were investigated in the FREEDOMS II trial [8]. Fingolimod-induced second-degree AV blocks usually occurred in the first six hours. The data indicated that nighttime second-degree AV blocks were infrequent and occurred in 0.6% of the patients receiving fingolimod and in 2.0% of the placebo patients. These results underpin the interpretation that the incidence of AV blocks during nighttime (>12 h after first dose) does not seem higher than in the healthy population. However, as the study cohorts differ, a valid comparison of incidence rates would require adjustment for variations in patient characteristics.

Except for one case accompanied by mild symptoms, AV blocks observed in the START study were not associated with cardiac symptoms. Thus, the pathologic ECG findings were usually not associated with any clinically relevant event. Conversely, none of the few mild cardiac symptoms observed showed a corresponding event in the Holter ECG. In summary, Holter ECG data provide scientifically valuable information of an in-depth understanding of the electrocardiographic effects of fingolimod, but does not help to identify patients at risk for clinically relevant cardiac symptoms.

As lower degree AV conduction abnormalities also occur in an otherwise healthy population without clinical significance, they are generally not considered harmful [18]. In general, type I second-degree AV blocks do not require intervention as long as they are asymptomatic [19]. On the contrary, third-degree and type II second-degree AV blocks usually warrant intervention and even constitute an indication for permanent pacemaker implantation, which indicates their prognostic relevance [19]. However, this approach does not apply to drug-induced lower degree AV blocks, which are associated with clinical concerns as they might predict more severe AV conduction disturbances [18]. Drugs like beta-blockers or calcium channel blockers are known for their potential to induce deleterious AV conduction abnormalities [18]. These disturbances can even relapse after discontinuation of the inducing drug and may require permanent use of pacemakers [20, 21].

The characteristics of second-degree AV blocks in the START study indicate that the nature of AV conduction effects of fingolimod might differ from other AV block inducing drugs. For example, drug-induced AV blocks are usually associated with significant slowing of heart rate. However, in fingolimod-induced second-degree AV

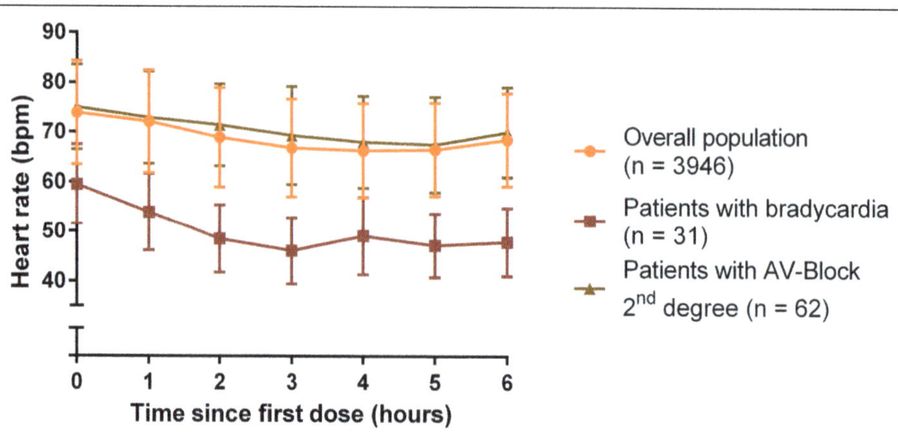

Fig. 3 Changes in heart rate after the first dose of fingolimod. The time course of heart rate during the first 6 hours after fingolimod intake is presented for the overall population, patients with bradycardia and patients with second-degree AV block (absolute values and SD)

Table 6 Most frequent (serious) adverse events

	Fingolimod 0.5 mg $N = 3951$	
	Number of patients, n (%)	Number of events, n
Summary of adverse events		
Any adverse event	1350 (34.17)	2207
Any serious adverse event	117 (2.96)	152
Any adverse event leading to discontinuation of study drug	38 (0.96)	69
Common adverse events (>1% in SOC/PT)		
Nervous system disorders	403 (10.20)	464
Headache	199 (5.04)	205
Dizziness	72 (1.82)	73
MS relapse	58 (1.47)	59
General disorders and administration site conditions	240 (6.07)	265
Fatigue	135 (3.42)	138
Cardiac disorders	231 (5.85)	263
AV block first degree	69 (1.75)	70
AV block second degree	65 (1.65)	67
Bradycardia	45 (1.14)	45
Gastrointestinal disorders	217 (5.49)	246
Nausea	91 (2.30)	92
Diarrhoea	52 (1.32)	52
Infections and infestations	170 (4.30)	178
Nasopharyngitis	78 (1.97)	78
Investigations	130 (3.29)	150
Blood and lymphatic disorders	115 (2.91)	140
Lymphopenia	73 (1.85)	74
Musculoskeletal and connective tissue disorders	94 (2.38)	102
Skin and subcutaneous tissue disorders	66 (1.67)	69
Psychiatric disorders	61 (1.54)	63
Vascular disorders	60 (1.52)	61
Respiratory, thoracic and mediastinal disorders	59 (1.49)	60
Ear and labyrinth disorders	47 (1.19)	49
Common serious adverse events (>0.1% in SOC/PT)		
Cardiac disorders	52 (1.32)	65
AV block second-degree	31 (0.78)	33
Bradycardia	15 (0.38)	15
AV block	5 (0.13)	5
Nervous system disorders	33 (0.84)	36
MS relapse	18 (0.46)	19
General disorders and administration site conditions	7 (0.18)	7
Infections and infestations	7 (0.18)	7
Gastrointestinal disorders	6 (0.15)	8
Vascular disorders	6 (0.15)	6
Symptoms that might have resulted from cardiac events (at Visit 2)		
Fatigue	68 (1.72)	
Dizziness	26 (0.66)	
Chest discomfort	8 (0.20)	
Vertigo	7 (0.18)	
Palpitations	7 (0.18)	
Dyspnea	5 (0.13)	
Angina pectoris	3 (0.08)	
Blurred vision	2 (0.05)	
Syncope	1 (0.03)	
Exertional dyspnoe	1 (0.03)	

PT preferred term, *SOC* system organ class

blocks no relevant decrease in heart rate was observed. The mean minimal heart rate over ten consecutive beats during AV block observed was 51.5 bpm. Furthermore, the Holter ECGs did not show relevant pauses. Usually, pauses are reported if they exceed 3 s in patients with sinus rhythm. The longest pause recorded in association with a second-degree AV block in this study was 2.6 s. The absence of relevant pauses is underlined by the fact that the events mostly remained asymptomatic. Finally, none of the AV blocks progressed to a complete block (third-degree AV block), as would have been expected for drugs known to induce AV blocks (e.g. calcium channel blockers).

Therefore, AV blocks associated with fingolimod treatment initiation can be considered as rather benign, self-limiting and associated with an either low or virtually non-existing propensity to progression to a complete AV block. Although affected by fingolimod, overall AV conduction, which is determined by several ion currents (i.e. particularly by calcium currents) [22, 23], remains preserved. In the present study, AV blocks were not preceded by excessive slowing of heart, what would be expected, but followed increases in heart rate. This suggests that slowing of AV conduction is due to a positive rate-dependent electrophysiological effect of fingolimod. A mild direct effect of fingolimod on the AV node was postulated in a rodent study, where S1P1 receptor mRNA expression was found to be high in the AV node. Fingolimod prolonged the cycle length in isolated AV node cells by 9% from 230 to 251 ms. Under pathological conditions (such as ischemia/reperfusion), fingolimod did not further prolong AV conduction. Fingolimod-induced AV node conduction abnormalities were discussed to be the result of a direct effect of the

Table 7 Study drug discontinuations due to adverse events

	Fingolimod 0.5 mg $N = 38$	
	Number of patients, n (%)	Number of events, n
Adverse events leading to discontinuation of study drug (<4% in SOC/PT)		
Cardiac disorders	16 (42.1)	20
AV block second-degree	9 (23.7)	10
Bradycardia	3 (7.9)	3
Gastrointestinal disorders	8 (21.1)	10
Nausea	4 (10.5)	4
Diarrhoea	3 (7.9)	3
Nervous system disorders	8 (21.1)	8
Dizziness	2 (5.3)	2
Headache	2 (5.3)	2
Vascular disorders	5 (13.2)	5
Hypertension	4 (10.5)	4
Investigations	5 (13.2)	5
QT prolongation	2 (5.3)	2
Skin and subcutaneous tissue disorders	5 (13.2)	5
Psychiatric disorders	4 (10.5)	4
General disorders and administration site conditions	3 (7.9)	4
Asthenia	2 (5.3)	2
Eye disorders	2 (5.3)	2
Vision blurred	2 (5.3)	2
Pregnancy, puerperium and perinatal conditions	2 (5.3)	2
Pregnancy	2 (5.3)	2

PT preferred term, *SOC* system organ class

drug on ion channels expressed in the AV node with mild prolongation of AV conduction time [24].

Generally speaking, the effects of fingolimod on AV conduction have to be interpreted and weighed in the broader context of its beneficial effects in a progressive disease such as MS [1–3].

Conclusions

The results presented here are derived from an interim analysis. The events identified by continuous ECG monitoring were associated neither with severe clinical symptoms nor with clinically relevant pauses or clinically relevant drops in heart rate. Furthermore, patients with clinical symptoms had no pathological findings on Holter ECG. Cardiac symptoms, if present, were rare, mild, and occurred independently of the expected benign AV conduction abnormalities and heart rate decline. ECG monitoring did not detect any otherwise unforeseen arrhythmias. In summary, clinically relevant cardiac events were not associated with abnormalities on continuous ECG monitoring and conduction abnormalities as demonstrated by Holter ECG usually remained clinically asymptomatic. Even without statistical evidence, the results presented here suggest that continuous Holter ECG monitoring after fingolimod first dose likely do not add clinically relevant value to patient safety with respect to bradycardia or conduction abnormalities in a general RRMS population without cardiovascular comorbidities.

Abbreviations

AE: Adverse event; AV: Atrioventricular conduction; DSMB: Data Safety Monitoring Board; ECG: Electrocardiogram; EDSS: Expanded Disability Status Scale; EU: European Union; EUDRACT: European Clinical Trials Database; FTY720: Fingolimod; RRMS: Relapsing remitting multiple sclerosis; S1P: Sphingosine-1-phosphate; SAE: Serious adverse event; SD: Standard deviation; US: United States

Acknowledgements

Editorial support was provided by Karin Eichele, www.mediwiz.de.

Funding

This study was sponsored by Novartis Pharma GmbH. Editorial support by a medical writing expert was also funded by Novartis Pharma GmbH.

Authors' contributions

VL: Design and conceptualization of the study, interpretation of the data; revising the manuscript for intellectual content; TZ, ML, SR, BW, JH, SS, KG, CL, LK, OH, CA: Revising the manuscript for intellectual content; KS: Design and conceptualization of the study, revising the manuscript for intellectual content; MB: Statistical Expert, interpretation of the data; revising the manuscript for intellectual content; GW, HS, SH, RD, WH: Interpretation of the data; revising the manuscript for intellectual content. All authors read and approved the final manuscript.

Competing interests

V. Limmroth has received speaker's honoraria, financial research support or consultancy fees from Antisence, Allergan, Almirall, Bayer, Biogen, Bionorica, Genzyme, Novartis, Roche, Sanofi, and Teva.

T. Ziemssen has received compensation for consulting services from Almirall, Biogen Idec, Bayer, Genzyme, GSK, MSD, Merck Serono, Novartis, Sanofi, Teva and Synthon, and has received research support from Bayer, Biogen Idec, Hertie Foundation, Roland Ernst Foundation, German Diabetes Foundation, Merck Serono, Novartis, Teva, and Sanofi Aventis.

M. Lang has received travel grants, speaker's honoraria, financial research support, consultancy fees from Teva, Merck Serono, Genzyme, Sanofi, Novartis, Bayer, and Biogen Idec.

S. Richter has received travel grants und compensation for scientific advisory boards from Novartis and travel grants from Biogen, Teva, Bayer, and Genzyme.

J. Haas has received compensation from Almirall, Biogen, Bayer, Octapharma, Teva, Allergan, and Novartis.

B. Wagner has received travel grants from Novartis, Biogen, Bayer, and Genzyme and speaker's honoraria from Biogen and Novartis.

S. Schmidt has received speaking honoraria and travel expenses from Bayer Vital, Biogen, Genzyme, Merck Serono, Novartis, and Teva. He has also served on advisory boards for Bayer Vital, Biogen, Genzyme, Merck Serono, Novartis, and Teva.

K. Gerbershagen has received speaker's honoraria, financial research support or consultancy fees from Bayer, Biogen, Genzyme, Novartis, Sanofi, and Teva.

C. Lassek has received travel grants, speaker's honoraria, financial research support, consultancy fees from Teva, Merck Serono, Genzyme, Sanofi, Novartis, Bayer, and Biogen Idec.
L. Klotz has received compensation for serving on scientific advisory boards for Genzyme and Novartis. She has received speaker's honoraria and travel support from Novartis, Merck Serono and CSL Behring. She receives research support from Novartis and Biogen Idec.
O. Hoffmann reports research grants from Biogen, Boehringer Ingelheim, Novartis, and Sanofi-Genzyme not pertaining to this study. He has received compensation for activities with Bayer Healthcare, Biogen, Daiichi-Sankyo, Merck-Serono, Novartis, Roche, Sanofi-Genzyme, and TEVA.
C. Albert has received travel grants from Novartis, Biogen, Genzyme, and Teva, compensation for scientific advisory boards from Novartis and Merck Serono, as well as speaker's honoraria from Biogen.
K. Schuh is employed by Novartis Pharma GmbH, Germany.
M. Baier-Ebert is employed by Novartis Pharma GmbH, Germany.
G. Wendt is employed by Novartis Pharma GmbH, Germany.
H. Schieb is employed by Novartis Pharma GmbH, Germany.
S. Hoyer is employed by Novartis Pharma GmbH, Germany.
R. Dechend has received speaker's honoraria, financial research support or consultancy fees from Berlin Chemie, Novartis, Alnylam, Boehringer Ingelheim, Bayer, and MSD.
W. Haverkamp is working as consultant to Novartis.

Author details

[1]Department of Neurology, Cologne General Hospitals, University of Cologne, Cologne, Germany. [2]Center of Clinical Neuroscience, University Clinic Carl Gustav Carus Dresden, Dresden, Germany. [3]NTD Study Group, Neurologische Praxis, Ulm, Germany. [4]NeuroMVZ, Stuttgart, Germany. [5]Jewish Hospital Berlin, Berlin, Germany. [6]NTD Study Group, Neurologische Gemeinschaftspraxis, Bonn, Germany. [7]Neurologische Gemeinschaftspraxis Kassel und Vellmar, Kassel, Germany. [8]Department of Neurology, University of Muenster, Muenster, Germany. [9]St. Josefs-Krankenhaus Potsdam-Sanssouci, Potsdam, Germany. [10]Novartis Pharma GmbH, Nuremberg, Germany. [11]Experimental and Clinical Research Center, Charité-Campus Buch, Berlin, Germany. [12]Charité Universitaetsmedizin Berlin, Campus Virchow Klinikum, Augustenburger Platz 1, Berlin 13353, Germany.

References

1. Cohen JA, Barkhof F, Comi G, Hartung HP, Khatri BO, Montalban X, et al. Oral fingolimod or intramuscular interferon for relapsing multiple sclerosis. N Engl J Med. 2010;362(5):402–15.
2. Calabresi PA, Radue EW, Goodin D, Jeffery D, Rammohan KW, Reder AT, et al. Safety and efficacy of fingolimod in patients with relapsing-remitting multiple sclerosis (FREEDOMS II): a double-blind, randomised, placebo-controlled, phase 3 trial. Lancet Neurol. 2014; 13(6):545–56.
3. Kappos L, Radue EW, O'Connor P, Polman C, Hohlfeld R, Calabresi P, et al. A placebo-controlled trial of oral fingolimod in relapsing multiple sclerosis. N Engl J Med. 2010;362(5):387–401.
4. Brinkmann V, Davis MD, Heise CE, Albert R, Cottens S, Hof R, et al. The immune modulator FTY720 targets sphingosine 1-phosphate receptors. J Biol Chem. 2002;277(24):21453–7.
5. Brinkmann V, Billich A, Baumruker T, Heining P, Schmouder R, Francis G, et al. Fingolimod (FTY720): discovery and development of an oral drug to treat multiple sclerosis. Nat Rev Drug Discov. 2010;9(11):883–97.
6. Chun J, Hartung HP. Mechanism of action of oral fingolimod (FTY720) in multiple sclerosis. Clin Neuropharmacol. 2010;33(2):91–101.
7. Camm J, Hla T, Bakshi R, Brinkmann V. Cardiac and vascular effects of fingolimod: mechanistic basis and clinical implications. Am Heart J. 2014; 168(5):632–44.
8. DiMarco JP, O'Connor P, Cohen JA, Reder AT, Zhang-Auberson L, Tang D, et al. First-dose effects of fingolimod: Pooled safety data from three phase 3 studies. Mult Scler Relat Disord. 2014;3(5):629–38.
9. Schmouder R, Serra D, Wang Y, Kovarik JM, DiMarco J, Hunt TL, et al. FTY720: placebo-controlled study of the effect on cardiac rate and rhythm in healthy subjects. J Clin Pharmacol. 2006;46(8):895–904.
10. Gold R, Comi G, Palace J, Siever A, Gottschalk R, Bijarnia M, et al. Assessment of cardiac safety during fingolimod treatment initiation in a real-world relapsing multiple sclerosis population: a phase 3b, open-label study. J Neurol. 2014;261(2):267–76.
11. Rolf L, Muris AH, Damoiseaux J, van Daele M, Hupperts R. Paroxysmal atrial fibrillation after initiation of fingolimod for multiple sclerosis treatment. Neurology. 2014;82(11):1008–9.
12. van Pesch V, Marchandise S, El Sankari S, Sindic C. Ventricular arrhythmia in a male MS patient on fingolimod. Acta Neurol Belg. 2015;115(1):77–9.
13. Castillo-Trivino T, Lopetegui I, Alarcon-Duque JA, Lopez de Munain A, Olascoaga J. Ventricular tachycardia on chronic fingolimod treatment for multiple sclerosis. J Neurol Neurosurg Psychiatry. 2015. doi:10.1136/jnnp-2014-310013.
14. Rosini JM, Rajasimhan S, Fellows SE, Nomura JT. Delayed cardiac dysrhythmias after fingolimod administration. Am J Emerg Med. 2015;33(7):987 e1-3.
15. Sellner J, Holl B, Wipfler P, Chroust V, Pilz G, Winhard M, et al. Delayed third degree atrioventricular block with pacemaker placement in a multiple sclerosis patient on fingolimod treatment. Neurology. 2014;82:10 Suppl 1.
16. Espinosa PS, Berger JR. Delayed fingolimod-associated asystole. Mult Scler. 2011;17(11):1387–9.
17. DePaula RS, Antelmi I, Vincenzi MA, Andre CD, Artes R, Grupi CJ, et al. Cardiac arrhythmias and atrioventricular block in a cohort of asymptomatic individuals without heart disease. Cardiology. 2007;108(2):111–6. doi:10.1159/000095950.
18. Nada A, Gintant GA, Kleiman R, Gutstein DE, Gottfridsson C, Michelson EL, et al. The evaluation and management of drug effects on cardiac conduction (PR and QRS intervals) in clinical development. Am Heart J. 2013;165(4):489–500.
19. Epstein AE, DiMarco JP, Ellenbogen KA, Estes 3rd NA, Freedman RA, Gettes LS, et al. 2012 ACCF/AHA/HRS focused update incorporated into the ACCF/AHA/HRS 2008 guidelines for device-based therapy of cardiac rhythm abnormalities: a report of the American College of Cardiology Foundation/American Heart Association Task Force on Practice Guidelines and the Heart Rhythm Society. Circulation. 2013;127(3):e283–352. doi:10.1161/CIR.0b013e318276ce9b.
20. Zeltser D, Justo D, Halkin A, Rosso R, Ish-Shalom M, Hochenberg M, et al. Drug-induced atrioventricular block: prognosis after discontinuation of the culprit drug. J Am Coll Cardiol. 2004;44(1):105–8. doi:10.1016/j.jacc.2004.03.057.
21. Osmonov D, Erdinler I, Ozcan KS, Altay S, Turkkan C, Yildirim E, et al. Management of patients with drug-induced atrioventricular block. Pacing Clin Electrophysiol. 2012;35(7):804–10. doi:10.1111/j.1540-8159.2012.03410.x.
22. Scheinman MM. Atrioventricular nodal conduction and refractoriness. Pacing Clin Electrophysiol. 1993;16(3 Pt 2):592–8.
23. Katz AM. Calcium channel diversity in the cardiovascular system. J Am Coll Cardiol. 1996;28(2):522–9.
24. Egom EE, Kruzliak P, Rotrekl V, Lei M. The effect of the sphingosine-1-phosphate analogue FTY720 on atrioventricular nodal tissue. J Cell Mol Med. 2015. doi:10.1111/jcmm.12549.

11

Pleocytosis in a patient with relapsing polychondritis accompanied by meningoencephalitis

Jie Cao and Min Zhang*

Abstract

Background: Relapsing polychondritis (RP) is an uncommon immune-related disease with unknown causes. It is characterized by inflammation of cartilaginous or non-cartilaginous structures, such as the ears, nose, respiratory tract, eyes, and joints. Neurological involvement is rare in RP.

Case presentation: We report a case of pleocytosis in a 64-year-old man diagnosed as having RP with meningoencephalitis. The patient's condition markedly improved following methylprednisolone treatment.

Conclusions: To our knowledge, this is the first report of recurrent pleocytosis in a patient with RP accompanied by meningoencephalitis. Steroid pulse therapy is effective in most cases, and early diagnosis is of importance.

Keywords: Cerebrospinal fluid, Meningoencephalitis, Relapsing polychondritis

Background

Relapsing polychondritis (RP) is a rare immune-related disease that primarily, but not exclusively, affects cartilaginous structures, such as the ears, nose, and laryngotracheobronchial tree. RP eventually leads to the deformation of these structures [1]. This disease has a wide array of clinical manifestations that can mimic other unrelated diseases, and it has no specific laboratory indicators. An involvement of the central nervous system (CNS) is rare in RP and is often not considered by physicians, which may result in delayed treatment.

Here, we report the case of a patient with pleocytosis who was initially considered to have tuberculous meningitis (TBM). However, further exploration finally led to a diagnosis of RP with meningoencephalitis.

Case presentation

A 64-year-old man with a history of headache for 4 months, dull responses, and gait disturbance for 3 months was admitted to our hospital. At admission, the patient had low-grade fever and replied very slowly (sometimes incorrectly) to questions. However, he was able to follow simple orders. The patient had symmetrical paralysis of both lower limbs, leaving him unable to walk without assistance. In addition, auricular swelling (Fig. 1) was observed upon physical examination. Bilateral Kernig's sign was positive and ankle clonus was present. Assessment with the Mini-Mental State Examination (MMSE) yielded a score of 20/30, indicating impaired cognitive function. It was noteworthy that the patient had difficulty performing simple mathematical tasks as he had been an accountant for decades.

We reviewed the patient's history and found that he had been in good health before the onset of symptoms. In particular, the patient had no history of trauma, smoking, alcohol abuse, allergy, recent vaccination, or hereditary factors. Headache and intermittent fever occurred after travelling, which led him to seek medical advice 4 months prior to his admission. At that time, TBM was suspected based on cerebrospinal fluid (CSF) tests, which revealed pleocytosis with a predominance of lymphocytes (Table 1). However, after a few weeks of antituberculous therapy, the patient developed several new symptoms, including ear swelling, tinnitus, dizziness, and gait disturbance.

Subsequently, the patient was hospitalized three times with complaints of recurrent headaches, worsening gait disturbance, and other new symptoms including eyelid swelling and arthralgia. Two months

* Correspondence: zhang_min_3464@126.com
Department of Neurology, Tongji Hospital, Tongji Medical College, Huazhong University of Science and Technology, No. 1095 Jiefang Avenue, Wuhan 430030, China

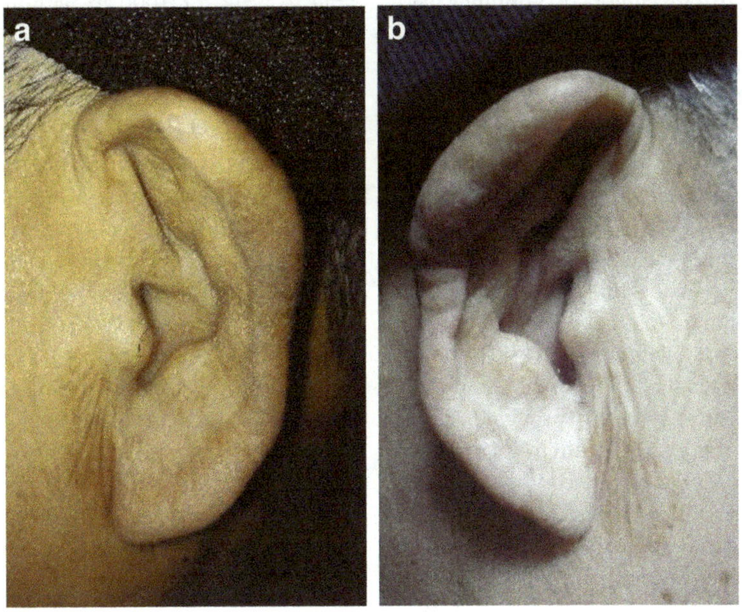

Fig. 1 Bilateral swelling of the auricles in our patient. Swelling of left (**a**) and right (**b**) side of the auricles in our patient

after his first admission, the patient was diagnosed as having RP based on the Damiani and Levine criteria [2], and was treated with low-dose steroids. Antituberculous therapy was continued simultaneously. However, he showed little symptomatic improvement with treatment.

At the time of admission to our hospital, the patient's CSF was assayed again. We detected pleocytosis (Table 1) and increased immunoglobulin G (IgG) levels (125 mg/L). CSF pathogen cultures and serologic tests for bacteria, viruses (such as human immunodeficiency virus, herpes simplex virus, Epstein-Barr virus, varicella-zoster virus, hepatitis viruses, and enteroviruses), fungi, parasites, and *Treponema* yielded negative results. The results of assays for tumor markers and paraneoplastic-related antibodies were also negative. In addition, assays for CNS vasculitis and autoimmune encephalitis yielded negative results.

Between the patient's first clinical visit and admission to our hospital, his erythrocyte sedimentation rate (ESR) increased from 40 mm/h to 111 mm/h. An anti-nuclear antibody (ANA) test indicated a particle pattern with a titer of 1: 100. The level of anti-cyclic citrullinated peptide antibody (anti-CCP) was 10 U/ml. The results of tests for other immune and rheumatoid biomarkers, such as anti-neutrophil cytoplasmic antibody, lupus anticoagulant, anti-phospholipid antibodies, and rheumatoid factors, were all negative or within the normal range. A Gene X-pert mycobacterium tuberculosis/rifampin detection test eliminated the possibility of a rifampin-resistant gene locus. Other indices were negative or within the normal ranges.

Table 1 Cerebrospinal fluid profile of the patient

CSF profile				
Date	Protein (mg/dL) (normal range: 15-45)	Cell count (per mm^3) (PMN/L/K)	Glucose (mmol/L) (normal range: 2.22-3.89)	Chlorides (mmol/L) (normal range: 120-132)
8/21/2016	77	52/208/260	2.74	117
9/3/2016	55	6/59/65	3.05	115
9/18/2016	66	–/–/8	3.66	117
9/28/2016	41	0/0/0	4.37	120
1/16/2017	43	–/–/42	3.79	117
2/4/2017	27	0/0/0	3.84	127

CSF cerebrospinal fluid, *PMN* polymorphonuclear cells, *L* lymphocytes, *K* karyocytes, –, no registry of cellular fraction

Spinal magnetic resonance imaging (MRI) findings were normal. However, brain MRI indicated brain atrophy, hydrocephalus, and abnormal signals in periventricular white matter. Brain MRI with gadolinium enhancement showed leptomeningeal enhancement mainly in the right occipitotemporal and posterior cingulate gyri (Fig. 2), but not in the basal cisternal area, which is often indicative of typical tubercular meningitis.

Based on the aforementioned examinations, we suspected that the patient had RP with meningoencephalitis. Subsequently, intravenous methylprednisolone pulse therapy (500 mg for 3 days) with methotrexate (MTX, 12.5 mg, once per week) was administered. Supportive and symptomatic treatments were also provided. Three weeks after treatment initiation, the patient's symptoms dramatically improved. We also observed a decrease in the ESR (20 mm/h), normalization of CSF assay results (Table 1), and an improved MMSE score of 28/30. Upon discharge, the patient had normal responses and was able to walk for 1000 m without help. No flare-up was reported at the 6-month follow-up visit.

Discussion and conclusion

Initially, the patient was suspected to have TBM, which has a relatively high incidence rate in China. The detection of mycobacterium tuberculosis is necessary for a diagnosis of TBM. However, in reality, CSF cultures for mycobacterium tuberculosis have a low positive rate in patients with TBM [3]. Therefore, empirical treatment for TBM is usually initiated in patients clinically suspected of having the disease. Unfortunately, following several months' treatment with standard antituberculous therapy, the patient's condition did not improve but rather deteriorated, although we did not detect mutations in rifampin-resistant genes. In addition, a transient normalization of the lymphocyte count in the CSF during therapy and an atypical enhancement pattern on brain MRI aroused suspicions of a potential diagnosis of

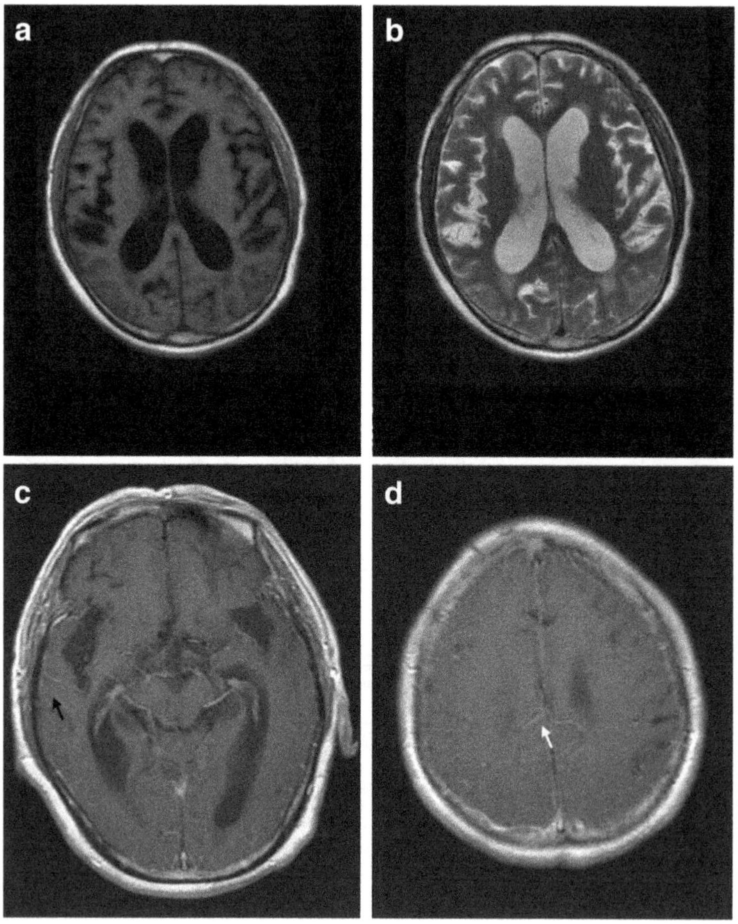

Fig. 2 Head MRI of the patient. **a**, **b** T1- and T2-weighted images indicate supratentorial ventricular enlargement and abnormal signals in periventricular white matter, respectively. **c**, **d** Head MRI with gadolinium enhancement indicated leptomeningeal enhancement mainly located in the right temporal lobe (black arrow) and posterior cingulate gyri (white arrow)

TBM. Moreover, the patient constantly complained of side effects of antituberculous therapy throughout the treatment course. Therefore, we cautiously stopped antituberculous treatment after a general discussion.

We considered a diagnosis of aseptic meningitis because repeated CSF gram stains and cultures were negative. Aseptic meningitis is a clinical syndrome characterized by meningeal inflammation not caused by pyogenic bacteria [4], but by some other factors such as infectious agents (e.g., viruses and parasites), neoplasms, anatomical structure-related events, vaccinations, drug-induced diseases, and autoimmune or inflammatory diseases. However, our patient likely did not have infectious aseptic meningitis because repeated CSF pathogen cultures and serologic tests were all negative. Negative results in tumor-related assays also indicated that the patient's condition was unlikely to be due to the presence of neoplasms. Furthermore, there was no history of trauma or recent vaccination for the patient. Drug-induced aseptic meningitis was deemed unlikely in our patient, especially as he denied the use of any drugs before symptom onset.

After ruling out the above possibilities, the cause underlying the patient's condition remained unknown. The signs and symptoms in our patient indicated the presence of both meningitis and encephalitis. To the best of our knowledge, prior to admission, the patient had only been diagnosed with RP, a rare autoimmune disease. We observed rheumatoid and immune-related abnormalities in our patient, such as elevated ESR, ANA, anti-CCP, and CSF IgG levels. Notably, CSF pleocytosis has previously been reported in patients with RP and, although rare, neurological involvement may be observed in RP [5]. Therefore, we suspected a correlation between RP and meningoencephalitis. Significant clinical improvement in our patient after treatment with a high-dose corticosteroid confirmed a diagnosis of RP with meningoencephalitis.

The etiology and pathophysiological mechanisms of RP remain largely unknown. The diagnostic criteria for RP are mainly clinical and no specific laboratory parameters have been confirmed to date. RP with meningitis or meningoencephalitis is rare, with approximately 3% of patients with RP having complications involving neurological symptoms [5].

Pleocytosis was detected in our patient. Vasculitis of the intracranial arteries, autoantibodies against the glutamate receptor GluRε2, and the presence of neutral glycosphingolipids in the CSF may explain CNS involvement in some cases of RP [6–8]. Although the pathogenesis of pleocytosis in RP is unclear, it seems to be associated with autoimmunity.

We observed a recurrent pattern of pleocytosis in 6 lumbar punctures from our patient. Karyocyte levels were normalized in the fourth CSF assay, which was conducted between adjacent assays with abnormalities before steroid treatment. To our knowledge, spontaneous normalization of karyocyte levels in CSF has not been previously reported in any other type of meningitis or meningoencephalitis. This may indicate a unique pattern of symptoms in this disease. Therefore, this is the first specific description of pleocytosis recurrence in a patient with RP. The marked normalization of karyocyte levels in CSF shortly after treatment may consequently invalidate previous diagnosis of TBM.

There are currently no randomized clinical trials of treatments for RP with meningitis or meningoencephalitis. Normally, empirical treatments are performed and steroid pulse therapy is preferred in most cases [7]. However, therapy may be ineffective or flare-ups may occur when an improper dosage is used or upon premature termination of therapy, as observed in our patient. The administration of immunosuppressive agents, such as azathioprine, MTX, cyclophosphamide, or cyclosporin A, may reduce the need for the long-term use of steroids and contribute to symptom control [9].

Meningoencephalitis is a rare complication of RP. Here, we report a case of RP with meningoencephalitis that was initially misdiagnosed as TBM. The patient recovered after steroid pulse therapy. This is also the first report of recurrent pleocytosis in a patient with RP accompanied by meningoencephalitis. Early diagnosis and steroid therapy are important in RP patients with meningoencephalitis. More case reviews and research are required to uncover the pathogenesis of RP and its rare neurological involvement.

Consent

Informed consent was obtained from the patient for publication of this case report and any accompanying images.

Abbreviations

ANA: Anti-nuclear antibody; Anti-CCP: Anti-cyclic citrullinated peptide antibody; CNS: Central nervous system; CSF: Cerebrospinal fluid; IgG: Immunoglobulin G; MMSE: Mini-Mental State Examination; MRI: Magnetic resonance imaging; MTX: Methotrexate; RP: Relapsing polychondritis; TBM: Tuberculous meningitis

Funding

National Natural Science Foundation of China.
Award Number: 81271406 | Recipient: Min Zhang.

Authors' contributions

JC: study concept and design, acquisition and analysis of data, drafting of the manuscript, interpretation of data. MZ: interpretation of data, critical revision of the manuscript for important intellectual content, study supervision, obtaining funding. Both authors read and approved the final manuscript.

Competing interests

The authors declare that they have no competing interests.

References

1. Longo L, Greco A, Rea A, Lo Vasco VR, De Virgilio A, De Vincentiis M. Relapsing polychondritis: a clinical update. Autoimmun Rev. 2016;15:539–43.
2. Emmungil H, Aydin S. Relapsing polychondritis. Eur J Rheumatol. 2015;2:155–9.
3. Erdem H, Ozturk-Engin D, Elaldi N, et al. The microbiological diagnosis of tuberculous meningitis: results of Haydarpasa-1 study. Clin Microbiol Infect. 2014;20:O600–8.
4. Lee BE, Davies HD. Aseptic meningitis. Curr Opin Infect Dis. 2007;20:272–7.
5. Mathian A, Miyara M, Cohen-Aubart F, et al. Relapsing polychondritis: a 2016 update on clinical features, diagnostic tools, treatment and biological drug use. Best Pract Res Clin Rheumatol. 2016;30:316–33.
6. Mihara T, Ueda A, Hirayama M, et al. Detection of new anti-neutral glycosphingolipids antibodies and their effects on Trk neurotrophin receptors. FEBS Lett. 2006;580:4991–5.
7. Lahmer T, Treiber M, von Werder A, et al. Relapsing polychondritis: an autoimmune disease with many faces. Autoimmun Rev. 2010;9:540–6.
8. Kashihara K, Kawada S, Takahashi Y. Autoantibodies to glutamate receptor GluRε2 in a patient with limbic encephalitis associated with relapsing polychondritis. J Neurol Sci. 2009;287:275–7.
9. Letko E, Zafirakis P, Baltatzis S, Voudouri A, Livir-Rallatos C, Foster CS. Relapsing polychondritis: a clinical review. Semin Arthritis Rheum. 2002; 31:384–95.

12

Low threshold unmyelinated mechanoafferents can modulate pain

Kathrin Habig[1*], Anne Schänzer[2], Wolfgang Schirner[1], Gothje Lautenschläger[1], Benjamin Dassinger[3], Håkan Olausson[4], Frank Birklein[5], Elke R. Gizewski[6] and Heidrun H. Krämer[1]

Abstract

Background: Human, hairy skin contains a subgroup of C-fibers, the C-low threshold mechanoreceptive afferents ((C-LTMR) C-tactile or C-touch (CT) fibers) that are linked with the signaling of affective aspects of human touch. Recent studies suggest an involvement of these afferents in the modulation of pain in healthy volunteers. Small fiber neuropathy (SFN) is associated with a damage of C-fibers. Therefore, an impairment of C-LTMRs can be assumed. We aimed to elaborate a possible role of CT-afferents in pain modulation by investigating healthy volunteers and SFN-patients.

Methods: Experiment I: 20 SFN-patients (12 women, median age 52.0 years) and 20 healthy controls (14 women, median age 43.0 years) participated in this prospective fMRI and psychophysical study. Heat-pain (HP), CT-targeted touch (slow brushing) and HP combined with CT-targeted touch were applied in randomized order to the left shank in a block design. The participants rated pain intensity on a visual analogue scale. Experiment II: We investigated a possible impact of pain intensity on CT induced pain modulation (10 healthy participants). The intensity of HP stimulation was chosen to induce pain intensity 50/100 (NRS). HP stimulation was applied with and without CT-targeted touch.

Results: Experiment I: CT-stimulation was sufficient to reduce heat pain in healthy participants ($p = 0.016$), but not in SFN-patients. HP induced pain intensity was significantly higher (32,2 vs 52,6) in SFN-patients. During HP, bold responses in pain associated areas were observed in both groups. Additional CT-stimulation elicited no significant difference of bold responses compared to HP. Experiment II: In healthy volunteers, we reproduced a significant reduction of HP intensity by CT-stimulation ($p = 0.038$).

Conclusions: CT input seems to be sufficient to modulate pain, independent of intensity of the pain stimulus. As a prerequisite, the CT fibers have to be intact as in healthy volunteers. If CT fibers are impaired – as in SFN -, CT-targeted touch does not modulate pain intensity. The location of CT-induced pain modulation might be attributed to the level of the dorsal horn since the cortical activation pattern of heat pain with and without CT-targeted touch did not differ in healthy subjects and in SFN-patients.

Keywords: CT afferents, Small fiber neuropathy (SFN), Pain perception, Pain inhibition, Spinal cord, fMRI

Background

In human hairy skin, pleasant touch is signaled by Aβ afferents and a subgroup of C fibers, the C-low threshold mechanoreceptive (C-LTMR; CT = C touch or C tactile) afferents. Those fibers were first detected using microneurography of the infraorbital nerve [1], but were then found to be distributed more widely in the arm and leg [2]. They do not appear in glabrous skin [2, 3]. Characterization of C-LTMR revealed that these afferents react to low mechanical indentation forces (<5 mN) [4] and to slowly moving stimuli [5, 6] as in gentle stroking. The pleasantness of touch is positively correlated with the firing rate of these fibers [6]. In mice, the cell bodies of the C-LTMRs are randomly distributed in the dorsal root ganglia, C-LTMRs terminate in Lamina II of the dorsal horn accompanied by Aδ and Aβ afferents [7]. They enter the lamina I/II spinothalamic pathway up to the ventromedial posterior thalamic nucleus [8, 9].

* Correspondence: kathrin.habig@neuro.med.uni-giessen.de
[1]Department of Neurology, Justus Liebig University, Klinikstr. 33, 35392 Giessen, Germany
Full list of author information is available at the end of the article

In humans, the main brain areas receiving C-LTMR information belong to the somatosensory system and affect processing brain networks like the contralateral posterior insular cortex [10] or the medial prefrontal cortex [11]. The intensity of CT targeted touch is encoded in the primary and secondary somatosensory cortex (S1 contralateral, S2 bilateral), whereas the pleasantness is encoded in the pregenual anterior cingulate cortex [12]. C-LTMRs also activate regions involved in reward processing (putamen and orbitofrontal cortex [13, 14]) and in processing of social stimuli (posterior superior temporal sulcus [15–17]).

Animal experiments indicate that CT activation reduces pain, but the precise anatomical localization of this phenomenon is still unknown [18–20]. In humans, slow and gentle touch is supposed to ease pain [21]. Recently a modulation of laser evoked pain by CT targeted touch on the contralateral extremity has been reported. The effect of CT targeted touch (attenuating/ increasing pain) was dependent on the attachment styles (attachment anxiety/ attachment avoidance) of the participants [22]. It needs to be further elucidated, whether an inhibition of nociceptive neurons by C-LTMRs exists in humans and additionally, where this is being processed. An ideal model to answer this question is the investigation of small fiber neuropathy (SFN) patients. SFN is defined as a neuropathy that exclusively affects the thin sensory (C and Aδ fibers) nerve fibers [23]. It is confirmed by thermal testing and skin biopsy. Although C-LTMRS cannot be easily tested, it can be assumed, that C-LTMRs as a subgroup of C fibers should be impaired as well.

In the present study, we examined healthy volunteers with intact C-LTMRs and SFN patients with supposedly impaired C-LTMRs to investigate the impact of C-LTMR signaling on pain modulation in humans. We compared heat pain intensity with and without CT targeted touch (gentle stroking with a soft brush) in both groups. CT targeted touch was proposed to attenuate pain in healthy volunteers and to a lesser extend in SFN patients. To search for possible CNS mechanisms, we performed fMRI.

Methods

Participants

Twenty patients with SFN (12 women, 8 men, median age: 52 years, age range: 35–71 years) and 20 healthy controls (14 women, 6 men, median age: 44 years, age range: 30–75 years) were included in the study. All participants were fully right handed according to a modified handedness score [24].

In all SFN patients, the medical history was recorded and a thorough neurological examination was performed. SFN was diagnosed according to the diagnostic criteria by Hoeijmakers et al. [25]. In brief, all patients suffered from length dependent neuropathic pain in the feet and lower legs. In all patients, cold (CDT) and warm detection thresholds (WDT) were determined using quantitative sensory testing (QST). Every SFN patient underwent a skin biopsy. The intraepidermal nerve fiber density (IENFD) in skin punch biopsies was analyzed according to the recommended guidelines to confirm the diagnosis of SFN [26, 27]. Electroneurography was performed to exclude large fiber involvement. SFN was diagnosed if the patients presented with typical clinical features [25], pathological thermal detection thresholds as well as decreased IENFD. Patients were excluded from the study if they showed abnormalities in the clinical neurological examination especially in vibration detection thresholds or pathological values in the motor and sensory nerve conduction studies. Patients that presented with allodynia were also excluded from the study since CT targeted touch would elicit pain in these patients [28].

In healthy volunteers, the medical history, the clinical neurological examination as well as the thermal testing had to be unremarkable.

All participants gave their informed written consent according to the latest revision of the Declaration of Helsinki. The study was approved by the local ethics committee of the Justus-Liebig-University, Gießen (105/11).

Skin biopsy

In SFN patients, skin punch biopsies (3 mm) were taken 10 cm above the malleolus lateralis in the innervation territory of the sural nerve and the tissue samples were analysed according to the recommended guidelines [26, 29]. In brief the tissue samples were fixed in 2% Zamboni solution and cut into 50 μm thick slices. Immunofluorescence staining was performed at free floating sections with antibody against PGP 9.5 (rabbit polyclonal anti-PGP 9.5 1:1000; zytomed) and a second antibody (goat anti-rabbit Alexa Fluor 488, 1:1000; invitrogen). In a minimum of six sections the intraepidermal nerve fibers (IENF) were analysed using a Leica Immunofluorescence Microscope DM 2000 at magnification 400fold. IENFD was calculated as the mean of IENF per millimetre.

Cold and warm detection thresholds

All participants were tested for cold and warm detection thresholds on the dorsum of the left foot. The exact procedure has been already described elsewhere [30]. In brief, warm and cold detection thresholds were determined using a TSA 2001-II (MEDOC, Israel; contact area of the thermode: 9 cm^2; baseline temperature: 32 °C; slope: 1 °C/s). The mean threshold temperature of 3 consecutive measurements was calculated.

Experiment I: stimulation protocol

During fMRI, three different conditions were applied at the left lower leg in a randomized order: 1. heat pain only, 2. heat pain and CT-targeted brushing and 3. CT targeted touch only. The heat pain elicited pain was rated on a computerized rating scale that was presented via a projector. Each condition was applied for 10 s alternating with rest for a total of 6 times each. The heat pain- and tactile stimulus were synchronized to the MR-images via an electrical trigger from the scanner. The trigger has been linked to a matlab-based program showing a time scale, which has been presented on a screen in the scanner room. The screen could be seen inside (CT stimulation) and outside (heat pain stimulation) of the scanner room. The timescale started with the sequence "rest" and a countdown signalizing stimulus onset, which has been additionally marked as a color change, so that the investigators were primed for the final optical trigger to start the stimulation manually. The rating period started 5 s after stimulus onset and was presented on the same screen. See Fig. 1. When an error of timing occurred, the sequence has been excluded.

We applied all conditions in randomized order to minimize order effects, all participants were blinded for the expected pain inhibition by CT stimulation. Participants were unaware of the aims of the study. They were only informed that central activation patterns and pain intensity during heat pain and touch are investigated in various combinations.

Heat pain stimulation

Heat pain thresholds (HPT) were determined in all participants at the left foot within the L5 dermatome. The mean HPT was calculated from 3 consecutive measurements according to the method of limits (for detail see: [31]. The individual heat pain threshold was determined directly before the subject entered the scanner, to obtain stable heat pain intensities the applied temperature was HPT + 1.5 °C. The intended pain intensity was characterized as "painful but bearable". Heat pain stimulation was carried out at the participants left foot.

Tactile stimulation

Repetitive strokes with a soft painter's brush (2 cm wide, stimulation force 0.8 N; stimulation velocity 3 cm/s) were applied in proximal to distal direction on the left lower leg (CT targeted touch). The stroking was performed over a length of 30 cm with a velocity of 3 cm/s on the lateral lower leg in the area of hairy skin in the dermatome L5. To avoid inter-investigator variability stroking was always performed by the same investigator (KH).

Pain rating

Subjects were asked to quantify the heat derived pain intensity on a numeric rating scale (NRS; 0–100) with the anchors 0 "no pain" on the left end and 100 "worst pain imaginable" on the right end. The rating started 5 s

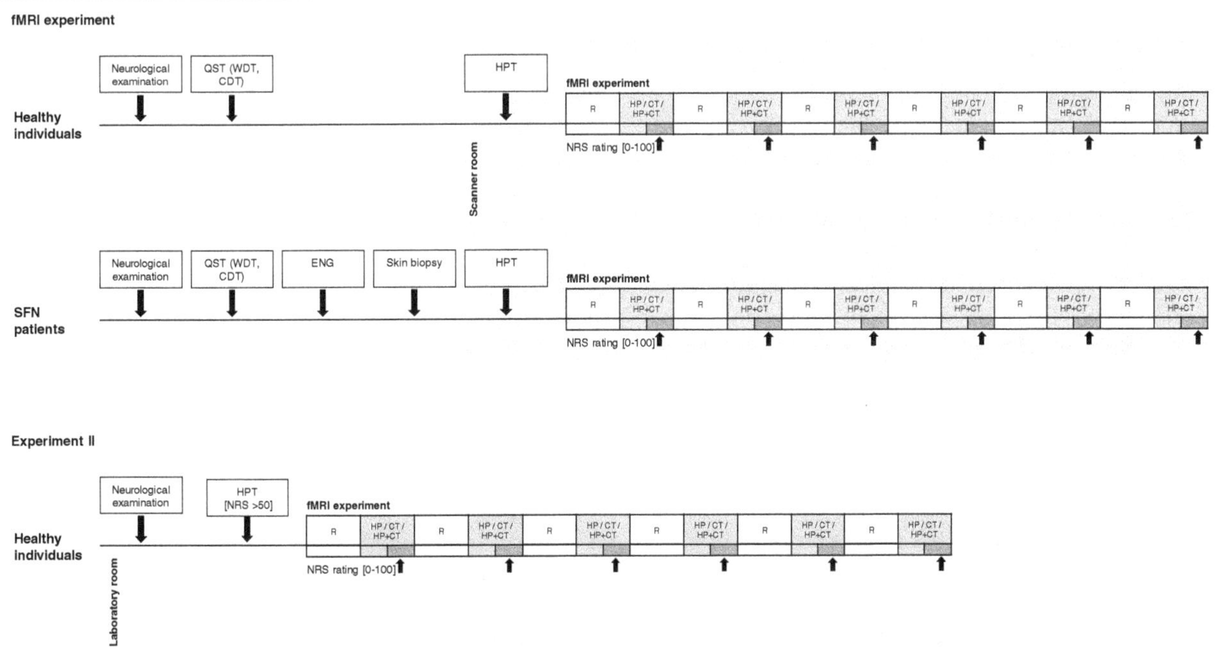

Fig. 1 Sequence of the neurophysiological pre-investigations (warm detection threshold (WDT), cold detection threshold (CDT), heat pain threshold (HPT), electroneurography (ENG)) and of the fMRI experiment (rest (R) alternating with the conditions "CT touch" (CT), "heat pain" (HP) and "heat pain with CT touch" (HP + CT), which were performed in randomized order) is demonstrated for both groups. The dark grey scaled boxes indicate the rating periods of pain intensity (on NRS), onsets are marked by black arrows. The big grey box demonstrates the tests performed in the scanner room

after the beginning of each trial and lasted for 5 s. The computerized NRS was presented via a projector. Pain ratings were assessed by operating a fiber optic response pad (Current Designs, Inc., Philadelphia, USA) which was connected to a computer. The pad was held in the dominant right hand by all subjects. The handling of the NRS was practiced before the scanning. See Fig. 1.

fMRI

Data acquisition

Functional and anatomical MR scans were performed in a 3 Tesla MR Scanner (Siemens Magnetom Verio, Siemens Medical Systems, Erlangen, Germany) using the 8 channel standard head coil. For structural images, a T1 weighted sequence (TR 1900 ms, TE 2.45 ms, bandwidth 170 Hz/Pixel, TI 900 ms, flip angle 9°, FOV 176 × 512 × 512 mm, orientation: sagittal, voxel size 1 × 1 × 1 mm) was acquired. Functional images consisted of EPI sequences (TR 2800 ms, TE 30 ms, bandwidth 2232 Hz/Pixel, flip angle 90°, FOV 240 × 240 × 120 mm, orientation: T > C-21.4, 40 slices, voxel size 3 × 3 × 3 mm^3, TA 5:43).

Data processing

For data processing, we used Statistical Parametric Mapping (SPM8, Welcome Department of Cognitive Neurology, London, UK). Prior to first level analysis, the images underwent preprocessing. This included realignment to the mean functional image (b-spline interpolation), segmentation of the structural image and normalization into Montreal Neurological Institute (MNI) space. Data were smoothed with full-width and half maximum (FWHM) of 6 mm of the Gaussian smoothing kernel.

A first level analysis was performed for each subject individually using the general linear model with a high-pass filter with a cutoff of 128 s. Contrasts were defined for the different stimuli (heat pain and heat pain combined with CT-targeted touch) vs rest. Subsequently mixed-effects group analyses were performed for healthy subjects and SFN patients separately with a one sample t-test. Additionally, two sample t-tests were used for the evaluation of group differences for the conditions "heat pain" versus "heat pain and CT targeted touch" between healthy participants and SFN patients.

Supplementary, we performed a region of interest (ROI) analyses using the small volume correction feature of SPM. As ROIs we chose the projection sides of CT fibers (insula, medial prefrontal cortex (MPFC) and pregenual ACC). The mask for the insulas were derived from the wfu pickatlas (human atlas, TD labels) for insula bilaterally. For masking the MPFC and pregenual ACC spheres with a diameter of 10 mm were placed according to Liljencrantz and Björnsdotter (medial frontal gyrus, MNI coordinates 11, 52, – 6; – 11, 52, – 6; [11]) and Case 2016 (pregenual ACC, MNI coordinates – 8, 50, 6; 8, 50, 6; [12]). These regions were saved as one image and used as inclusive mask for an additional ROI analysis.

Analysis was performed on a voxel-level and corrected for multiple testing by random field theory with a family-wise error rate of $\alpha = 0.05$.

For anatomical labelling, FSL based atlases were used (Harvard-Oxford Cortical Structural Atlas; Harvard-Oxford Subcortical Structural Atlas; Juelich Histological Atlas (http://fsl.fmrib.ox.ac.uk/fsl/fslwiki/Atlases)).

For visualization of the results, we used a standard template (SPM 8 template avg152T2), only showing significant activations.

Experiment II

In the second experiment, we investigated 10 healthy individuals in our laboratory rooms. "Heat pain" and "heat pain with CT targeted touch" were applied to the left foot (within the L5 dermatome), CT stimulation was performed on the left shank by slow brushing (3 cm/s), according to the setup in our first experiment during fMRI. The stimulations were applied in a randomized order lasting 10 s each with 10 s of rest in between stimulations. Heat pain stimulation was chosen to elicit pain intensities >50 on a NRS (0–100; anchors 0 "no pain" and 100 "worst pain imaginable"). The rating started 5 s after the beginning of each trial and lasted for 5 s. NRS rating was performed with the same computerized NRS which we used during the experiment in the scanner room, but was presented on a laptop. Pain ratings were delivered by pressing a computer key.

Statistics

Psychophysical data were analyzed using the SPSS Statistics (IBM, Version 23.0 for Windows) software package. Kolmogorov-Smirnov tests of normality were run for all data sets and parametric or non-parametric statistics were used accordingly as described in the experiment-specific results. All values are given as medians and interquartile range (IQR) in the case of a non-normal distribution and as means ± standard deviation (SD) in the case of a normal distribution. Values were considered significant if $p<0.05$.

Results

Skin biopsies

The mean intraepidermal nerve fiber density (IENFD) in all SFN patients was decreased compared to normal control values (mean IENFD: 2.46 (SD 1.65); norm: 4.0 to 7.8 [27]).

Cold and warm detection thresholds (CDT and WDT)

SFN patients had significantly higher warm detection thresholds (SFN patients: median 43 °C, IQR 5.3; healthy participants: 39.8 °C, IQR 6.3; $p<0.001$) and lower cold detection threshold (SFN patients: median 24.1 °C, IQR 5.7; healthy controls: median 29.0 °C, IQR 2.9; $p = 0.003$). These findings support the impairment of Aδ- (CDT) and C-fibers (WDT) in accordance with diagnosis of SFN.

Heat pain thresholds (HPT)

SFN patients had significantly higher heat pain thresholds compared to the controls (HPT healthy participants: median 46 °C, IQR 3; HPT SFN patients: median 47 °C, IQR 1; $p = 0.045$).

Pain ratings during fMRI

In healthy subjects, heat pain intensity was significantly reduced by the addition of CT targeted touch (NRS heat pain only: mean 32.2, SD 22.35; NRS heat-pain and CT targeted touch: 28.6, SD 21.86; $p = 0.016$, paired t-test). For details see Fig. 2.

In SFN patients, heat pain intensity was not altered by the addition of CT targeted touch (NRS heat pain only: mean 52.6, SD 20.2; NRS heat-pain and CT targeted touch: 57.2, SD 23.08; $p = 0.139$, paired t-test). For details see Fig. 2.

Pain ratings for the conditions heat pain ($p = 0.005$) and heat pain with CT stimulation ($p<0.001$) were significantly higher in SFN patients compared to controls. For details see Fig. 2.

fMRI

Bold responses for "CT targeted touch" only

CT targeted touch in healthy subjects showed bold responses in the left postcentral gyrus and the right parietal operculum (supramarginal gyrus). In SFN patients, CT-targeted touch resulted in activation of the right parietal operculum (supramarginal gyrus). For details see Fig. 3 and Table 1.

No significant difference of bold responses could be detected between healthy controls and SFN patients in the condition "CT targeted touch" only.

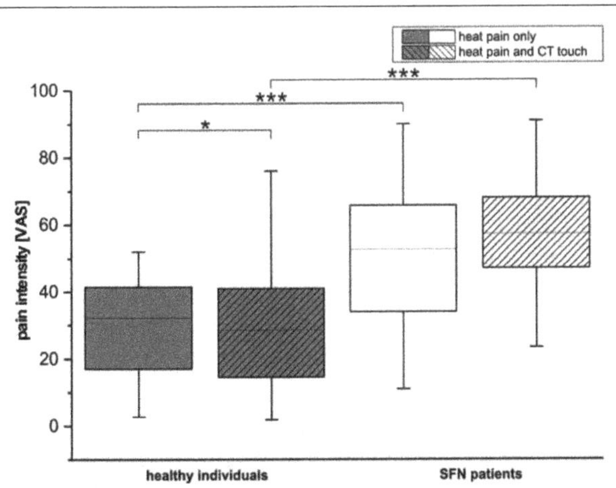

Fig. 2 Visual analogue scale (NRS) ratings for the conditions "heat pain only" and "heat pain combined with CT stimulation" in healthy subjects and SFN patients. CT stimulation significantly reduced of heat pain intensity in healthy subjects ($p = 0.016$) but not in SFN patients (* $p≤0.05$, ** of p≤0.01, *** of p≤0.005). The overall rating of pain intensity for both conditions was significantly higher in the SFN patients (heat pain only: $p = 0.005$; heat pain combined with CT targeted touch: $p<0.001$)

Bold responses for "heat pain" only

In healthy subjects, the heat pain stimulus evoked activations of areas known to be associated with pain processing: anterior insular cortices bilaterally (right 33,23,1; T 10.0; left – 30,23,1; T 10.1) and the anterior cingulate cortex (cluster peak 9,20,31; T 7.2). For details see Fig. 3 and Table 1. In SFN patients the condition "heat pain" also evoked activations in cortical areas associated with pain processing (e.g. anterior cingulate cortex bilaterally (cluster peak at 3,11,46; T 8.7), the insular cortex bilaterally (right anterior-middle insular cortex: 42,17,-2; T 7.2 and left anterior insular cortex: –27,20,-5; T 8.3). For details see Fig. 3 and Table 1.

No differences in the cortical activation could be detected between healthy controls and SFN patients for the condition "heat pain" only.

Bold responses for "heat pain and CT touch"

In healthy volunteers, heat pain and CT targeted stimulation evoked significant bold responses in the anterior insula bilaterally, the ACC and the supramarginal gyrus. Right hemispherical activations correspond to the putamen, frontal opercular cortex, middle frontal gyrus, anterior intra-parietal sulcus, inferior parietal lobule, inferior frontal gyrus and activation of less specified brain regions. There were no supplementary bold responses in the left hemisphere. For details see Fig. 3 and Table 1.

In SFN patients, heat with CT touch elicited bilateral bold responses of the insula, ACC, supramarginal gyrus, the opercular cortex and the anterior intra-parietal sulcus. In addition, the right paracingulate gyrus showed a significant bold response. For details see Fig. 3 and Table 1.

There was no difference of bold responses comparing the conditions "heat pain only" and "heat pain with CT targeted touch" in both groups.

A sensitive ROI analysis for all performed tests detected no additional bold responses in the predefined areas (insula, medial frontal gyrus and pregenual ACC).

Experiment II

Since heat induced pain intensity was higher in SFN patients compared to our controls, we performed an additional psychophysical experiment (experiment II) in healthy subjects to investigate a possible impact of pain intensity on CT mediated pain modulation. The heat stimuli were set to induce pain intensity NRS 50 from

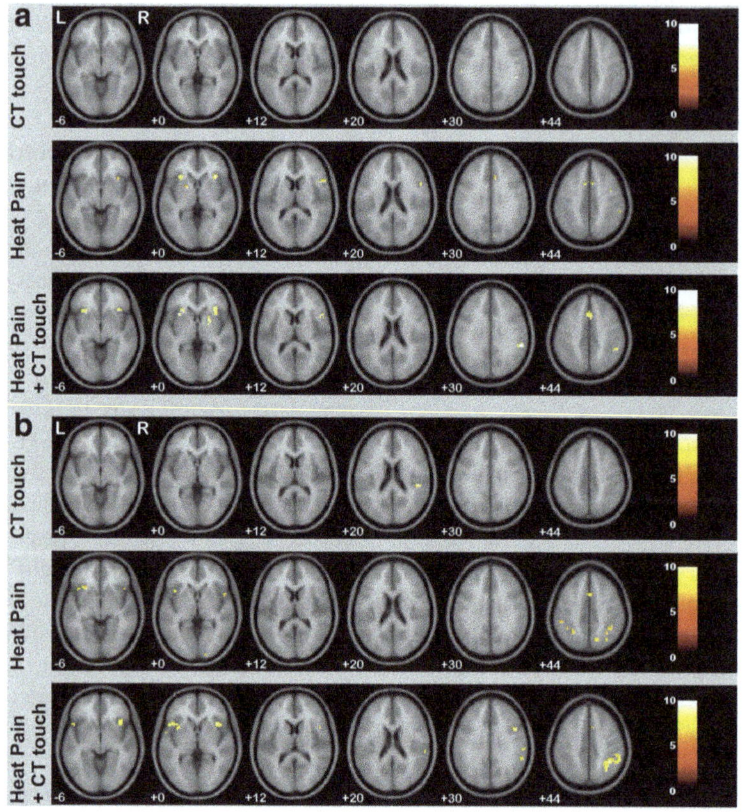

Fig. 3 fMRI images for **a** healthy subjects and **b** SFN patients, showing neuronal activation for the main effect of "CT touch", "heat pain only" and "heat pain combined with CT targeted touch". The right side of the images corresponds to the right hemisphere. Bold responses are shown with FWE correction, $p<0.05$ and cluster size >3 voxel. Results are shown on SPM template avg152T2

100 (applied temperature median 47.0 °C, IQR 3.25). With this setup, we reproduced the significant reduction of heat pain by CT stimulation despite high pain intensities (NRS heat pain only: mean 55.9, SD 15.26; NRS heat-pain and CT targeted touch: 48.4, SD 16.97; p = 0.038, paired t-test).

Discussion

We provide psychophysical evidence that C-LTMR activation modulates experimental heat pain in humans. This notion is largely independent of the stimulus induced pain intensity. In SFN, in which CT fibers are presumed to be impaired, CT activation does not alter heat pain. Since the thick myelinated Aβ fibers were intact in both groups, these afferents were assumed to be less involved in pain reduction. The mechanisms how CT modulated pain relief is being processed remain unclear. We did not detect significant differences in cortical activation patterns between heat stimulation with and without CT targeted touch.

Pain modulation

Heat pain intensity was significantly reduced by CT targeted touch in healthy volunteers. This finding holds true for different pain intensities. It is known from animal experiments that C-LMTRs have pain inhibiting capacities [19]. Our results show that this can also be confirmed in humans. Thus, C-LMTRs are not only important for the mediation of pleasantness [6, 10] and social aspects of touch [32] but also for the modulation of heat pain under physiological conditions. This assumption is supported by the missing effect of brushing hairy skin in SFN patients with probable C-LTMR degeneration.

The question arises whether the findings can be attributed to Aβ-afferent activation. We used a velocity and intensity of brushing that was shown to reliably activate C-LMTRs [6] and to induce a feeling of pleasant touch with a poor spatial localization in two patients with a complete Aβ fibre loss [10, 33]. Coding of pleasantness is one of the major functions of CT afferents [6, 10]. Stroking with a velocity of 3 cm/s has also been shown to correlate with the highest pleasantness ratings [33], substantiating a primary activation of CT afferents. Morrison and coworkers investigated patients with hereditary sensory and autonomic neuropathy type V (HSAN V) with a reduction of thin myelinated nerve fibers. The HSAN V patients did not perceive pleasantness of touch by stimulation with a soft brush even though they have

Table 1 Summary of bold responses for "heat pain only", "heat pain combined with CT targeted touch" and "CT touch", versus control condition showing MNI coordinates, cluster size and peak T-value for healthy subjects (A) and SFN patients (B)

H	Brain region	MNI coordinate (x, y, z)	cluster size	peak T-value
A. Bold responses (healthy subjects)				
Heat pain				
R	Insula (ant)	33, 23, 1	25	10.0226202
R	Middle frontal gyrus, BA 40	45, 35, 25	16	9.40863228
R	Middle frontal gyrus	33, − 1, 55	13	8.20184994
R	Supramarginal gyrus, posterior division	57, − 37, 43	3	7.02497864
R	Inferior frontal gyrus, pars opercularis	48, 14, 13	21	8.32530499
R	Angular gyrus; S2*	45,- 49, 46	9	7.82689619
R	ACC	3, 26, 37	4	7.43887186
R	Paracingulate gyrus	6, 14, 46	58	8.13667107
L	Paracingulate gyrus	-6, 26, 34	8	7.75460911
L	Insula (ant)	− 30, 23, 1	21	10.1233358
L	Lateral globus pallidus*	− 18, 2, 1	4	8.00571537
Heat pain combined with CT targeted touch				
R	Insula (ant.)	36, 26, − 5	63	8.555808067
R	ACC	0, 17, 49	45	7.733303547
R	Putamen	24, 2, 1	8	7.900562286
R	Supramarginal gyrus, BA 40; S2*	57, − 40, 31	19	8.539946556
R	Middle frontal gyrus, BA 40	36, 2, 49	8	7.389503002
R	Anterior intra-parietal sulcus hIP1	42, − 49, 46	10	7.324296474
R	Inferior frontal gyrus, BA 47	42, 20, − 11	3	7.169946671
R	Cerebellum	30, − 58, − 32	24	7.958759308
L	Insula (ant)	− 30, 23, − 2	38	8.298020363
L	Supramarginal gyrus, BA 40	− 42, − 34, 34	5	7.888269424
CT targeted touch				
R	Parietal operculum	48, − 34, 31	3	7.85348225
L	Postcentral gyrus	− 57, − 25, 34	3	6.73631382
B. Bold responses (SFN patients)				
Heat pain				
R	Insula (med.-ant.)*	42, 17, − 2	7	7.24895525
R	ACC	3, 11, 46	42	8.66720772
R	Angular gyrus, BA 40; S2*	45,-46, 49	30	10.2263985
R	Precuneous cortex	15,-67, 43	20	8.95573997
R	Lateral occipital cortex	33, − 67, 40	8	8.75775337
R	Lateral occipital cortex	33, − 58, 46	18	8.02260399
R	Broca's area, BA 44	54, 11, 1	4	8.00252247
R	Cerebellum, anterior lobe	27, − 55, − 20	4	7.94967175
R	Visual cortex, BA 17	18, − 97, 4	4	7.3528986
L	Insula (ant.)*	− 27, 20, − 5	5	8.33598518
L	Superior parietal lobule	− 30, − 52, 49	40	8.32214737
L	Anterior intra-parietal sulcus	− 36, − 43, 37	3	7.88397264
L	Supramarginal gyrus	− 51, − 37, 46	5	7.11958122
L	Frontal operculum	− 42, 17, − 2	13	9.18519974

Table 1 Summary of bold responses for "heat pain only", "heat pain combined with CT targeted touch" and "CT touch", versus control condition showing MNI coordinates, cluster size and peak T-value for healthy subjects (A) and SFN patients (B) *(Continued)*

H	Brain region	MNI coordinate (x, y, z)	cluster size	peak T-value
L	Cerebellum, posterior lobe	− 27, − 62, − 29	42	10.7323313
L	Cerebellum, posterior lobe	− 6, − 76, − 23	22	8.34745884
L	Inferior cerebellum*	− 24, − 61, − 50	21	10.6803532
Heat pain combined with CT targeted touch				
R	Supramarginal gyrus, BA 40; S2*	42, − 46, 46	168	9.750800133
R	Insula (mid-ant)	39, 17, − 2	48	9.569821358
R	Parietal operculum	60, − 28, 22	13	9.502679825
R	Precentral gyrus; S1*	48, 11, 31	14	8.683162689
R	Paracingulate gyrus	9, 14, 40	9	7.428187847
R	Cerebellum, anterior lobe (culmen)	9, − 49, − 17	3	6.953028679
R	Cerebellum, anterior lobe (culmen)	30, − 49, − 26	28	8.335325241
R	Broca's area BA44	48, 14, 16	4	7.146142006
R	Visual cortex, BA 17	18, − 79, 10	4	6.931876659
L	Frontal operculum	− 48, 17, − 2	40	8.466537476
L	Paracingulate gyrus, premotor cortex BA 6	0, 8, 52	11	7.569615841
L	Precentral gyrus	− 57, 5, 4	8	9.12651825
L	Superior parietal lobule, anterior intra-parietal sulcus; S2*	− 36, − 49, 46	3	7.223741531
L	Supramarginal gyrus, postcentral gyrus	− 42, − 34, 4	12	8.600948334
L	Cerebellum, posterior lobe	− 33, − 64, − 44	12	8.533157349
L	Cerebellum, posterior lobe (Pyramis)	− 9, − 76, − 29	15	9.127865791
L	Cerebellum posterior lobe (Uvula)	− 21, − 67, − 26	6	7.966376305
L	Cerebellum, anterior lobe	− 36, − 55, − 29	32	8.700092316
CT targeted touch				
R	Parietal operculum	48, − 31, 19	8	10.0452766

All activations are shown with p (peak, FWE-corr) < 0.05 and cluster size ≥ 3
*anatomical correspondence in SPM using template
All activations are shown with $p<0.05$ (peak, FWE-correction) and cluster size$\geq$3. Regions marked with * are named after their anatomical correspondence in SPM using the template avg152T2

intact Aβ afferents [34]. Using this stimulation protocol, we acted on the assumption to mainly observe effects of CT afferents. Moreover, our SFN patients did not show indications of large fibre neuropathy according to the definition of the disease [25]. We performed electroneurography and measured vibration detection thresholds in all patients in order to minimise large fiber involvement. Nevertheless, as we could not directly measure CT fiber activity, we cannot fully exclude possible Aβ fiber involvement in both groups. An example of Aβ fiber mediated heat pain reduction has been reported by Staud et al. with vibro-tactile in healthy individuals and patients with chronic musculoskeletal pain [34].

Very recently published research by Liljencrantz et al. demonstrated that CT targeted touch (using the same stimulation technique as in our study) but not fast brushing (Aβ targeted touch) nor vibration stimuli reduced heat pain intensity in healthy volunteers [35], confirming our argumentation above.

Suffering from chronic neuropathic pain central sensitization can be expected in SFN patients that might lead to altered transmission of sensory input. We would expect soft stroking to increase pain intensity, since light sensory stimuli can enter the pain pathway. Since we did not observe a significant modification of heat pain (neither increase nor decrease) by CT stimulation in the patient group we suggest that rather CT fiber loss than alteration of sensory stimuli by central sensitization causes the unaltered pain perception during stroking.

Site of pain modulation

The cortical activation patterns elicited by pain combined with "CT targeted touch" did not differ between SFN patients and the control group, even though during "CT targeted touch only" we observed significant activations in brain areas processing somatosensory information. Therefore, the major site of C-LTMR pain modulation might not be the brain, but the dorsal horn.

In the original gate control theory, the spinal cord was considered the site were skin perceptions were modulated before entering the cerebral sensory and affective systems [36]. Many histological studies show a large variety of interneurons and synaptic contacts implying multiple connections of C-LTMRs within the dorsal horn. In mice about 25% of the neurons in lamina I and II in the dorsal horn, known to be the projection side of C-LTMRs, are inhibitory interneurons [37]. These histological observations are already indicative for a modulation of afferent input in the dorsal horn of the spinal tract. Lu and Perl showed in rats that C-LTMR signaling reduces nociceptive C-fiber signaling at the level of the dorsal horn in Lamina I and II [19]. They reported distinct but overlapping projection areas within the dorsal horn of C-LTMRs, Aβ-LTMRs and Aδ-LTMRs, further supporting an interaction on the spinal level.

Besides these histo-morphological implications of spinal mechanisms in rodents Mancini et al. presented data with laser evoked potentials in humans, showing a pain relief by touch with von Frey hairs on a segmental level [21]. Recently they added new information, showing, that touch during laser evoked pain changed the laser-evoked potentials (cortical effect) but also the laser evoked blink reflex [38], implying a pain modulation by non-CT targeted touch at the level of the brainstem or below e.g. the spinal cord.

As we did not perform fMRI analysis of the spinal cord, we are not able to report a change of bold responses by CT stimulation there. A further investigation would be needed to examine a spinal activation pattern by CT stimulation and heat pain, even though a possible extinction of counteracting effects might occur as well on the spinal level.

Limitations of the study

We did not find significant differences in fMRI activation between the condition "heat pain" and "heat pain combined with CT targeted touch" in both groups. Besides the implications arguing for a spinal mechanism of CT modulated pain inhibition, another possible explanation could be lack of statistical power, even though a prior power calculation was positive. During the fMRI session, the participants had to evaluate their intensity of pain and perform a motor task (rating). Therefore, the subtle stimulus of CT activation might be suppressed. But sole CT targeted touch was performed under the same conditions and elicited significant activations of somatosensory brain areas in both groups. We might have achieved a stronger CT stimulation by using a stroking device with skin temperature instead of a brush with neutral temperature [39]. Case and coworkers found different neural processes for coding intensity (posterior insula, primary and secondary somatosensory cortex) and pleasantness of soft touch (pregenual ACC) [12]. These areas are also involved in pain processing [40] which might explain the similarity of the conditions "heat pain" and "heat pain combined with CT targeted touch". Hypothetically, CT targeted touch reduces the heat pain derived activation of the posterior insular and primary sensory cortex by spinal inhibition, but since these areas are not pain specific and activated by sensory stimuli (e.g. CT targeted touch) as well, they might extinct each other (activation and deactivation in the same region) so that there is no resulting difference of bold responses.

The stimulation protocol has not been fully computerized, we relied on an optical trigger to start the stimulation sequences. Therefore, an inaccuracy of synchronism (manual stimulation and start of the MRI acquisition) needs to be taken into account. Because of the preprocessing (e.g. realignment to the mean) we assume no significant interference.

Pain ratings were significantly higher in the SFN patients group. Obviously, SFN patients, which suffer from neuropathic pain have thermal hyperalgesia. To control for a possible effect of pain intensity on CT mediated heat pain modulation we performed an additional experiment (heat pain with and without CT stimulation) on healthy individuals with higher pain intensities, according to those rated by SFN patients (NRS = 50). We also observed a significant reduction of heat pain by CT stimulation which renders a major effect of the different pain intensity on the MRI findings less likely. Nevertheless, high pain intensities in healthy individuals do not control for possible alteration of pain pathways in SFN patients (e.g. central or peripheral sensitization in SFN patients).

To better control against possible Aβ fiber involvement in pain reduction by soft stroking, we should have performed tests with different stroking velocities and pleasantness ratings. But the present protocol included fMRI analysis, hence we had to obey limited investigation times to overcome movement artefacts.

Conclusion

This study provides new evidence that CT fibers own the ability to reduce heat pain perception in healthy subjects. In a next step, it needs to be investigated if C-LTMRs are able to reduce other forms of pain, and how this works. This might open an avenue to new therapy concepts in different pain disorders.

Abbreviations

CDT: Cold detection threshold; C-LTMR: C-low threshold mechanoreceptive afferents; CNS: Central nervous system; CT: C-tactile, C-touch; fMRI: Functional magnetic resonance imaging; HP: Heat pain; HPT: Heat pain threshold; IENFD: Intraepidermal nerve fiber density; NRS: Numeric rating scale;

QST: Quantitative sensory testing; ROI: Region of interest; SFN: Small fiber neuropathy; VAS: Visual analogue scale; WDT: Warm detection threshold

Acknowledgements
We would like to thank the members of the department for Neuroradiology of the Justus-Liebig-University Giessen and Marion Roß for their technical assistance.

Funding
This work was supported by the Forschungsförderung §2 of the Justus Liebig University, Giessen to HHK.

Authors' contributions
HHK and KH are responsible for the conception and design of the study. HHK, WS, GL and KH were responsible for acquisition of data (e.g. recruitment of patients, electroneurography, quantitative sensory profiles and execution of the experiments). AS was responsible for evaluation of the skin biopsies. BD and ERG supervised the technical settings for fMRI and attended the fMRI experiments. HHK, HO and FB were constantly involved in the analysis and interpretation of data. KH drafted the article. All authors revised the article critically for important intellectual content and approved to the final version of the manuscript.

Competing interests
The authors declare that they have no competing interests.

Author details
[1]Department of Neurology, Justus Liebig University, Klinikstr. 33, 35392 Giessen, Germany. [2]Institute of Neuropathology, Justus Liebig University, Arndtstr. 16, 35392 Giessen, Germany. [3]Department of Radiology, Justus Liebig University, Klinikstr.33, 35392 Giessen, Germany. [4]Center for Social and Affective Neuroscience, Linköping University, Linköpings Universitet, 58183 Linköping, Sweden. [5]Department of Neurology, University Medical Center, Johannes Gutenberg-University, Langenbeckstr. 1, 56101 Mainz, Germany. [6]Department of Neuroradiology, Medical University Innsbruck, Innrain 52, 6020 Innsbruck, Austria.

References

1. Johansson RS, Trulsson M, Olsson KA, Westberg KG. Mechanoreceptor activity from the human face and oral mucosa. Exp Brain Res. 1988;72(1): 204–8.
2. Vallbo A, Olausson H, Wessberg J, Norrsell U. A system of unmyelinated afferents for innocuous mechanoreception in the human skin. Brain Res. 1993;628(1–2):301–4.
3. Bessou P, Burgess PR, Perl ER, Taylor CB. Dynamic properties of mechanoreceptors with unmyelinated (C) fibers. J Neurophysiol. 1971;34(1): 116–31.
4. Vallbo AB, Olausson H, Wessberg J. Unmyelinated afferents constitute a second system coding tactile stimuli of the human hairy skin. J Neurophysiol. 1999;81(6):2753–63.
5. Nordin M. Low-threshold mechanoreceptive and nociceptive units with unmyelinated (C) fibres in the human supraorbital nerve. J Physiol. 1990;426:229–40.
6. Loken LS, Wessberg J, Morrison I, McGlone F, Olausson H. Coding of pleasant touch by unmyelinated afferents in humans. Nat Neurosci. 2009;12(5):547–8.
7. Li L, Rutlin M, Abraira VE, Cassidy C, Kus L, Gong S, Jankowski MP, Luo W, Heintz N, Koerber HR, et al. The functional organization of cutaneous low-threshold mechanosensory neurons. Cell. 2011;147(7):1615–27.
8. Craig AD. How do you feel? Interoception: the sense of the physiological condition of the body. Nat Rev Neurosci. 2002;3(8):655–66.
9. Andrew D. Quantitative characterization of low-threshold mechanoreceptor inputs to lamina I spinoparabrachial neurons in the rat. J Physiol. 2010;588(Pt 1):117–24.
10. Olausson H, Lamarre Y, Backlund H, Morin C, Wallin BG, Starck G, Ekholm S, Strigo I, Worsley K, Vallbo AB, et al. Unmyelinated tactile afferents signal touch and project to insular cortex. Nat Neurosci. 2002;5(9):900–4.
11. Liljencrantz J, Bjornsdotter M, Morrison I, Bergstrand S, Ceko M, Seminowicz DA, Cole J, Bushnell MC, Olausson H. Altered C-tactile processing in human dynamic tactile allodynia. Pain. 2013;154(2):227–34.
12. Case LK, Laubacher CM, Olausson H, Wang B, Spagnolo PA, Bushnell MC. Encoding of touch intensity but not pleasantness in human primary somatosensory cortex. J Neurosci. 2016;36(21):5850–60.
13. Sailer U, Triscoli C, Häggblad G, Hamilton P, Olausson H, Croy I. Temporal dynamics of brain activation during 40min of pleasant touch. NeuroImage. 2016;139:360–7.
14. Olausson H, Lamarre Y, Backlund H, Morin C, Wallin B, Starck G, Ekholm S, Strigo I, Worsley K, Vallbo Å. Unmyelinated tactile afferents signal touch and project to insular cortex. Nat Neurosci. 2002;5(9):900–4.
15. Voos AC, Pelphrey KA, Kaiser MD. Autistic traits are associated with diminished neural response to affective touch. Soc Cogn Affect Neurosci. 2013;8(4):378–86.
16. Bennett RH, Bolling DZ, Anderson LC, Pelphrey KA, Kaiser MD. fNIRS detects temporal lobe response to affective touch. Soc Cogn Affect Neurosci. 2013;9(4):470–6.
17. Gordon I, Voos AC, Bennett RH, Bolling DZ, Pelphrey KA, Kaiser MD. Brain mechanisms for processing affective touch. Hum Brain Mapp. 2013;34(4):914–22.
18. Le Bars D. The whole body receptive field of dorsal horn multireceptive neurones. Brain Res Brain Res Rev. 2002;40(1–3):29–44.
19. Lu Y, Perl ER. A specific inhibitory pathway between substantia gelatinosa neurons receiving direct C-fiber input. J Neurosci. 2003;23(25):8752–8.
20. Delfini MC, Mantilleri A, Gaillard S, Hao J, Reynders A, Malapert P, Alonso S, Francois A, Barrere C, Seal R, et al. TAFA4, a chemokine-like protein, modulates injury-induced mechanical and chemical pain hypersensitivity in mice. Cell Rep. 2013;5(2):378–88.
21. Mancini F, Nash T, Iannetti GD, Haggard P. Pain relief by touch: a quantitative approach. Pain. 2014;155(3):635–42.
22. Krahe C, Drabek MM, Paloyelis Y, Fotopoulou A. Affective touch and attachment style modulate pain: a laser-evoked potentials study. Philos Trans R Soc Lond Ser B Biol Sci. 2016;371(1708):20160009. doi:10.1098/rstb.2016.0009.
23. Lacomis D. Small-fiber neuropathy. Muscle Nerve. 2002;26(2):173–88.
24. Varney NR, Benton AL. Tactile perception of direction in relation to handedness and familial handedness. Neuropsychologia. 1975;13(4):449–54.
25. Hoeijmakers JG, Faber CG, Lauria G, Merkies IS, Waxman SG. Small-fibre neuropathies-advances in diagnosis, pathophysiology and management. Nat Rev Neurol. 2012;8(7):369–79.
26. Lauria G, Hsieh ST, Johansson O, Kennedy WR, Leger JM, Mellgren SI, Nolano M, Merkies IS, Polydefkis M, Smith AG, et al. European Federation of Neurological Societies/Peripheral Nerve Society Guideline on the use of skin biopsy in the diagnosis of small fiber neuropathy. Report of a joint task force of the European Federation of Neurological Societies and the Peripheral Nerve Society. Eur J Neurol. 2010;17(7):903–12. e944-909
27. Bakkers M, Merkies IS, Lauria G, Devigili G, Penza P, Lombardi R, Herrmans MC, van Nes SI, De Baets M, Faber CG. Intraepidermal nerve fiber density and its application in sarcoidosis. Neurology. 2009;73(14):1142–8.
28. Nagi SS, Rubin TK, Chelvanayagam DK, Macefield VG, Mahns DA. Allodynia mediated by C-tactile afferents in human hairy skin. J Physiol. 2011;589(Pt 16):4065–75.
29. Bakkers M, Merkies IS, Lauria G, Devigili G, Penza P, Lombardi R, Hermans MC, van Nes SI, De Baets M, Faber CG. Intraepidermal nerve fiber density and its application in sarcoidosis. Neurology. 2009;73(14):1142–8.
30. Rolke R, Baron R, Maier C, Tolle TR, Treede RD, Beyer A, Binder A, Birbaumer N, Birklein F, Botefur IC, et al. Quantitative sensory testing in the German Research Network on Neuropathic Pain (DFNS): standardized protocol and reference values. Pain. 2006;123(3):231–43.
31. Rolke R, Magerl W, Campbell KA, Schalber C, Caspari S, Birklein F, Treede RD. Quantitative sensory testing: a comprehensive protocol for clinical trials. Eur J Pain. 2006;10(1):77–88.
32. Morrison I, Loken LS, Olausson H. The skin as a social organ. Exp Brain Res. 2010;204(3):305–14.

33. Loken LS, Evert M, Wessberg J. Pleasantness of touch in human glabrous and hairy skin: order effects on affective ratings. Brain Res. 2011;1417:9–15.
34. Staud R, Robinson ME, Goldman CT, Price DD. Attenuation of experimental pain by vibro-tactile stimulation in patients with chronic local or widespread musculoskeletal pain. Eur J Pain. 2011;15(8):836–42.
35. Liljencrantz J, Strigo I, Ellingsen DM, Kramer HH, Lundblad LC, Nagi SS, Leknes S, Olausson H. Slow brushing reduces heat pain in humans. Eur J Pain. 2017;21(7):1173–85.
36. Melzack R, Wall PD. Pain mechanisms: a new theory. Science. 1965;150(3699):971–9.
37. Polgar E, Durrieux C, Hughes DI, Todd AJ. A quantitative study of inhibitory interneurons in laminae I-III of the mouse spinal dorsal horn. PLoS One. 2013;8(10):e78309.
38. Mancini F, Beaumont AL, Hu L, Haggard P, Iannetti GD. Touch inhibits subcortical and cortical nociceptive responses. Pain. 2015;156(10):1936–44.
39. Ackerley R, Backlund Wasling H, Liljencrantz J, Olausson H, Johnson RD, Wessberg J. Human C-tactile afferents are tuned to the temperature of a skin-stroking caress. J Neurosci. 2014;34(8):2879–83.
40. Garcia-Larrea L, Peyron R. Pain matrices and neuropathic pain matrices: a review. Pain. 2013;154(Suppl 1):S29–43.

Anterior sacral meningocele infected with Fusobacterium in a patient with recently diagnosed colorectal carcinoma

Anne K. Braczynski[1*], Marc A. Brockmann[2], Torben Scholz[3], Jan-Philipp Bach[1], Jörg B. Schulz[1] and Simone C. Tauber[1]

Abstract

Background: Anterior sacral meningoceles are rare, and usually occur with other malformations of the posterior lower spine. While these are more frequently reported in pediatric cohorts, we report a case in an elderly woman.

Case presentation: We report on a 71 year-old woman with a recently diagnosed colorectal adenocarcinoma who presented with a severe bacterial meningitis. The cerebrospinal fluid cell count revealed a pleocytosis of 80,000 cells/μl and a severe disturbance of the blood-brain-barrier. *Fusobacterium nucleatum* was cultured as the causing pathogen. A lumbar MRI showed, in addition to contrast-enhancing meninges as sign of inflammation, a presacral mass. In the next step, the mass was diagnosed as an anterior sacral meningocele connected to the gut. An adequate antibiotic was used to treat the leptomeningitis. The connection between gut and meningocele was closed surgically and the patient recovered well and underwent further treatment of her colorectal adenocarcinoma.

Conclusion: We report on a case of meningitis with an anterior sacral meningocele that was connected to the gut in a patient with a infiltrative colorectal adenocarcinoma. Anatomic variants have to be considered as rare causes of meningitis with typical intestinal germs.

Keywords: Meningitis, Colorectal carcinoma, Anterior sacral meningocele, Occult spinal dysraphism

Background

Usually, a sacral meningocele develops from an incomplete closure of the neuroporus posterior. This so-called dysraphism is subcategorized according to its content: It is termed meningocele if it contains parts of the meninges; or myelocele, if spinal cord tissue is part of the herniated tissue and meningomyelocele, if it contains boths. These structures are usually dorsal deformations located at the posterior part of the lower back [1]. Nevertheless, anterior also termed pre-sacral myeloceles are described. Data on the incidence of anterior sacral myeloceles is not available. Clinically, patients present with bladder dysfunction and constipation. Most often, patients get already diagnosed during childhood.

* Correspondence: abraczynski@ukaachen.de
[1]Department of Neurology, RWTH University Hospital, Pauwelsstr. 30, 52074 Aachen, Germany
Full list of author information is available at the end of the article

Case presentation

We report on a 71 year-old female patient who presented with fever, worsening of her general condition, neck stiffness, impaired vigilance and strong pain in the lower lumbar spine. Two weeks before, the patient had presented with weight loss and blood in her stool at a regional hospital. In a subsequent colonoscopy, a colorectal adenocarcinoma was diagnosed histologically. Staging consisting of a computed tomography (CT)-scan revealed infiltration into the uterus and also into *Os sacrum*. A CT-guided biopsy from the mass infiltrating Os sacrum also confirmed the carcinoma. The caregivers opted for a neo-adjuvant treatment plan including radio- and chemotherapy with capecitabine. Irradiation had been applied once. The neurologic examination at admission to our hospital revealed a somnolent patient with nuchal rigidity and bilateral positive Babinski sign, all of which had developed in less than 12 h.

Due to the clinical presentation, meningitis in the course of a spondylodiscitis was suspected. An antibiotic treatment with ceftriaxone and ampicilline was started, which lead to a rapid improvement of the patient's consciousness. Extensive imaging including spinal magnetic resonance imaging (MRI), lumbar MRI, small pelvis MRI and CT scans of the lumbar spine and the brain were performed (results see Neuroradiological findings) and could rule out several differential diagnoses. There was no sign of spondylodiscitis. Analysis of the cerebrospinal fluid (CSF) revealed a pleocytosis of 80,000 cells/µl, dominated by neutrophilic granulocytes. Microbiologic work-up of CSF found the typical gastrointestinal germ *Fusobacterium nucleatum* as the causative agent of the bacterial infection, no other germs, e.g. *E. coli*, were detected. The antibiotic treatment was changed to ceftriaxone and vancomycine and continued for 14 days (see also Fig. 1).

Neuroradiological findings

Neuroradiological diagnostics including CT scans and MRI of the lumbar spinal column and the pelvis were performed. The CT-scan showed multiple spots of gas accumulation in the region of the lumbar vertebral disk between the vertebral bodies L4 and L5. MRI (Fig. 2) revealed, in addition to contrast-enhancing meninges illustrating the severe leptomeningits, a presacral mass filled with CSF isointens content. This mass could not be discriminated from necrotic cell debris. Initially, either necrotic tumor tissue of the adenocarcinoma or a malformation of the spinal dural sac seemed possible. Further anatomic abnormalities were an unusually low ending of conus of the spinal cord at L3/4 and a partial agenesis of the left sacral bone. A comprehensive work-up of the neuroradiological images revealed evidence of the presence of an anterior sacral meningocele. The carcinoma had infiltrated neighboring structures in the lower pelvis including bladder, and the sacral bone. Furthermore, a connection between the distended rectum and the spinal canal was visible. Through this pathway, bacterial invasion may have occurred and lead to a meningeal infection with typical gastrointestinal germ *Fusobacterium*. An interdisciplinary tumor board opted for surgical treatment to close the connection between gut and the anterior meningocele, which would prevent further pathogen invasion.

Neurosurgical treatment

To avoid recurrent meningitis, neurosurgical treatment was necessary. Since surgical therapy of the colorectal carcinoma after a neoadjuvant treatment would include creating terminal stomas of both bowel and urinary tracts, we opted for detachment of the local structures and closure of the thecal sac and amputation of the meningocele as far distal as possible. This was achieved distal of the S2-roots via a dorsal laminectomy from S1 to S3 (Fig. 3). We detached the cauda equina intradurally and sectioned and closed the thecal sac. Around and between adherent roots of the cauda equina postinflammatory debris was found. Moreover we could visualize the connection of the meningocele through the ventral defect of the *Os sacrum* into the small pelvis extra- and intradurally. The patient recovered well after surgery. Motor function was unchanged postoperatively. Bladder function could not be assessed due to an inserted urinary catheter. Histology of the surgical specimen showed meningeal cell layers invaded by leucocytes and macrophages.

Oncologic treatment and follow up

Oncologic treatment consisting of radio- and chemotherapy resumed three weeks after the initial surgery. Radiotherapy of pelvis and *os sacrum* was applied in fractions of 1.8 Gy leading to a total of 54 Gy. In parallel, capecitabine was administered twice daily (825 mg/m^2 body surface). At a clinical follow up 3 months later, the patient's gait was normal, she denied abnormal functions of bladder or rectum. An abdominal CT-scan 24 weeks after initial admission showed necrotic consolidation of the tumor mass but a mild progression of lymph node size. In week 25, total mesorectal excision and ultralow anterior resection of the colon was performed. The patient had no children; there were no additional family history details. Siblings and

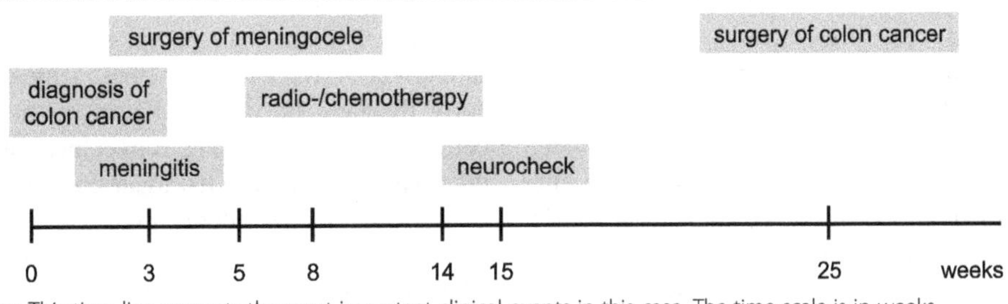

Fig. 1 Case time line. This time line presents the most important clinical events in this case. The time scale is in weeks

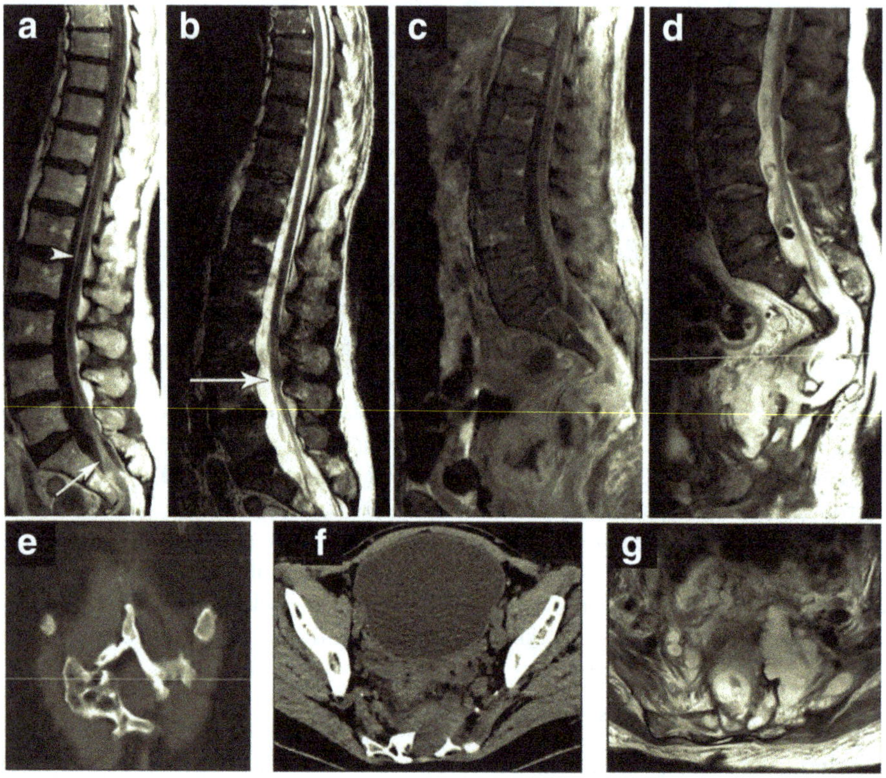

Fig. 2 Neuroradiological Imaging. MRI imaging (**a** sagittal T1-SE post-contrast; **b** sagittal T2-TSE: sagittal fat-saturated T1-SE post-contrast; **d** sagittal T2-TSE, **e** coronally reconstructed CT; **f** axially reconstructed CT at the level marked by a line in **d**; **g** axial T2-TSE sequence at the level marked by a line in **c**). (**a**, **c**) Strong contrast enhancement of the meningeal structures due to the meningitis are shown in the post-contrast MRI series. The arrowhead in A exemplarily points at the strongly enhancing surface of the spinal cord. The arrow in A points at the contrast-enhancing filum terminale. (**b**) The level of the medullary cone is at the level of the vertebrates L3 and L4, which is unusually low, see arrow. (**c**) The distended rectum and a connection to the spinal canal are visible. The meningocele cannot be unequivocally delineated from the rectal carcinoma. (**d**, **e**) CT at the level marked by a line in **d**; (**f**) axial sequence at the level marked by a line in **c**) demonstrating a sacral menigocele with tethering of the spinal cord and bony dysraphism

parents were reported to be healthy. There were no other cutaneous or orthopedic stigmata pointing to a dystrophic condition. The patient had no foot deformities. The patient reported voiding problems, which had been present for many years. Unfortunately, the patient refused further genetic testing or urodynamic investigations (see also Fig. 1).

Discussion and conclusion

We reported on a patient with known bladder dysfunction who developed severe leptomeningitis caused by *Fusobacterium nucleatum* shortly after the diagnosis of a colorectal adenocarcinoma. Neuroradiologic imaging lead to the diagnosis of a pre-existing anterior sacral meningocele. A presacral mass during staging via CT-scans at the time of the diagnosis of the colorectal cancer was first interpreted as extensive tumor mass. The anterior sacral meningocele and a connection into the colon was confirmed during surgery. The meningocele was accompanied by a tethered cord and partial agenesis of the left lower sacrum, thereby pointing to a complex developmental malformation.

Finding a gut germ in the CSF was rather unusual. Different scenarios might explain its presence. First, a contamination of the biopsy needle during the CT-guided biopsy could have inoculated the germ into the CSF, therefore being an iatrogenic event. Still, a delay of three weeks between the biopsy and the onset of the meningitis leaves this option less probable. Second, in patients with the given malformations preformed colon-to-spinal fistulas are described. If such fistulas are preexisting, meningitis can occur and need a surgical closure, as a case in a one-month old girl infected with *E. coli* illustrates [2]. If a fistula might have been present in our patient, we postulate, that it might have gotten symptomatic at an earlier time point in live. Third, a hematogenic distribution of the germ through the venous plexus in the pelvis, that may contain anastomoses between colorectal veins and peridural veins, could have led to an infection. Lastly, we think that the colorectal adenocarcinoma formed an artificial connection between the meningocele and the colon, which was reported to exist during surgery. Unfortunately, the tumor invasion into the meningocele could not be

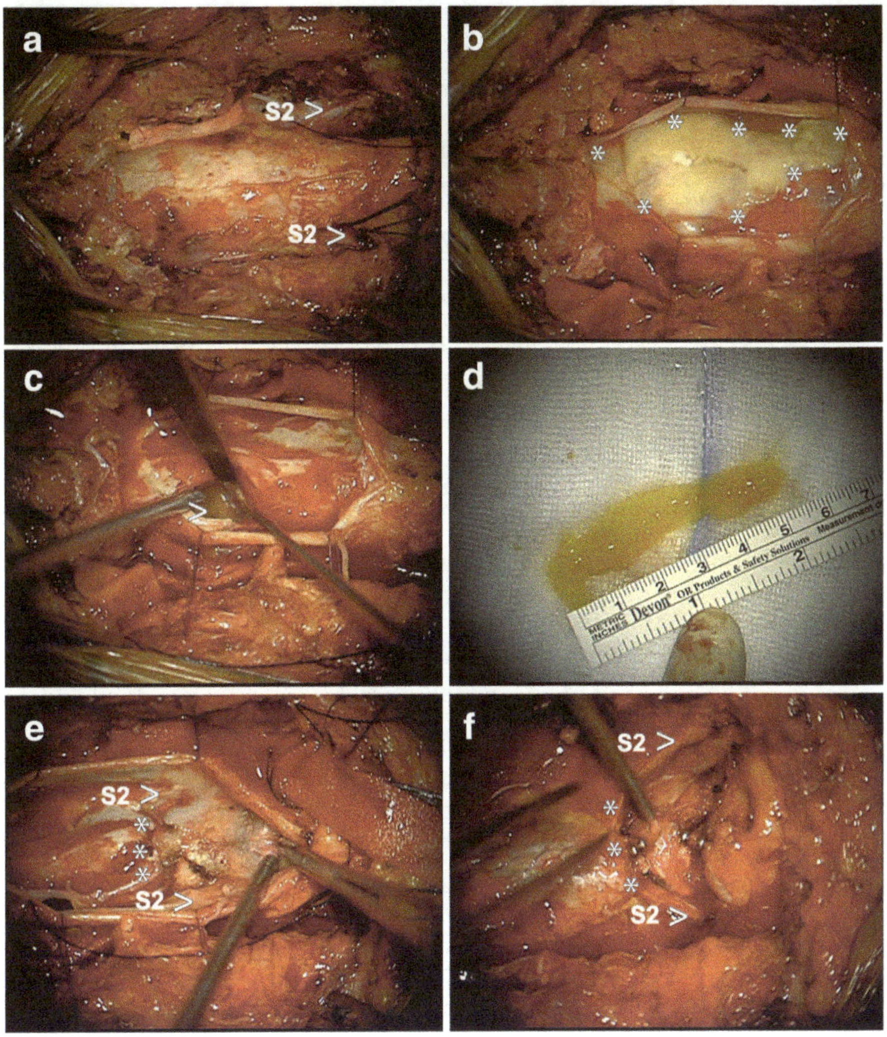

Fig. 3 Neurosurgical intraoperative situs. Intraoperative findings. (**a**) Opening of the dural sac with spinal root of S2 (arrow). (**b**) Pus and necrotic cell debris (stars indicate the borders) were visible upon opening of the dural sac. (**c**) Cauda fibers adhered to each other due to the necrotic cell debris (arrow). (**d**) Extracted necrotic cell debris without any indication of tumor infiltration in the neuropathologic examination. (**e**, **f**) The intradural spinal root of S2 (arrow) and amputated cauda equina below S2 is visible (stars indicate amputation line)

proven histologically (Fig. 4), which might be explained by a sampling error. Both last options can explain the acute onset of the meningitis.

The patient admitted a bladder dysfunction being present a long time before the onset of the colorectal adenocarcinoma. Unfortunately, no further diagnostics had been performed earlier, and she denied urodynamic investigation after recovery. Patients with anterior sacral meningocele can suffer from pollakisuria because of bladder compression leading to a small capacity and can lead to obstetrical hindrance during pregnancy and delivery [2]. From a surgical and oncologic perspective, the presence of a postoperative bladder dysfunction is likely.

In patients with bladder dysfunction, sacral meningoceles were described in a pediatric cohort of 175 patients [3]. In 60% of the patients, they were associated with defects of the bone as present in our adult patient. Meningoceles can be part of the Currarino syndrome, which consists of a sacrococcygeal defect, a presacral mass (anterior meningocele and/or tumor, often teratoma) and an anorectal malformation. Currarino proposed this triad as a persistent neuroenteric malformation transmitted autosomal dominantly [4]. A mutation in the homeobox gene HLXB9 can be causative [5] and is found in about 50% of these patients [6]. A few reports describe case series with Currarino triad predominantly in pediatric cohorts [2, 7]. Nevertheless, while more than 80% of the cases are diagnosed within the first to third decade, Currarino syndrome may be diagnosed in older adults, especially if single features of the triad are missing due to incomplete penetrance [8]. The embryonic development of anterior sacral meningoceles also in the

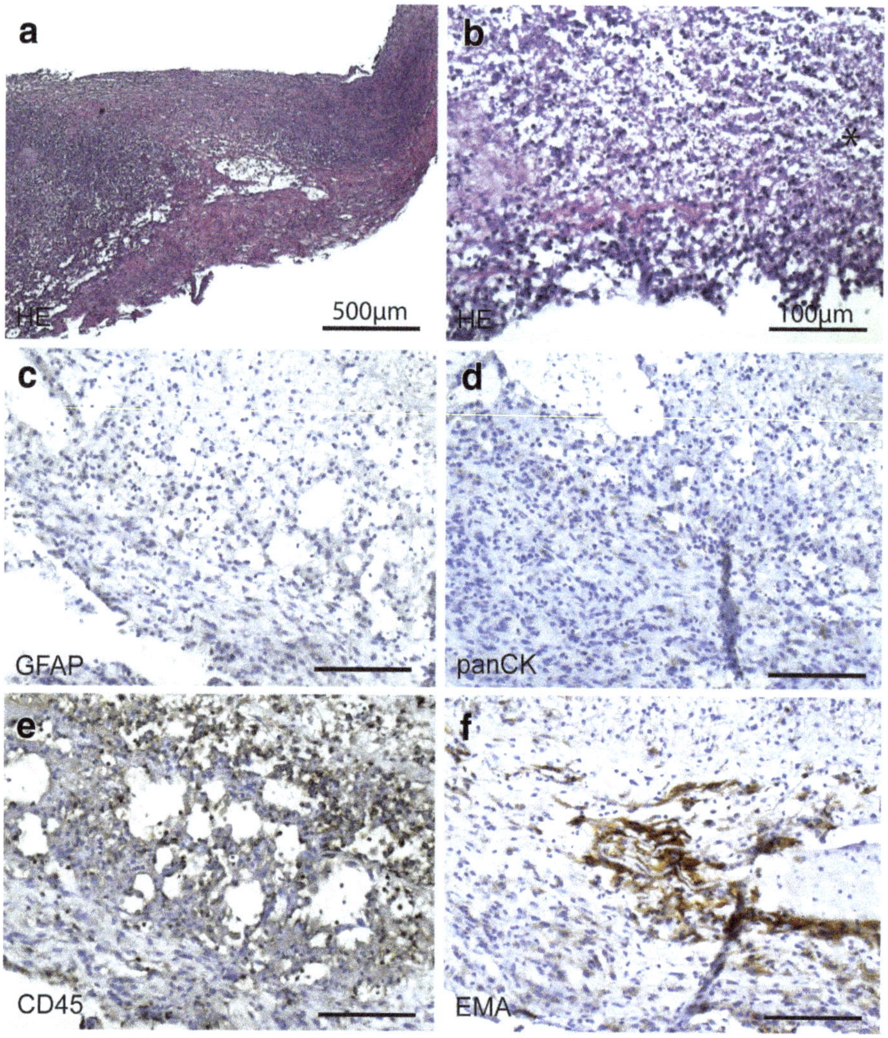

Fig. 4 Neuropathologic findings. Histology of the tissue sample. (**a**) Overview of the tissue consisting of cell debris with sparse organisation (scale bar 500 µm, HE) and (**b**) detail (scale bar 100 µm). (**c**) Central nervous tissue (scale bar 100 µm, GFAP) as well as (**d**) infiltrative carcinoma cells (scale bar 100 µm, panCK) were absent. (**e**) The specimen were infiltrated by leukocytes and macrophages (scale bar 100 µm, CD45). (**f**) There were few EMA positive flat cells indicating presence of meningeal cell layer as a wall of the meningocele (scale bar 100 µm, EMA)

context of Currarino syndrome is not fully understood, it most probably results from a complex formation disorder. It is thought to develop in the course of the split notochord syndrome, a gastrulation defect, where persisting tissue parts are supposed to prevent the sufficient development of the vertebral bodies [9]. Given the triad of meningocele, sacral malformation and tethered cord, our patient possibly had suffered from Currarino syndrome. She reached a relatively old age at the time of diagnosis. Unfortunately, she refused further genetic testing to clarify the diagnosis. Genetic testing is advisable in such patients more importantly with respect to its autosomal-dominant inheritance. Evidence on the treatment of anterior meningoceles is very rare as well and a consensus on neurosurgical treatment is missing. In the case of a meningitis, surgery is well accepted [2]. Lower spinal imaging is advisable in patients which neurogenic bladder dysfunction, and a comprehensive presurgical neuroradiologic work-up is necessary in patients with this malformation.

In summary, anterior sacral meningoceles are underdiagnosed and account for differential diagnosis of anterior sacral masses. These anatomic variants have to be considered as rare causes of meningitis with typical intestinal germs. They need detailed neuroradiologic description, and lack established therapy strategies. We report on the distal sectioning of the thecal sac to close the anterior sacral meningocele for the prevention of recurrent meningitis.

Abbreviations

CSF: Cerebrospinal fluid; CT: Computed tomography; MRI: Magnetic resonance imaging

Acknowledgments
We thank the patient for letting us publish her case and all contributors for their input and work. We thank Christoph Bernhard Hoog Antink for language editing.

Funding
AKB received funding the START program of the Medical Faculty of RWTH Aachen University.

Authors' contributions
AKB treated the patient, performed the neuropathologic analysis, drafted the manuscript and participated in the conception and design of the case report. TS has performed the surgery and wrote the neurosurgical part of the case report. MB performed the neuroradiologic examinations and helped in the discussion of the case. JPB helped interpreting the findings and drafted the manuscript JBS treated the patient and gave input into the discussion and interpretation of all neuroradiological, neuropathological and neurological findings. SCT treated the patient, supervised the study, helped interpreting the findings and drafted the manuscript. All authors read and approved the final manuscript.

Competing interests
AKB received funding the START program of the Medical Faculty of RWTH Aachen University. All other authors declare no competing interests.

Author details
[1]Department of Neurology, RWTH University Hospital, Pauwelsstr. 30, 52074 Aachen, Germany. [2]Department of Diagnostic and Interventional Neuroradiology, RWTH University Hospital, Aachen, Germany. [3]Department of Neurosurgery, RWTH University Hospital, Aachen, Germany.

References

1. Copp AJ, Greene ND. Neural tube defects–disorders of neurulation and related embryonic processes. Wiley Interdiscip Rev Dev Biol. 2013;2(2): 213–27.
2. Emans PJ, van Aalst J, van Heurn EL, Marcelis C, Kootstra G, Beets-Tan RG, Vles JS, Beuls EA. The Currarino triad: neurosurgical considerations. Neurosurgery. 2006;58(5):924–9. discussion 924-929
3. Sadiq S, Faiq SM, Idrees MK. Lumbosacral dysraphism as cause of neurogenic bladder: magnetic resonance imaging based study from SIUT Pakistan. J Pak Med Assoc. 2015;65(5):501–5.
4. Currarino G, Coln D, Votteler T. Triad of anorectal, sacral, and presacral anomalies. AJR Am J Roentgenol. 1981;137(2):395–8.
5. Ross AJ, Ruiz-Perez V, Wang Y, Hagan DM, Scherer S, Lynch SA, Lindsay S, Custard E, Belloni E, Wilson DI, et al. A homeobox gene, HLXB9, is the major locus for dominantly inherited sacral agenesis. Nat Genet. 1998;20(4):358–61.
6. Riebel T, Kochling J, Scheer I, Oellinger J, Reis A. Currarino syndrome: variability of imaging findings in 22 molecular-genetically identified (HLXB9 mutation) patients from five families. Rofo. 2004;176(4):564–9.
7. Lee SC, Chun YS, Jung SE, Park KW, Kim WK. Currarino triad: anorectal malformation, sacral bony abnormality, and presacral mass–a review of 11 cases. J Pediatr Surg. 1997;32(1):58–61.
8. Kochling J, Pistor G, Marzhauser Brands S, Nasir R, Lanksch WR. The Currarino syndrome–hereditary transmitted syndrome of anorectal, sacral and presacral anomalies. Case report and review of the literature. Eur J Pediatr Surg. 1996;6(2):114–9.
9. Kaplan KM, Spivak JM, Bendo JA. Embryology of the spine and associated congenital abnormalities. Spine J. 2005;5(5):564–76.

The humanistic burden of Pompe disease: are there still unmet needs?

Benedikt Schoser[1*], Deborah A. Bilder[2], David Dimmock[3], Digant Gupta[4], Emma S. James[5] and Suyash Prasad[5]

Abstract

Background: Humanistic burden considers the impact of an illness on a patient's health-related quality of life (HRQoL), activities of daily living (ADL), caregiver health, and caregiver QoL. Humanistic burden also considers treatment satisfaction and adherence to treatment regimens. Pompe disease is an autosomal recessive, progressive, multisystemic neuromuscular disease. Approval of enzyme-replacement therapy (ERT) markedly improved prognosis for patients, but considerable morbidity and a substantial humanistic burden remain. This article characterizes the humanistic burden of Pompe disease through a systematic literature review.

Methods: A systematic search of MEDLINE® and Embase® with back-referencing and supplementary literature searches was performed to retrieve data from interventional and non-interventional studies on the humanistic burden of Pompe disease. Publications were screened according to predefined criteria, extracted, and assessed for quality. Extracted data were narratively synthesized.

Results: No publications on the humanistic burden of infantile-onset Pompe disease (IOPD) were identified. As such, of 17 publications included here, all are in patients with late-onset Pompe disease (LOPD). Thirteen publications were initiated after approval of ERT, two were initiated before, and two overlapped the approval of ERT. The review shows that LOPD patients have a significantly lower HRQoL than the general population, even if treated with ERT. On transitioning to ERT, treatment was associated with improvement in the physical component score of the SF-36 and fatigue, although the SF-36 mental component score remained stable. Physical HRQoL remained below population norms after 4 years of ERT. Significantly more ERT-treated patients reported pain than controls, and bodily pain worsened in later years following ERT initiation. Treatment-naïve LOPD patients had significantly poorer ADL functioning compared with the general population, although ERT stabilized deteriorating functioning impairment. ERT studies showed caregivers provide 17.7 h/week informal care on average. Fifty percent, 40% and <20% of caregivers reported mental health, physical health, and financial/relational problems, respectively. In ERT-naïve patients, wheelchair use and home ventilatory support was associated with lower physical HRQoL and ADL functioning. In ERT-treated patients, key factors predicting worse HRQoL and ADL functioning were higher respiratory distress, poorer sleep quality, greater pain, and more fatigue.

Conclusions: Pompe disease has a substantial humanistic burden, with strong inter-relationships among and between humanistic burden parameters and clinical progression.

Keywords: Pompe, Humanistic burden, Quality of life, Daily living, Caregiver burden

* Correspondence: Benedikt.Schoser@med.uni-muenchen.de
[1]Friedrich-Baur-Institut, Neurologische Klinik und Poliklinik, Klinikum der Universität München, Ludwig-Maximilians-Universität München, Ziemssenstr, D-80336 Munich, Germany
Full list of author information is available at the end of the article

Background

The humanistic burden considers the impact of an illness on a patient's health-related quality of life (HRQoL), activities of daily living (ADL), caregiver health, and caregiver QoL. The humanistic burden also takes into account patients' treatment satisfaction and adherence to their specific treatment regimen.

Pompe disease is an autosomal recessive, progressive, debilitating disease in which acid α-glucosidase (GAA) deficiency leads to intralysosomal accumulations of glycogen in all tissues. All muscle groups are affected, including ventilatory, cardiac, and skeletal muscles, and there is some evidence of motor neuron dysfunction and pathology of the central and peripheral nervous systems [1–3], with resultant effects on cognitive function, hearing loss, speech muscle pathology, and fine motor dysfunction in patients with classic-infantile Pompe disease.

Pompe disease presents as a wide spectrum of phenotypes, ranging from the severe, rapidly progressive infantile-onset Pompe disease (IOPD) to the more slowly progressing late-onset Pompe disease (LOPD) that can manifest any time from early childhood to late adulthood [4–6].

Clinically, infants with IOPD typically present during the first few weeks of life with hypotonia, progressive weakness, macroglossia, hepatomegaly, and hypertrophic cardiomyopathy. This presentation usually facilitates identification of the disorder [7, 8]; however, identifying LOPD can be more challenging as these patients generally present with slowly progressive limb girdle-type weakness and ventilatory insufficiency without significant cardiomyopathy. Cardiac involvement in LOPD has been described, and may manifest as Wolff-Parkinson-White syndrome, left ventricular hypertrophy, and dilatation of the ascending aorta [9, 10]. Rigid spine syndrome, scoliosis, and low body weight have also been reported in some patients with LOPD that have onset in adolescence, resulting in postural anomalies [7–9]. The laboratory diagnosis of Pompe disease depends on the measurement of GAA activity in the blood or tissues, or the detection of disease-causing variants in the *GAA* gene.

Pompe disease is a rare condition. The reported prevalence estimates vary widely depending on ethnicity and diagnostic approach used [5, 11], and there is a lack of accurate, consistent estimates for both IOPD and LOPD in the published literature; however, for Europe the estimated prevalence of Pompe disease is about 1 in 283,000 [11]. Based on predictions from carrier frequencies, newborn screening data, and retrospectively registered data, the frequency of IOPD has been estimated between 1 in 8684 to 138,000 worldwide [12–14].

Currently, the only specific drug treatment for Pompe disease is ERT with recombinant human GAA (rhGAA), which was approved for use in the United States (US) and Europe in 2006 [15]. A recent systematic review and meta-analysis demonstrated a nearly five-fold reduction in mortality rates over an average study duration of approximately 46 months in patients treated with ERT compared with untreated patients (rate ratio: 0.21; 95% credible interval [CrI]: 0.11–0.41) [6]. This meta-analysis also reported a benefit of ERT in terms of slowing pulmonary functioning decline and improving 6-min walk test (6MWT; the distance an individual is able to walk in 6 min) results. While ERT as the principal treatment targeting the underlying pathology in Pompe disease has transformed the lives of patients, supportive care has an important ongoing role in the management of the condition.

Several limitations of ERT remain, including (1) dependency on high infusion volume, time-consuming infusions at least every other week [4, 15], (2) associated adverse infusion reactions in some patients [4, 15], (3) the inability to clear neuronal glycogen, with subsequent pathology progression and functional decline [16–18]; (4) the reappearance of glycogen in satellite cells [16–18]; (5) continued autophagic buildup in tissue [19]; and (6) antibody responses to ERT that mitigate the efficacy of ERT [20]. These limitations, along with the non-recoverable muscle function loss from Pompe disease, lead to a substantial burden of illness, both for treated and untreated patients.

When investigating the overall burden of a disease, clinical manifestations and economic costs tend to capture the greatest interest of clinicians and payers and garner the focus of most research effort. However, the humanistic burden of a disease, rather than its clinical and economic burden, is typically of greatest concern to patients and their caregivers. Although several reviews have previously been published on the clinical burden of Pompe disease [4–6, 8], the overall humanistic burden has been neglected. This article aims to characterize all aspects of the humanistic burden of Pompe disease and of ERT through a systematic review of the relevant literature for both IOPD and LOPD.

Methods

No ethical approval was required because no individual patient identifiers were disclosed in the publications contained in this systematic literature review. A PRISMA 2009 Checklist [21] and a review protocol summary are provided as Additional Information.

The following research questions were formulated by the authors at the start of this analysis:

- What is the impact of Pompe disease on humanistic burden in patients receiving ERT throughout the course of clinical studies (both observational and interventional), and in patients transitioning from supportive treatment to ERT during the course of a clinical study?

- What inter-relationships exist among humanistic burden parameters in Pompe disease?
- How does the humanistic burden change as the disease progresses?
- What is the impact of ERT on the humanistic burden of Pompe disease?

Search strategy

Systematic searches were performed in Embase®/MEDLINE® using Embase.com® to identify relevant articles published through July 2016 on the humanistic burden (patient HRQoL, ADL, caregiver burden, treatment satisfaction and adherence) of Pompe disease. Each search was conducted using controlled vocabulary and key words, and was limited to articles published in English and involving human subjects (as is standard practice for literature reviews of this kind). The specific search terms used are provided as Additional Information. Additional publications were identified through bibliography reviews of relevant articles as well as supplementary searches using Google, Google Scholar and other web-based sources.

Selection criteria

Titles and abstracts of articles identified were carefully screened by the authors in the initial review for relevance to the topic. Articles were selected for inclusion based on predefined acceptance criteria, which included patient population (adults/children diagnosed with Pompe disease), outcome measures of interest (HRQoL, ADL, caregiver burden, treatment satisfaction, and treatment adherence), and study design (quantitative and/or qualitative data collection). Articles exclusively reporting clinical and/or economic outcomes were excluded, along with those in a non-English language and with an absence of peer-review for articles, editorials, correspondence, and conference abstracts.

Potentially relevant articles were obtained in full-text for further evaluation. Each was screened and its eligibility confirmed by two reviewers. Inconsistencies were resolved through consensus.

Quality assessment

A descriptive analysis of each publication was conducted during data extraction. Each publication was assessed for quality by considering characteristics that could introduce bias, using the following tools: 1) Newcastle-Ottawa Scale for cohort studies and case-control studies [22]; 2) Adapted Newcastle-Ottawa Scale for cross-sectional studies [22]; 3) AMSTAR measurement tool for reviews [23]; 4) Cochrane risk of bias assessment tool for randomized controlled trials [24].

Data extraction

Data from the included studies were extracted into a predefined extraction grid by a single reviewer. Information was recorded for study design, setting, patient characteristics, outcome measures, key results, and conclusions. A description of the outcome scales used in the studies included in this review is provided in Table 1. Given the descriptive nature of this systematic review, the extracted data were narratively synthesized.

Results

Overview

Titles and abstracts of a total of 352 citations were screened following the initial searches, 36 of which were included for full-text screening. Seventeen articles were subsequently selected for final inclusion in the narrative synthesis (Fig. 1). The basic characteristics and quality ratings of the included studies reporting data on the humanistic burden of Pompe disease are shown in Table 2. All 17 publications included patients with LOPD. Importantly, no studies on the humanistic burden of IOPD were identified, demonstrating a gap in the literature. The 17 LOPD publications included six prospective cohort studies [25–30], one randomized controlled trial (RCT) [31], eight cross-sectional studies [32–39], and two case series [40, 41].

Five of the 17 publications are based on separate analyses of the International Pompe Survey, a long-term prospective natural history study initiated 4 years prior to the approval of ERT and continuing today [29, 30, 32, 33, 36]. This survey was established to collect information on the course of the disease and its burden on patients, and includes patients from Australia, Germany, the Netherlands, the United Kingdom (UK), and the United States of America (US).

Thirteen publications included in this systematic review are based on clinical studies that were initiated after the approval of ERT [25–28, 31, 34–41]; consequently, all participants were receiving open-labeled ERT throughout the course of these studies. Two publications published before ERT approval describe participants treated in the absence of ERT [32, 33]. Finally, two publications [29, 30] are based on studies that were initiated before ERT approval and continued into the ERT era; therefore, these studies include patients who were not receiving ERT at study onset but transitioned to ERT during the study.

In addition to the complete absence of publications reporting on the humanistic burden of IOPD, this review did not identify any LOPD studies describing treatment satisfaction or adherence. Therefore, the following

Table 1 Description of outcome scales used in studies in this review

Scale	Description	Range	Interpretation
Brief pain inventory (BPI)	Measures both the intensity of pain (sensory dimension) and interference of pain in the patient's life (reactive dimension); it also queries the patient about pain relief, pain quality, and patient perception of the cause of pain	Scores range from 0 (no pain) to 10 (pain as bad as you can imagine)	A higher score indicates greater pain
Pain interference score (PIS)	Average score of four items on the BPI devoted to severity of pain	Scores range from 0 (does not interfere) to 10 (completely interferes)	A higher score indicates greater interference of pain
Pain severity score (PSS)	Calculated on the basis of the average interference of pain (assessed on the BPI) with the following seven activities: general activities, mood, walking ability, normal work, relations with other people, sleep, and enjoyment of life	Scores range from 0 (no pain) to 10 (pain as bad as you can imagine)	A higher score indicates greater pain
CarerQoL	Measure of care-related QoL in informal care givers; comprising two parts: a description of the care situation on seven burden dimensions (CarerQoL-7D) and a valuation component in terms of general QoL using a Visual Analog Scale (CarerQol-VAS)	Assesses the overall well-being of the caregiver on a 0–10 scale, ranging from "completely unhappy" (0) to "completely happy" (10)	A higher score indicates greater happiness
Fatigue severity scale (FSS)	Self-reported nine-item questionnaire concerning the respondent's fatigue; for example, how fatigue affects motivation, exercise, physical functioning, carrying out duties, interfering with work, family or social life	Participants grade each question on a Likert scale from 1 to 7, where 1 indicates strong disagreement and 7 indicates strong agreement	A higher score indicates more severe fatigue. Scores above 4 indicate significant fatigue and scores above 5 indicate severe fatigue
Hospital anxiety and depression scale (HADS)	14-item self-rated scale. Seven of the items relate to anxiety and seven relate to depression. Each item is rated from 0 to 3, where 0 = not at all to 3 = most severe	Depression and anxiety scores can each range from 0 to 21	Higher scores indicate greater anxiety or depression
Nottingham health profile (NHP)	Assesses subjective health status	Ranges from 0 (good) to 100 (poor)	Higher scores indicate poorer health status
Pittsburgh sleep quality index (PSQI)	19 self-rated questions and five questions rated by the partner. The latter five questions are used for clinical information only and are not tabulated in the scoring of the PSQI. The 19 self-rated questions assess a wide variety of factors relating to sleep quality, including estimates of sleep duration and latency, and the frequency and severity of specific sleep-related problems	Global PSQI score is calculated from the responses given using a predefined algorithm, and ranges from 0 to 21	A higher score indicates worse sleep quality
Rotterdam handicap scale (RHS)	Used to measure a patient's functional ability and level of handicap, and can be used to monitor a patient's status over time as well as to evaluate the effectiveness of interventions	Scores per item range from 1 ('unable to fulfill the task or activity') to 4 ('complete fulfillment of the task or activity'). The total score is derived by adding individual component scores and ranges from 9 ('unable to fulfill any task/activity') to 36 ('able to fulfill all applicable tasks or activities')	A higher score indicates better functional ability
Short-form-36 (SF-36)	Multidimensional HRQoL instrument comprising four physical health scales (physical functioning, role limitations due to physical problems, bodily pain, and general health perceptions) and four mental health scales (vitality, social functioning, role limitations due to emotional problems, and mental health). These eight scales can be aggregated into two summary measures: the physical (PCS) and mental (MCS) component summary scores	Each scale is directly transformed into a 0–100 scale on the assumption that each question carries equal weight	A lower score indicates greater disability (i.e., a score of zero is equivalent to maximum disability and a score of 100 is equivalent to no disability)

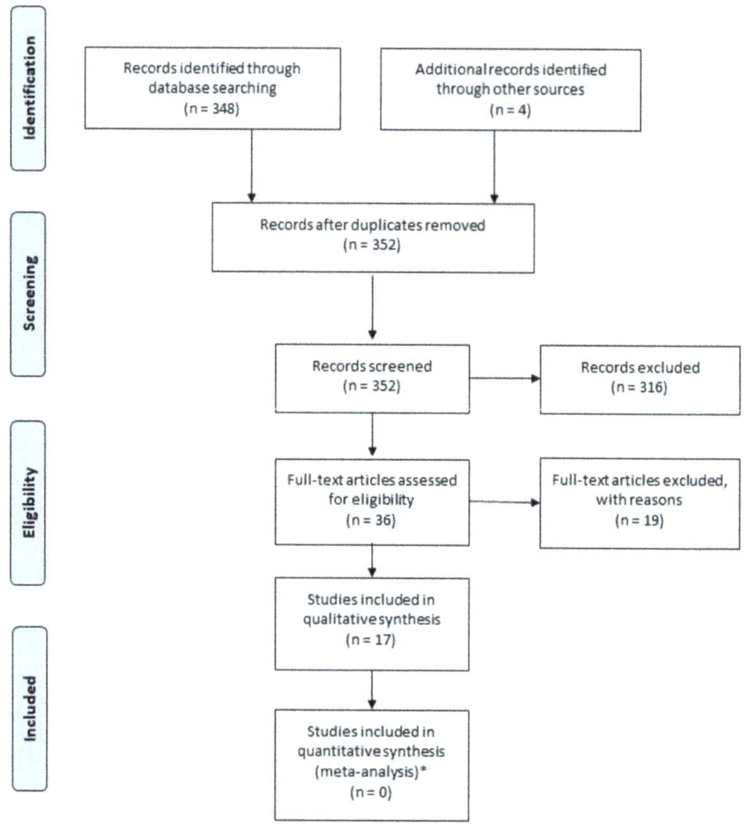

Fig. 1 Flowchart of screening and identification process

analysis focuses on the impact of LOPD on humanistic burden, and is structured according to the predefined research questions outlined above.

LOPD is associated with substantial humanistic burden

This section focuses on the overall reported humanistic burden of LOPD, both in the absence and presence of ERT.

HRQoL

Overall HRQoL burden was described in four studies; one in the absence of ERT [32], two among patients treated with ERT [26, 34], and one RCT in which patients were randomized to either placebo or ERT [31]. HRQoL was typically measured using the 36-item Short-Form Survey (SF-36) (Table 1).

Hagemans et al. [32] reported a cross-sectional analysis of the International Pompe Survey in 210 patients with LOPD, prior to approval of ERT. Patients presented with a wide range of disease severity, from the mildly affected to wheelchair- and ventilator-dependent, and reported significantly poorer HRQoL on the physical functioning, physical role functioning, general health, vitality, and social functioning subscales of the SF-36 than the general population ($p < 0.001$ on all scales). The difference was most profound for the physical functioning scale, with an adjusted mean score among patients of 29.3, compared with 83.1 (standard deviation [SD] not reported) in the general population. No significant differences were found for the bodily pain, emotional role functioning, or mental health scales, which, the authors speculated may have reflected the slow progression of limitations in daily activities, allowing patients to adapt over time to their situation and adjust their expectations. In a subset of 38 Dutch patients, the authors compared SF-36 scores at baseline and after 1 year; participants were asked on a 5-point scale whether their physical situation had improved a lot, improved a little, remained the same, deteriorated a little, or deteriorated a lot. Twenty-seven of the 38 participants reported deterioration in their physical situation, while none reported improvement. No significant differences were seen for any of the SF-36 subscales between the two time points. The authors suggested that either changes in the physical situation were not always accompanied by changes in QoL or that, as a generic QoL instrument, the SF-36 was insufficiently sensitive to capture such changes.

van der Ploeg et al. [31] reported data from the Late Onset Treatment Study (LOTS), an RCT of 90 LOPD

Table 2 Basic characteristics of studies reporting on humanistic burden of LOPD

Publication	Quality rating	Study design	Geographic region	Population (sample size)	Disease severity	ERT status
Angelini 2009 [25]	5/9	Prospective cohort	Italy	Symptomatic LOPD patients recruited from three collaborating University Centers ($n = 11$)	Symptomatic (≥2 on the Gardner-Medwin and Walton functional scale)	ERT
Aslan 2016 [26]	6/9	Prospective cohort	Turkey	Subjects with a genetically confirmed diagnosis of LOPD ($n = 8$)	Not stated	ERT
Boentert 2015 [34]	7/9	Cross-sectional	Germany	LOPD patients recruited from specialized outpatient clinics at three neuromuscular centers ($n = 65$)	Not stated (outpatients)	ERT
Freedman 2013 [35]	3/9	Cross-sectional	Australia	LSD patients selected through purposive criterion sampling representing patients receiving ERT to treat a LSD, siblings and parents (9 parents, 4 patients, 3 siblings)	Not stated	ERT
Furusawa 2012 [40]	NA	Case series	Japan	Patients with LOPD who had undergone ERT at the National Center Hospital ($n = 5$)	Wheelchair bound (n = 4) or able to stand for a few minutes (n = 1)	ERT
Güngör 2013 [36]	8/9	Cross-sectional	Germany, Netherlands	LOPD patients recruited through the German patient organization or through Erasmus MC in The Netherlands ($n = 124$)	Full range of severities (mild to fully wheelchair/ ventilator dependent)	ERT
Güngör 2016 [29]	3/9	Prospective cohort	Australia, Canada, France, Germany, Netherlands, US, UK, others	Child and adult Pompe disease patients included through national support groups ($n = 174$)	Full range of severities (mild to fully wheelchair/ ventilator dependent)	ERT-transition (minimum 6 months follow-up before and after ERT)
Hagemans 2007 [33]	5/9	Cross-sectional	Multiple countries	LOPD patients recruited through patient organizations affiliated with the IPA ($n = 257$)	Full range of severities (mild to fully wheelchair/ ventilator dependent)	No ERT
Hagemans 2004 [32]	5/9	Cross-sectional	Australia, Germany, the Netherlands, the UK, the US	LOPD ($n = 210$)	Full range of severities (mild to fully wheelchair/ ventilator dependent)	No ERT
Kanters 2013 [37]	5/9	Cross-sectional	Netherlands	All patients at the Center for Lysosomal and Metabolic diseases in Rotterdam receiving informal care plus one caregiver per patient (67 patients; 67 informal caregivers)	Range	ERT
Karabul 2014a [38]	3/9	Cross-sectional	UK	Adult LOPD patients ($n = 25$)	Not stated	ERT
Karabul 2014b [39]	6/9	Cross-sectional	Germany	Adult LOPD patients ($n = 73$)	Not stated	ERT
Regnery 2012 [27]	5/9	Prospective cohort	Germany	Adult LOPD patients from university-based centers ($n = 38$)	Various	ERT
Strothotte 2010 [28]	6/9	Prospective cohort	Germany	LOPD patients treated in participating German university-based centers ($n = 44$)	Various	ERT
	5/9	Case series	Netherlands			ERT

Table 2 Basic characteristics of studies reporting on humanistic burden of LOPD *(Continued)*

Publication	Quality rating	Study design	Geographic region	Population (sample size)	Disease severity	ERT status
Van Capelle 2008 [41]				Two severely affected LOPD patients and one moderately affected LOPD patient ($n = 3$)	Moderate ($n = 1$) to severe ($n = 2$)	
van der Meijden 2015 [30]	7/9	Prospective cohort	Australia, Canada, France, Germany, Netherlands, US, UK, others	Child and adult Pompe disease patients included through national support groups ($n = 408$)	Full range of severities (mild to fully wheelchair/ventilator dependent)	ERT-transition
van der Ploeg 2010 [31]	7/9	RCT	US and Europe (eight centers)	LOPD patients, 8 years of age or older, ambulatory, and free of invasive ventilation ($n = 90$)	Range (excluded if invasive ventilation or if required noninvasive ventilation while awake and upright)	ERT

'ERT-transition' studies refer to those initiated before the approval of ERT but continuing into the post-ERT era

Quality rating refers to a quality score assigned to each publication considering characteristics that could introduce bias, using the following tools: 1) Newcastle-Ottawa Scale for cohort studies and case-control studies [22]; 2) Adapted Newcastle-Ottawa Scale for cross-sectional studies [22]; 3) AMSTAR measurement tool for reviews [23]; 4) Cochrane risk of bias assessment tool for randomized controlled trials [24]. The maximum score for the Newcastle-Ottawa Scale is 9

IPA: International Pompe Association; LOPD: Late-onset Pompe disease; LSD: Lysosomal storage disorders; MC: Medical center; RCT: Randomized controlled trial patients aged 8 years or older, ambulatory, and free of invasive ventilation, who received ERT or placebo for 78 weeks. All patients had substantially diminished SF-36 physical component summary (PCS) scores at baseline (ERT-treated patients, 34.3 ± 8.9; placebo-treated patients, 34.9 ± 7.2), which were more than 1.5 SD below the norm for the US general population (50 ± 10). Importantly, despite treatment with ERT, the mean SF-36 PCS score did not increase significantly over the 78-week study ([35.1 ± 9.9], change [95% CI], 0.80 [−1.22 to 2.82]).

Boentert et al. [34] presented a cross-sectional analysis in which 60 of 65 German patients received ERT (mean ERT duration, 5 years), while Aslan et al. [26] described a prospective cohort study of nine Turkish LOPD patients receiving ERT, who participated in an inspiratory muscle training (IMT) program to improve QoL. Boentert et al. stated (without providing quantitative data) that despite ERT, LOPD patients had significantly lower HRQoL than the general population, based on the SF-36 subscales for physical functioning, physical role limitation, general health perception, vitality and social functioning. Aslan et al. also reported impaired HRQoL despite ERT, using the Nottingham Health Profile (NHP), which assesses subjective health status on a scale from 0 (good) to 100 (poor). At baseline, subscales of the NHP ranged from 15.7 for emotional reaction to 82.8 for physical ability. Following implementation of IMT, this study reported improvement in social isolation from 22.5 (interquartile range, 53.8–100.0) to 0.0 (0.0–16.9) ($p = 0.02$), but no other HRQoL subscale demonstrated a treatment response. This led the authors to speculate that participation in the IMT program and the associated weekly telephone contact may have been responsible for the improved social isolation scores.

Patient-reported symptoms

This section describes patient-reported symptoms (PRS) that were reported alongside HRQoL, ADL, caregiver burden, treatment satisfaction and adherence. This is included because studies reporting on humanistic parameters frequently also describe common symptoms of Pompe disease (most notably pain, fatigue, and sleep disorders) with a considerable negative impact on humanistic burden. A systematic review of PRS was beyond the protocol-defined objectives of this review because PRS is typically classified under clinical burden.

Patient-reported symptoms were discussed in two publications in the absence of ERT [30, 32], and five publications in the presence of ERT [26, 34, 36, 38, 39]. In Hagemans et al. [32], where no ERT was available, excessive daytime sleepiness (EDS) was reported in approximately 25% of patients and sleep disturbances were reported in more than 40% of patients. In a later analysis of the same study, van der Meijden et al. [30] found that 78% of patients experienced fatigue (Fatigue Severity Scale [FSS] score ≥ 4), and 67% reported severe fatigue (FSS score ≥ 5).

Patients receiving ERT also had poor sleep quality, as assessed by Aslan et al. [26] using the Pittsburgh Sleep Quality Index (PSQI) to measure the quality and patterns of sleep during the previous four weeks. Among these patients, there was a median (interquartile range) total score of 5.0 (2.0–10.5; a cut off score of 5 or more distinguishes 'bad sleepers'). Introduction of IMT did not improve sleep quality. Boentert et al. [34] also reported sleep symptoms, noting that 45.2% of patients were bad sleepers according to the PSQI (mean PSQI global score, 6.2 ± 3.7). Scores for sleep disturbances, sleep quality impairment and reduced daytime performance were the highest of the PSQI component scales. EDS was reported by 24.6% of patients (mean ESS, 6.9 ± 4.3).

In addition, Boentert et al. also presented respiratory symptoms, reporting that morning headache was reported by 40.0% of patients ('occasional' 35.4%; 'often' 4.6%) [34]. Nocturnal dyspnea was specified as 'occasional' by 18.5% of patients and as 'often' by 6.2%. Orthopnea was reported by 60.0% of patients, resting dyspnea in the upright position by 4.6%, and exertional dyspnea by 93.8% of patients. Dyspnea was reported in 29.2%, 40.0% and 24.6% of patients on mild, moderate and heavy exercise, respectively.

A cross-sectional study in 57 German adult LOPD patients (84% on ERT) and 57 controls reported the impact of urge incontinence and gastrointestinal symptoms [39]. In this study, stool urgency, diarrhea, and urinary urge incontinence were reported significantly more frequently in patients compared with the age- and gender-matched controls (55%, 56%, 33% vs. 20%, 18%, 7%).

In a cross-sectional analysis from Germany and the Netherlands from the International Pompe Survey, Güngör et al. [36] assessed the presence and severity of pain in 124 adult LOPD patients, 101 of whom were receiving ERT (median ERT duration, 4 years). They noted that a significantly greater proportion of ERT-treated LOPD patients reported pain compared with unaffected controls (45% vs. 27%, respectively; $p = 0.004$) on the Brief Pain Inventory (BPI) (Short-Form). In this study, the median pain severity score (PSS) – calculated from the BPI (Table 1) – was higher (worse) among patients than controls reporting pain in the previous 24 h (median PSS 3.1 [range 0.75–8] vs. 2.6, [range 0.75–5.25], respectively; $p = 0.06$). Similarly, the pain interference score (PIS; also calculated from BPI), was significantly higher (worse) in patients than controls (median PIS 3.3 [range 0–8.4] vs. 1.3 [range 0–4.4] respectively; $p = 0.001$). Pain particularly interfered (PIS score ≥ 4) with patients' general activities, walking, and normal work, and showed a mild interference (PIS score ≥ 3) with mood, sleep, and enjoyment of life. For each of the seven domains of daily life, PIS scores were significantly worse in LOPD patients than controls, except for interference with sleep. The authors concluded that while pain is not the most prominent symptom of Pompe disease, it is a common and debilitating aspect of the disease that merits identification and management in this population.

In a follow-up to this study, the same group surveyed 25 patients from the UK using the long-form of BPI, which assesses pain over the previous 7 days [38]. This study reported that 88% of patients reported pain in the last week, a considerably higher proportion than the 45% reporting current pain in Güngör et al. [36]. Median PSS (3.9 [0.5–7.5] vs 3.1 [0.75–8.0]) and median PIS (3.9 [0–7.5] vs 3.3 [0–8.4]) were only slightly higher (worse) in this paper than in the publication by Güngör et al. [36, 38]. These data reinforce the troublesome nature of pain in LOPD.

ADL

The International Pompe Survey is the primary source of data on ADL burden [33]. This cross-sectional analysis was conducted in 257 patients with treatment-naïve LOPD (across a broad range of severity) with a median age of onset of 38 years. The impact of LOPD on participation in ADL was assessed using the Rotterdam Handicap Scale (RHS). The mean RHS score among patients in this study was 25.9 ± 6.5 (median, 27), compared with a maximum of 36, which would be scored by a healthy person. Mean RHS scores ranged from 25.5 in Germany to 27.7 in France, but the differences between countries were not statistically significant. Highest scores (reflecting least restrictions) were found for 'mobility indoors' and 'leisure activities indoors', while the lowest scores were found for 'domestic tasks indoors', 'domestic tasks outdoors', and 'work/study'. The authors suggested that their findings demonstrate the considerable impact of Pompe disease on patients' everyday life experiences.

Caregiver burden

One publication so far examined caregiver burden in LOPD [37]. This Dutch study was conducted among 67 patients with LOPD and their caregivers. Caregivers were most often partners (92%), while for children, parents were generally the primary caregivers (94%). Fifty-nine of the 67 patients were receiving ERT.

Caregivers provided about 17.7 h per week of informal care, with some variation (SD 27.5) [37]. Adults primarily received maintenance for household activities (48% of time) and only limited for personal care (18%). In pediatric patients, informal care given as personal care (32% of time) and social activities (36%) was most significant. No caregiver time was spent on specific nursing activities in both age groups. Informal care was provided at the expense of the caregiver's leisure or work time. The majority (97%) of caregivers gained 'some satisfaction', while up to 60% gained a 'lot of fulfillment' for providing care. 50% of caregivers reported mental health problems, while 40% had physical health problems. The average burden for caregivers was 3.2 (range, 0.0 to 8.9), measured on a self-rated Visual Analog Scale (VAS, ranging from 0 [not at all straining] to 10 [too much straining]). The mean burden of caregiving for patients below the age of 18 years was higher than for adults (4.1 versus 2.9 respectively; $p = 0.075$). Caregiver burden for patients with LOPD was relatively mild and well-being was not far below the population norms.

Strong inter-relationships exist among humanistic burden parameters

Beyond humanistic burden overall, the association between individual parameters of humanistic burden was also investigated. Data on these relationships in the absence and presence of ERT are taken primarily from the four studies, previously described [33, 34, 36, 37].

Poorer HRQoL is associated with increased fatigue, reduced sleep quality, and increased pain

In Boentert et al. [34], fatigue among ERT-treated LOPD patients was assessed using the FSS and sleep quality was measured using the PSQI. In this analysis, the PCS and MCS of the SF-36 were both inversely correlated with the FSS score (PCS, $r = -0.46$, $p < 0.001$; MCS, $r = -0.44$, $p < 0.01$) and the PSQI global score (PCS, $r = -0.38$, $p < 0.001$; MCS, −0.47, p < 0.001). In terms of the impact of pain on HRQoL, Güngör et al. [36] reported that ERT-treated patients with pain had significantly lower physical (median PCS score 30 [range, 11–45] vs. 35 [range, 17–58], respectively; p < 0.001) and mental HRQoL (median MCS scores 54 [range, 29–74] vs. 58 [range, 29–71], respectively; $p = 0.049$) than those without pain.

Poorer HRQoL (except the mental health domain) is associated with greater functional disability

The relationship between the RHS and the SF-36 was investigated in the absence of ERT by Hagemans et al. [33]. The RHS correlated significantly with all SF-36 subscales except for the mental health domain. The largest positive correlation of RHS ($r = 0.83$, $p < 0.001$) was found with the physical functioning subscale of SF-36.

Poorer HRQoL is associated with greater caregiver burden

Kanters et al. [37] reported a significant, inverse correlation between patient HRQoL and both caregiver burden and the volume of care provided (rho = −0.430

and rho = −0.465, respectively; $p < 0.001$ in both cases) in ERT-treated patients. Patients with the lowest HRQoL (lowest quartile) received 35.1 h of care per week, with a caregiver burden of 5.3 on the self-rated burden scale, whereas patients with HRQoL in the highest quartile received only 3.9 h of care per week, with a lower caregiver burden of 2.3 on the self-rated scale.

Greater functional disability is associated with greater fatigue, poorer sleep quality, and increased pain

Boentert et al. [34] found that the functional ability of ERT-treated patients (measured using RHS) was inversely correlated with fatigue (FSS, $r = -0.40$, $p < 0.01$) and sleep disturbance, (PSQI, $r = -0.46$, p < 0.001). Similarly, Güngör et al. [36] reported that ERT-treated patients with pain had lower functional abilities based on median RHS scores than those without pain (26 [range, 15–36] vs. 28 [range, 16–36], respectively; $p = 0.02$).

Greater sleep disturbance is correlated with increased fatigue

Boentert et al. [34] reported, unsurprisingly, that PSQI global score was positively correlated with FSS score ($r = 0.33$, $p = 0.01$) in the presence of ERT, indicating that fatigue increased with greater sleep disturbance.

Increased pain is associated with increased depression and anxiety

Güngör et al. [36] found that ERT-treated patients with pain had significantly higher levels of depression and anxiety than those without pain. Anxiety and depression were measured using the median Hospital Anxiety and Depression Scale (HADS), with higher scores indicating greater anxiety or depression. HADS anxiety score among patients reporting pain was 5 (range, 0–15) compared with 3 (range, 0–12) among patients with no pain ($p = 0.003$), while the HADS depression score was 5 (range, 0–13) and 3 (range, 0–12) for patients with and without pain, respectively ($p = 0.005$).

Clinical progression of disease is strongly associated with greater humanistic burden

We investigated the impact of clinical progression on humanistic burden using data from four studies described previously [32–34, 37].

Wheelchair use is associated with decreased HRQoL, greater functional disability, and greater caregiver burden

Hagemans et al. [32] found that wheelchair use is associated with lower HRQoL and ADL scores. In their 2004 study, untreated patients who used a wheelchair scored on average 23.6 points lower on the physical functioning scale and 15.1 points lower on the social functioning scale of the SF-36 than patients who did not need a wheelchair (regression coefficient (B) = −23.6 and −15.1, $p < 0.001$) [32]. In their 2007 study, Hagemans et al. [33] reported significantly lower mean RHS scores in patients who used a wheelchair than those who did not (20.9 vs. 29.5, respectively; p < 0.001).

Kanters et al. [37] reported that ERT-treated wheelchair users received significantly more hours of informal care than patients who were not wheelchair-dependent (25.6 h vs. 14.0 h, respectively; p < 0.001). As such, caregiver burden was significantly higher (self-rated scale, 5.1 vs. 2.4, respectively; $p = 0.002$) and caregiver well-being was significantly lower (CarerQoL-VAS, 6.4 vs. 7.5, respectively; $p = 0.024$) for patients who used a wheelchair than those who did not.

Increased respiratory distress is associated with poorer HRQoL, greater functional disability, and greater sleep disturbance and fatigue

An association between increased respiratory symptoms and poorer HRQoL (both physical and mental components) among ERT-treated patients was reported by Boentert et al. [34]. Respiratory symptoms were quantified using the respiratory symptoms questionnaire (RSQ), in which a low score indicates less frequent respiratory symptoms. Both the PCS score and the MCS score were negatively correlated with the RSQ score (PCS, $r = -0.25$, $p < 0.05$; MCS, $r = -0.46$, $p < 0.001$). This finding is consistent with data from untreated patients reported by Hagemans et al. [32], in which reduced respiratory distress was significantly associated with higher HRQoL.

Boentert et al. [34] also found that higher levels of respiratory distress were associated with greater sleep disturbance, as demonstrated by a positive correlation between PSQI and RSQ scores ($r = 0.43$, $p < 0.0001$). Fatigue, measured using the FSS, was also positively associated with respiratory distress, assessed using the RSQ ($r = 0.58$, p < 0.0001), while respiratory distress and functional ability were inversely related, with RHS scores strongly associated with both upright and supine forced vital capacity (FVC) ($r = 0.62$ and $r = 0.69$, respectively, $p < 0.001$). Similar findings were observed in the absence of ERT, with Hagemans et al. [32] reporting that the need for home ventilatory support was associated with lower physical functioning scores (B = −8.4, $p = 0.004$), and that mean RHS scores were significantly lower in patients receiving respiratory support than those without it (22.9 vs. 28.5, p < 0.001). Among the patients who used respiratory support, the correlation between the number of hours of ventilation and the RHS score was −0.59 (p < 0.001), suggesting a reduction in functional ability with increasing use of ventilation. Consistent with this, in this study, almost all patients requiring more than 12 h of ventilation per day required a wheelchair.

Cardiopulmonary distress is associated with increased fatigue in male patients

Boentert et al. [34] assessed the relationship between fatigue and "cardiopulmonary distress" in patients receiving ERT, as measured using the 6MWT and FVC. It should be noted that 6MWT and FVC are not direct measures of cardiopulmonary distress; the 6MWT in particular reflects various aspects of physical functioning and may be influenced by cardiac function, walking ability, and respiratory muscle strength. The FSS score was inversely correlated with the 6MWT ($r = -0.35$, $p < 0.01$) (meaning that patients with more severe fatigue performed less well on the 6MWT), but surprisingly, this negative correlation was only apparent in the male subgroup ($r = -0.53$, $p < 0.01$), indicating that fatigue in female patients may be independent of motor performance.

ERT is associated with short-term stabilization of humanistic burden

Here, we consider the impact of ERT on the principal aspects of humanistic burden. No data describing the impact of ERT on caregiver burden were identified.

HRQoL

Seven articles describe the impact of ERT on HRQoL in LOPD (Table 2) [25, 27–29, 31, 35, 39]: van der Ploeg et al. (2010) reported results from LOTS [31] (discussed above); Güngör et al. [29] evaluated 174 untreated patients who transitioned to ERT during the study; Angelini et al. [25] describe clinical response and changes in functional ability in a prospective cohort study of 11 adult patients; Strothotte et al. [28] and Regnery et al. [27] report data from an open-label observational trial in 44 and 38 adult patients, respectively, in Germany over periods of 12 and 36 months Freedman et al. [35] present a cross-sectional analysis of seven families of young patients (age not specified) with LOPD in Australia, using semi-structured interviews; and van Capelle [41] reports a case series of two children and one adult with LOPD treated with ERT in the Netherlands.

As reported earlier, van der Ploeg et al. found that untreated patients with LOPD had lower SF-36 scores at baseline, which did not improve significantly over 78 weeks' treatment with ERT [31]. Similarly, Güngör et al. [29], evaluated PCS and MCS components of the SF-36 during three time periods: pre-ERT, first 2 years of ERT, and after more than 2 years of ERT. Before ERT, the PCS decreased significantly by 0.73 score points per year (sp/y). This was followed in the first 2 years after treatment by a significant increase of 1.49 sp./y, and by stabilization thereafter. The MCS was generally stable during the entire follow-up period. Throughout treatment follow-up, the physical functioning, physical role, general health and vitality domains improved, with particularly large increases during the first 2 years of ERT in physical role (9 sp./y), general health (5 sp./y) and vitality (4 sp./y), and a renewed decline thereafter. Mental health domain scores increased in the first 2 years of ERT (2 sp./y), and then declined, while social functioning and emotional role did not improve with treatment. The authors noted that the initiation of ERT halted the progressive decline in physical health status observed in the pre-treatment period, and argued that improvements in the physical functioning and physical role domains may be attributed to the positive effect of ERT on muscle function and strength reported in other studies.

A small prospective Italian study [25], described the clinical response and changes in functional ability in 11 adult patients (age at onset 15–42 years), although results of SF-36 testing are reported in only three patients: one had a mild improvement of mental health but not of bodily pain; the second had no improvement in mental health or role physical; and no HRQoL data are available for the third patient who stopped treatment after 3 months following ERT-related adverse events. These limited data are consistent with the open-label observational study of adult patients (mean age at onset 36 years) in Germany [27, 28]. Here, patients showed no significant longitudinal changes in HRQoL over the course of either 12 or 36 months of ERT treatment [27, 28]. The authors concluded that ERT stabilizes the chronic progressive natural disease course of LOPD in some patients, although motor performance and lung function still appear to decline in up to a third [27, 28].

Freedman et al. [35] reported on a cross-sectional study that used qualitative interviews to assess ERT response. They concluded that improved physical health resulted in increased psychosocial well-being. A benefit of ERT was also found by van Capelle et al. [41] in SF-36 sub-domains for two of three patients for whom these data were reported: one patient showed improvements on the physical health and, to a lesser extent, on the mental health domains, while the other showed particular improvements on the bodily pain and general health domains (no further details provided). The methodology of these studies (e.g., small sample size and reliance on qualitative interviews) limits interpretation and generalizability of their results.

Patient-reported symptoms

Data on the impact of ERT on fatigue and pain were identified from the following four publications on humanistic burden, as described above [25, 29, 30, 41].

Fatigue In a 10-year analysis of the International Pompe Survey evaluating 163 patients who transitioned to ERT during the study [30], the proportion of patients reporting fatigue (FSS ≥4) fell from 85% at baseline to 79% at the last follow-up (*p*-value not reported); the proportion who were severely fatigued (FSS ≥5) fell from 68% to 55% (p-value not reported). Fatigue improved mainly in women, patients aged 45 years or older, and those with a disease duration less than 15 years. Improvement in fatigue with length of ERT treatment was also reported by van Capelle et al. [41] among two of three patients studied.

Pain Güngör et al. [29] found that bodily pain worsened in the years prior to ERT initiation, then improved for 2 years during ERT, before declining again after 2 years. Interestingly, the authors also calculated the expected bodily pain scores at three timepoints (4 years before ERT, at start of ERT, and after 4 years of ERT) and reported that the scores were more favorable than population norms at all timepoints. No further details of this analysis are provided. Data from Angelini et al. [25] were available for two of the three patients who completed SF-36 questionnaires; one reported mild improvement in bodily pain on ERT initiation, while the second reported no improvement.

In a clinical survey study, 45% of 124 LOPD patients receiving long-term ERT (median ERT duration, 4 [0.07–12] years) reported having had pain in the previous 24 h, versus 27% of healthy adult controls ($p = 0.004$) [36]. Among patients who reported pain, the median PSS was 3.1 (indicating mild pain) and the median PIS was 3.3 (indicating mild interference); these compare with scores of 2.6 ($p = 0.06$) and 1.3 ($p = 0.001$) for PSS and PIS, respectively, in controls. Relative to patients without pain, those with pain had lower RHS scores ($p = 0.02$), lower SF-36 Physical and Mental component summary scores ($p < 0.001$ and $p = 0.049$), and higher levels of depression and anxiety ($p = 0.005$ and $p = 0.003$). In this largest study on pain, nearly one in two LOPD patients had experienced pain in the previous 24 h. Although pain severity and its interference with daily life was mild, pain was related to a lower QoL, reduced participation in daily life, and greater depression and anxiety. Pain management should therefore be seen as part of clinical practice involving Pompe patients [36].

ADL

The impact of ERT on patients' ability to perform ADL was reported in three studies, including Güngör et al. [29] and van Capelle et al. [41] described previously. In addition, information is taken from a Japanese case series of five long-term, ventilator-dependent patients with advanced LOPD (mean age of onset, 22 years), which examined the efficacy of ERT over a 2-year period [40].

In the International Pompe Survey [29], RHS scores decreased significantly by a mean of 0.49 sp./y (95% CI, −0.63 to −0.34) before ERT initiation and stabilized during ERT treatment (−0.02 sp./y; 95% CI, −0.17 to 0.13). No formal statistical comparisons between the two time periods were provided for ADL. Subgroup analyses showed that overall, RHS scores were better in less severely affected than in more severely affected patients, but the effects of ERT on the ADL of these subgroups did not differ. Van Capelle et al. [41] reported improved RHS scores over time for two of three adults receiving ERT (from 16 and 18 after 3 years of ERT to 25 and 20, respectively, after 8 years). Finally, Furusawa et al. [40] assessed the impact of ERT on patient ADL through interviews with patients and their families. Qualitatively, the authors reported that all patients showed some improvements in ADL and in muscle function, while they also argued that ERT elicited improvements in walking distance and stabilization of pulmonary function. The authors speculated that the improved muscle strength resulted in the better ADL and HRQoL during the follow-up period; however, no quantitative analysis was provided to support this.

Discussion

Overview

Pompe disease is a rare and devastating condition for both patients and their families. The clinical burden of Pompe disease, including impact on survival and physical function, has been reviewed elsewhere [4–6, 8]; however, no systematic review on the humanistic burden of Pompe disease has been published. Here, we present the findings from 17 published papers and systematically describe the humanistic burden of Pompe disease.

A major finding of this review is the complete absence of data on the humanistic burden of IOPD, precluding any discussion in this area. Further, although 17 publications describe the humanistic burden of LOPD, only two of these report studies conducted in the absence of ERT, leaving a deficiency in information on untreated patients. However, the association of LOPD with the many measures of clinical, functional, social and emotional well-being that comprise the humanistic burden is reasonably well documented, confirming the impact of LOPD on the everyday life of patients and their caregivers. Although the overall burden of LOPD is substantial for patients, it is interesting to note that the impact on caregivers reported in an isolated study [37] appears to be relatively modest. This may be because families do not consider it burdensome to care for loved ones [42–44], or it may reflect adaptation to their family condition; LOPD is a slowly progressive, heterogeneous disease, and the context may be similar to other chronic disorders or neuromuscular diseases, where caregivers and patients adjust their expectations and priorities over time. This reinforces the need to robustly study the impact of caring on families, and underscores the importance of examining and understanding patients' and caregivers' perspectives on the burden of illness, alongside traditional clinical and economic investigations.

Our review demonstrates that clinical disease progression is strongly associated with greater humanistic burden, and also shows strong correlations among individual humanistic burden parameters such as HRQoL, ADL, and caregiver burden. Importantly, ERT does not substantially improve this. Figure 2 (and its accompanying key) provides a graphical illustration of correlations between humanistic and clinical burden parameters in LOPD patients receiving ERT. Unsurprisingly, deterioration in one parameter is strongly linked to deterioration in another, and continues despite ERT. Although ERT provides some benefit, the results appear to be modest, and patients remain below population norms.

This ongoing burden of Pompe disease despite ERT may be partly due, not only to the variety of muscle groups affected, but also to pathology of the CNS and PNS [1–3]. However, presently only brain autopsies in untreated patients have shown clear evidence of glycogen storage in the CNS [45, 46], and periventricular white matter abnormalities on brain magnetic resonance imaging (MRI) have been seen in children receiving ERT [1]. Measuring the effects of CNS pathology on cognitive function is confounded by co-occurring hearing loss, speech muscle pathology, and fine motor dysfunction; however, it is clear from emerging signs and symptoms, which may be caused by neuronal glycogen deposition, that ERT is unable to address all aspects of the disease at least in infants with Pompe disease [3, 47–51]. While ERT clearly slows disease progression for many patients, available data demonstrate that it is limited in its ability to improve and maintain clinical symptomatology and associated disease burden in the long term. The reasons for this are not fully understood, but given that improvements in one facet of the disease burden are expected to positively influence others, there is still substantial potential for enriching patients' lives beyond the response currently achieved with ERT.

Evidence indicates that ERT leads to short-term improvement and a mid-term stabilization of HRQoL, although results have not been shown to persist in the long-term so far. For example, in one study, there was no improvement in mean SF-36 PCS scores over 78 weeks of treatment with ERT [31], while another found that although ERT reversed a decline in SF-36 PCS, the benefit plateaued after 2 years without

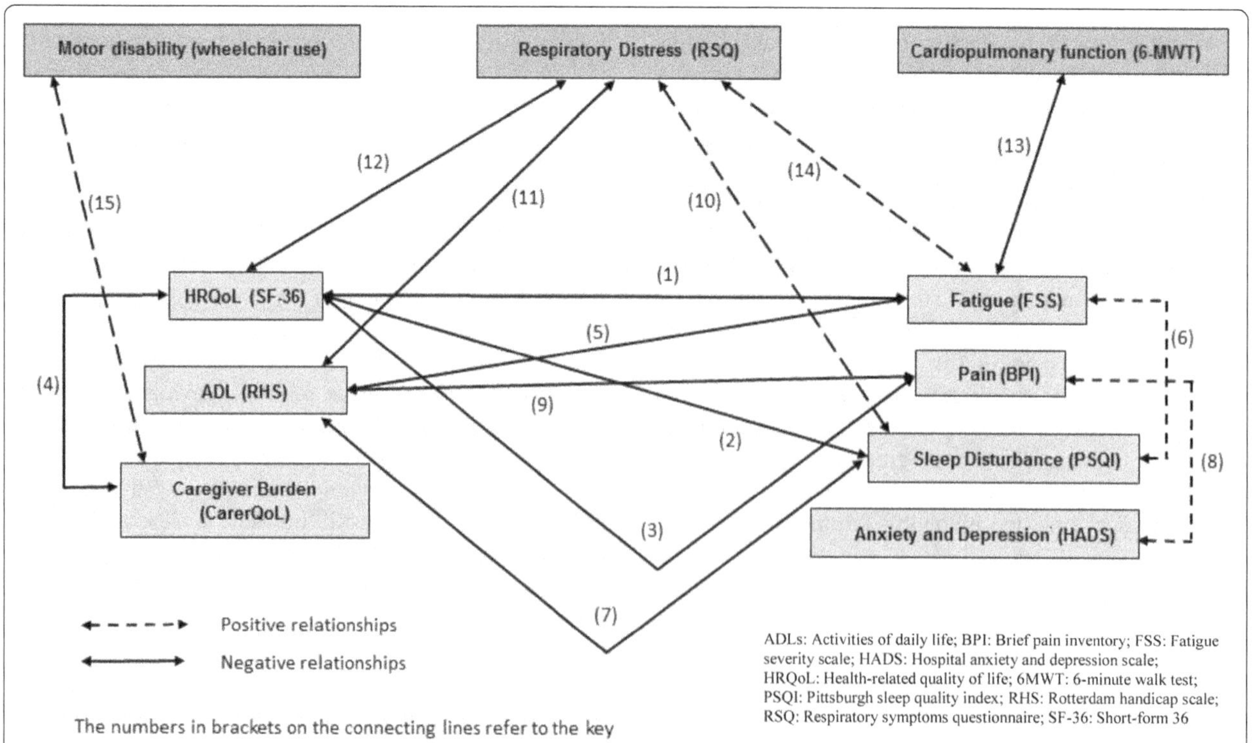

Fig. 2 Inter-relationships between clinical, humanistic and economic burden parameters in LOPD patients receiving ERT

normalizing; ERT appears to halt the decline in patients' ability to perform ADL, but reports on ERT's association with improved functioning are mixed [29, 40, 41]. As such, gaps remain in providing treatment options that treat the underlying disease, improve clinical symptomatology, and positively affect patients' abilities to lead normal lives.

It is interesting to note that pain was reported by a number of patients and interfered with their general activities, walking, and normal work, as well as mood, sleep and enjoyment of life [36]. While ERT temporarily stabilized bodily pain, it did not reverse it; in fact, after 2 years of ERT, pain began to worsen once again [29]. The reason for this is not clear, but could be due to neuronal deposition of glycogen, which cannot be cleared by ERT [16, 17]. Given the substantial impact pain has on people's lives, further investigation is warranted.

Gaps and limitations

Orphan diseases are hampered by lack of information within the medical community and the scientific literature [52], and this is also true for our topic of review, the humanistic burden of Pompe disease. For the most severely affected patients – those with IOPD – the humanistic burden of is unexplored, preempting any comparisons between IOPD and LOPD. For LOPD, data on the humanistic burden are comparatively extensive, although significant gaps remain. Data were most robust for HRQoL, the majority of which were generated after ERT approval in 2006. There were very limited longitudinal data on the progression of HRQoL, ADL and caregiver burden in LOPD in both the presence and absence of ERT, and no data on change in caregiver burden on the introduction of ERT. In addition, across the entire spectrum of disease severity, there are no data on patient adherence and satisfaction with ERT.

Few studies examining humanistic burden parameters were conducted before marketing approval was granted for ERT, and their limited depth and breadth merit consideration when interpreting this analysis. Similarly, there is no published literature on patients who discontinued ERT therapy, resulting in a lack of understanding of how this affects patients. Data quality also limits this systematic review; due to the rarity of Pompe disease, many of the published studies are small, cross-sectional, and lack the statistical robustness required to draw firm conclusions. In addition, based on the screening criteria employed, publications including relevant data only in the body of the report but not in the title or the abstract may have been overlooked, although attempts were made to mitigate this through back-referencing and supplementary searches. Finally, the possibility of double or triple reported subjects cannot be excluded.

Avenues for future research

The introduction of ERT into the Pompe disease treatment paradigm has reduced mortality and progression. Nonetheless, the burden of the disease remains high, and while the improved survival of many patients has led to a shift in the 'natural history' to modified disease stages and phenotypes, it has not led to a cure [6, 53]. Indeed, it is clear that ERT is unable to address all aspects of this disease, particularly in terms of those etiologies associated with neuronal glycogen deposition [3, 47–51]. Crucially, substantial morbidity persists, and, particularly in infants, mortality rates remain high at 28–43% [53–56]. Beyond an initial improvement, most patients continue to decline, albeit at a slower rate than untreated patients, and remain below population norms [29]. Due to the time required to administer infusions, ERT by itself is considered burdensome to patients and caregivers [57]; whether this affects patient adherence and satisfaction would also provide more context to the understanding of the overall burden of Pompe disease.

Retrospective studies are generally inadequate for collection of patient-reported humanistic data, such as HRQoL, which are associated with significant recall bias and limited to the preceding few weeks. It is important to note that the young ages of patients with IOPD necessitates the use of caregiver-reported instruments to accurately reflect the range and severity of the burden across the spectrum of the disease; however, such 'observer-reported outcomes' are themselves associated with bias. In addition, as the delay from diagnosis to treatment shortens, it is becoming increasingly difficult to capture the experience of untreated patients; in order to do this; it is likely to be necessary to study patients in countries that do not have access to ERT. Future collaborations with existing prospective studies, such as the International Pompe Survey and the Pompe Registry, may possibly enable further investigation of the impact of ERT on the overall disease burden. However, to understand the humanistic burden in detail, a long-term observational study, focused specifically on the humanistic burden of Pompe disease, may be necessary.

Alternative therapeutic approaches

There are alternative therapies under development for Pompe disease that, if successful, may help address the unmet medical need and the ongoing burden on the everyday lives of patients and their families. These include second generation ERTs that aim to improve targeting and extracellular uptake of the recombinant protein, either alone or in combination with pharmacological chaperones, to improve bioavailability and reduce immunogenicity. Oligonucleotide therapeutics in the form of mRNA-delivered GAA or exon-including antisense RNA (for c.32-13 T > G splice site mutations in late-onset patients) are in development [58–60]. Furthermore, gene therapies (in vivo adeno-associated virus [AAV] and Adenovirus, and ex vivo Lentivirus) are another route of treatment, seeking to continuously and endogenously produce GAA in target tissues and possibly minimize anti-GAA immunogenicity [61–64].

Thus, these new approaches may have the potential to substantially improve patients' clinical and humanistic burden of disease, by resolving signs, symptoms and progression previously resistant to treatment and thereby improving patients' HRQoL and ability to perform ADL. Given the increasing recognition of the importance of understanding and capturing the patient experience from patient and medical communities, as well as regulatory and reimbursement authorities, it will be key for new therapies to demonstrate not only their ability to treat the clinical signs and symptoms, but also to improve the day-to-day lives of patients and their families [65–68].

Conclusions

This systematic review demonstrates that LOPD has a substantial humanistic burden that is clearly associated with clinical disease progression; patients with more severe disease have increased fatigue, more pain, poorer QoL, and less ability to perform ADL. Although ERT has been shown to provide some benefit, patients remain well below population norms. While there is a reasonable amount of research published for LOPD, gaps remain, including a complete absence of information on treatment satisfaction or adherence, and little information on the humanistic burden in the absence of ERT. For IOPD, the lack of any published articles on the humanistic burden represents a significant gap in the understanding of the most severely affected patients. As such, these findings point to an ongoing unmet need in the understanding of Pompe disease. As new therapies are developed, it will be critical to capture patients' experiences and to further study the effect that the disease, as well as the treatment, has on both the clinical and humanistic aspects of Pompe disease [69]. Only in this way, will we be able to fully understand the effect that Pompe disease – and any potential treatments – have on the overall lives of patients and their families.

Abbreviations

6-MWT: 6-min walking test; AAV: Adeno-associated virus; ADL: Activities of daily living; BPI: Brief pain inventory; CNS: Central nervous system; EDS: Excessive daytime sleepiness; ERT: Enzyme-replacement therapy; FSS: Fatigue severity scale; FVC: Forced vital capacity; GI: Gastrointestinal; GSDII: Glycogen storage disease type II; HADS: Hospital anxiety and depression scale; HRQoL: Health-related quality of life; ICIQ-B-LF: International Consultation on Incontinence Questionnaire Bowel-Long Form; ICIQ-UI-SF: International Consultation on Incontinence Questionnaire Urinary Incontinence-Short Form; IMT: Inspiratory muscle training; IOPD: Infant onset Pompe disease; IPA: International Pompe Association; LOPD: Late-onset Pompe disease; LOTS: Late Onset Treatment Study; LSD: Lysosomal storage disease; MC: Medical center; MCS: Mental component score; MRI: Magnetic resonance imaging; NHP: Nottingham Health Profile; PCS: Physical component score; PIS: Pain interference score; PSQI: Pittsburgh Sleep Quality Index; PSS: Pain severity score; RCT: Randomized controlled trial; RHS: Rotterdam Handicap Scale; RSQ: Respiratory symptoms questionnaire; SD: Standard deviation; SF-36: Short-form 36; sp./y: score points per year; UK: United Kingdom; US: United States; VAS: Visual analog scale

Acknowledgements

The authors would like to thank Rachel Danks for assistance with the preparation of this manuscript, and Graeme Fielder and Kendra Bolt for their assistance in describing emerging therapies.

Funding

The literature review and editorial assistance for the manuscript was funded by Audentes Therapeutics. The funding body was not involved in the design of the study and the data collection and data interpretation.

Authors' contributions

The initial systematic review was performed by DG and reviewed by BS. BS made substantial contributions to conception and design, and interpretation of data. BS, DAB, DD, DG, ESJ, and SP have been involved in data interpretation, drafting of the manuscript and revising it critically for important intellectual content throughout all phases and versions. All authors gave their final approval of the version to be published.

Competing interests

BS is member of the Audentes Therapeutics Board of Scientific and Clinical Advisors. BS has received unrestricted research support, honoraria, and travel funding from Sanofi Genzyme during the past 5 years. BS received honoraria and travel funding as member of the Global Advisory Boards from Biomarin Pharmaceutical, Amicus Therapeutics, and Audentes Therapeutics. DB is a member of the Audentes Therapeutics Board of Scientific and Clinical Advisors. DD is member of the Audentes Therapeutics Board of Scientific and Clinical Advisors. DD has received consulting fees and related expenses from Biomarin, Demeter Therapeutics, Complete Genomics and Illumina during the past 5 years. DD received, through his institution, restricted research grants and related travel funding from Biomarin, Genzyme Sanofi, Hyperion, Alexion and Demeter Therapeutics. EJ and SP are employed by and own stock in Audentes Therapeutics.

Author details

[1]Friedrich-Baur-Institut, Neurologische Klinik und Poliklinik, Klinikum der Universität München, Ludwig-Maximilians-Universität München, Ziemssenstr, D-80336 Munich, Germany. [2]Department of Psychiatry, Division of Child and Adolescent Psychiatry, University of Utah School of Medicine, Salt Lake City, UT, USA. [3]Rady Children's Institute for Genomic Medicine, San Diego, CA 92123, USA. [4]Bridge Medical Consulting Ltd, Gainsborough House, 2 Sheen Road, Richmond, London TW9 1AE, UK. [5]Audentes Therapeutics, 600 California Street, Floor 17, San Francisco, CA 94104, USA.

References

1. Ebbink BJ, Aarsen FK, van Gelder CM, van den Hout JM, Weisglas-Kuperus N, Jaeken J, et al. Cognitive outcome of patients with classic infantile Pompe disease receiving enzyme therapy. Neurology. 2012;78:1512–8.
2. Ebbink BJ, Aarsen FK, van Gelder CM, van den Hout JMP, Weisglas-Kuperus N, Jaeken J, et al. Cognitive outcome of classic infantile Pompe patients receiving enzyme therapy. BMC Musculoskelet Disord. 2013;14(Suppl 2):14.
3. van Gelder CM, van Capelle CI, Ebbink BJ, Moor-van Nugteren I, van den Hout JM, Hakkesteegt MM, et al. Facial-muscle weakness, speech disorders and dysphagia are common in patients with classic infantile Pompe disease treated with enzyme therapy. J Inherit Metab Dis. 2012;35:505–11.

4. Bhengu L, Davidson A, du Toit P, Els C, Gerntholzt T, Govendrageloo K, et al. Diagnosis and management of Pompe disease. S Afr Med. 2014;104:273–4.
5. Chien Y-H, Hwu W-L, Lee N-C. Pompe disease: early diagnosis and early treatment make a difference. Pediatr Neonatol. 2013;54:219–27.
6. Schoser B, Stewart A, Kanters S, Hamed A, Jansen J, Chan K, et al. Survival and long-term outcomes in late-onset Pompe disease following alglucosidase alfa treatment: a systematic review and meta-analysis. J Neurol. 2017;264:621–30.
7. van den Hout HM, Hop W, van Diggelen OP, Smeitink JA, Smit GP. Poll-the BT, et al. the natural course of infantile Pompe's disease: 20 original cases compared with 133 cases from the literature. Pediatrics. 2003;112:332–40.
8. Dasouki M, Jawdat M, Almadhoun O, Pasnnor M, McVey AL, Abuzinadah A, et al. Pompe disease: literature review and case series. Neurol Clin. 2014;32:751–76.
9. Schüller A, Wenninger S, Strigl-Pill N, Schoser B. Toward deconstructing the phenotype of late-onset Pompe disease. Am J Med Genet C Semin Med Genet. 2012;160C:80–8.
10. Boentert M, Florian A, Dräger B, Young P, Yilmaz A. Pattern and prognostic value of cardiac involvement in patients with late-onset Pompe disease: a comprehensive cardiovascular magnetic resonance approach. J Cardiovasc Magn Reson. 2016;18:91.
11. Schoser B, Laforêt P, Kruijshaar ME, Toscano A, van Doorn PA, van der Ploeg AT. European POmpe consortium (EPOC). Minutes of the European POmpe consortium (EPOC) meeting march 27 to 28, 2015, Munich, Germany. Acta Myol. 2015;34:141–3.
12. Ausems MG, Verbiest J, Hermans MP, Kroos MA, Beemer FA, Wokke JH, et al. Frequency of glycogen storage disease type II in The Netherlands: implications for diagnosis and genetic counselling. Eur J Hum Genet. 1999;7:713–6.
13. New 15, Lin CY, Hwang B, Hsiao KJ, Jin YR. Pompe's disease in Chinese and prenatal diagnosis by determination of alpha-glucosidase activity. J Inherit Metab Dis. 1987;10:11–7.
14. Bashan N, Potashnik R, Barash V, Gutman A, Moses SW. Glycogen storage disease type II in Israel. Isr J Med Sci. 1988;24:224–7.
15. Cupler EJ, Berger KI, Leshner RT, Wolfe GI, Han JJ, Barohn RJ, et al. Consensus treatment recommendations for late onset Pompe disease. Muscle Nerve. 2012;45:319–33.
16. ElMallah MK, Falk DJ, Nayak S, Federico RA, Sandhu MS, Poirier A, et al. Sustained correction of motor neuron histopathology following intramuscular delivery of AAV in Pompe mice. Mol Ther. 2014;22:702–12.
17. Falk DJ, Soustek MS, Todd AG, Mah CS, Cloutier DA, Kelley JS, et al. Comparative impact of AAV and enzyme replacement therapy on respiratory and cardiac function in adult Pompe mice. Mol Ther Method Clin Develop. 2015;2:15007.
18. DeRuisseau LR, Fuller DD, Qui K, DeRuisseau KC, Donnelly WH Jr, Mah C, et al. Neural deficits contribute to respiratory insufficiency in Pompe disease. Proc Natl Acad Sci U S A. 2009;106:9419–24.
19. Shea L, Raben N. Autophagy in skeletal muscle: implications for Pompe disease. Int J Clin Pharmacol Ther. 2009;47(Suppl 1):S42–7.
20. Patel TT, Banugaria SG, Case LE, Wenninger S, Schoser B, Kishnani PS. The impact of antibodies in late-onset Pompe disease: a case series and literature review. Mol Genet Metab. 2012;106:301–9.
21. Moher D, Liberati A, Tetzlaff J, Altman DG, PRISMA group. Preferred reporting items for systematic reviews and meta-analyses: the PRISMA statement. PLoS Med. 2009;6:e1000097.
22. Wells G, Shea B, O'Connell D, Peterson J, Welch V, Losos M, et al. The Newcastle-Ottawa scale (NOS) for assessing the quality of nonrandomised studies in meta-analyses. 2013, http://www.ohri.ca/programs/clinical_epidemiology/oxford.asp. Accessed 05 June 2017.
23. Shea BJ, Grimshaw JM, Wells GA, Boers M, Andersson N, Hamel C, et al. Development of AMSTAR: a measurement tool to assess the methodological quality of systematic reviews. BMC Med Res Methodol. 2007;7:10.
24. Higgins JP, Altman DG, Gøtzsche PC, Jüni P, Moher D, Oxman AD, et al. The Cochrane Collaboration's tool for assessing risk of bias in randomised trials. BMJ. 2011;343:d5928.
25. Angelini C, Semplicini C, Tonin P, Filosto M, Pegoraro E, Sorarù G, et al. Progress in enzyme replacement therapy in glycogen storage disease type II. Ther Adv Neurol Disord. 2009;2:143–53.
26. Aslan GK, Huseyinsinoglu BE, Oflazer P, Gurses N, Kiyan E. Inspiratory muscle training in late-onset Pompe disease: the effects on pulmonary function tests, quality of life, and sleep quality. Lung. 2016;194:555–61.
27. Regnery C, Kornblum C, Hanisch F, Vielhaber S, Strigl-Pill N, Grunert B, et al. 36-months observational clinical study of 38 adult Pompe disease patients under alglucosidase alfa enzyme replacement therapy. J Inherit Metab Dis. 2012;35:837–45.
28. Strothotte S, Strigl-Pill N, Grunert B, Kornblum C, Eger K, Wessig C, et al. Enzyme replacement therapy with alglucosidase alfa in 44 patients with late-onset glycogen storage disease type 2: 12-month results of an observational clinical trial. J Neurol. 2010;257:91–7.
29. Güngör D, Kruijshaar ME, Plug I, Rizopoulos D, Kanters TA, Wens SC, et al. Quality of life and participation in daily life of adults with Pompe disease receiving enzyme replacement therapy: 10 years of international follow-up. J Inherit Metab Dis. 2016;39:253–60.
30. van der Meijden JC, Güngör D, Kruijshaar ME, Muir ADJ, Broekgaarden HA, Van Der Ploeg AT. Ten years of the international Pompe survey: patient reported outcomes as a reliable tool for studying treated and untreated children and adults with non-classic Pompe disease. J Inherit Metab Dis. 2015;38:495–503.
31. Van der Ploeg AT, Clemens PR, Corzo D, Escolar DM, Florence J, Groenveld GJ, et al. A randomized study of Alglucosidase alfa in late-onset Pompe's disease. N Engl J Med. 2010;362:1396–406.
32. Hagemans MLC, Janssens ACJW, Winkel LPF, Sieradzan KA, Reuser AJJ, Van Doorn PA, et al. Late-onset Pompe disease primarily affects quality of life in physical health domains. Neurology. 2004;63:1688–92.
33. Hagemans MLC, Laforêt P, Hop WJC, Merkies ISJ, Van Doorn PA, Reuser AJJ, et al. Impact of late-onset Pompe disease on participation in daily life activities: evaluation of the Rotterdam handicap scale. Neuromuscul Disord. 2007;17:537–43.
34. Boentert M, Karabul N, Wenninger S, Stubbe-Dräger B, Mengel E, Schoser B, et al. Sleep-related symptoms and sleep-disordered breathing in adult Pompe disease. Eur J Neurol. 2015;22:369–76.
35. Freedman R, Sahhar M, Curnow L, Lee J, Peters H. Receiving enzyme replacement therapy for a lysosomal storage disorder: a preliminary exploration of the experiences of young patients and their families. J Genet Couns. 2013;22:517–32.
36. Güngör D, Schober AK, Kruijshaar ME, Plug I, Karabul N, Deschauer M, et al. Pain in adult patients with Pompe disease: a cross-sectional survey. Mol Genet Metab. 2013;109:371–6.
37. Kanters TA, Van Der Ploeg AT, Brouwer WBF, Hakkaart L. The impact of informal care for patients with Pompe disease: an application of the CarerQol instrument. Mol Genet Metab. 2013;110:281–6.
38. Karabul N, Kruijshaar ME, Schober A, Güngör D, Hanisch F. Pain in adult patients with Pompe disease. Mol Genet Metab Rep. 2014;2:139–40.
39. Karabul N, Skudlarek A, Berndt J, Kornblum C, Kley RA, Wenninger S, et al. Urge incontinence and gastrointestinal symptoms in adult patients with Pompe disease: a cross-sectional survey. JIMD Rep. 2014;17:53–61.
40. Furusawa Y, Mori-Yoshimura M, Yamamoto T, Sakamoto C, Wakita M, Kobayashi Y, et al. Effects of enzyme replacement therapy on five patients with advanced late-onset glycogen storage disease type II: a 2-year follow-up study. J Inherit Metab Dis. 2012;35:301–10.
41. van Capelle CI, Winkel LPF, Hagemans MLC, Shapira SK, Arts WFM, Van Doorn PA, et al. Eight years' experience with enzyme replacement therapy in two children and one adult with Pompe disease. Neuromuscul Disord. 2008;18(6):447–52.
42. Matsumoto H, Clayton-Krasinski DA, Gomez JA, Booker WA, Hyman JE, Roye DP Jr, et al. Development and initial validation of the assessment of caregiver experience with neuromuscular disease. J Pediatr Orthop. 2011;31:284–92.
43. Payot A, Barrington KJ. The quality of life of young children and infants with chronic medical problems: review of the literature. Curr Probl Pediatr Adolesc Health Care. 2011;41:91–101.
44. Chou KR. Caregiver burden: a concept analysis. J Pediatr Nurs. 2000;15:398–407.
45. Shotelersuk V, Shuangshoti S, Chotivitayatarakorn P, Chouwsrikul W, Wattanasirmkit V, Maneesri S, et al. Clinical, pathological, and electron microscopic findings in two Thai children with Pompe disease. J Med Assoc Thail. 2002;85(Suppl 1):S271–9.
46. Martini C, Ciana G, Benettoni A. Intractable fever and cortical neuronal glycogen storage in glycogenosis type 2. Neurology. 2001;57:906–8.
47. Prater SN, Banugaria SG, DeArmey SM, Botha EG, Stege EM, Case LE, et al. The emerging phenotype of long-term survivors with infantile Pompe disease. Genet Med. 2012;14:800–10.

48. Tan QKG, Cheah SM, Dearmey SM, Kishnani PS. Low anal sphincter tone in infantile-onset Pompe disease: an emerging clinical issue in enzyme replacement therapy patients requiring special attention. Mol Genet Metab. 2013;108:142–4.
49. Ebbink BJ, Poelman E, Plug I, Lequin MH, van Doorn PA, Aarsen FK, et al. Cognitive decline in classic infantile Pompe disease: an underacknowledged challenge. Neurology. 2016;86:1260–1.
50. van Capelle CI, Goedegebure A, Homans NC, Hoeve HLJ, Reuser AJ, van der Ploeg AT, et al. Hearing loss in Pompe disease revisited: results from a study of 24 children. J Inherit Metab Dis. 2010;33:597–602.
51. Matsuoka T, Miwa Y, Tajika M, Sawada M, Fujimaki K, Soga T, et al. Divergent clinical outcomes of alpha-glucosidase enzyme replacement therapy in two siblings with infantile-onset Pompe disease treated in the symptomatic or pre-symptomatic state. Mol Genet Metab Rep. 2016;9:98–105.
52. Prasad S, James E. The challenges associated with developing therapies for rare diseases. Br J Med Procur. 2009;1:42–8.
53. Hahn A, Praetorius S, Karabul N, Dießel J, Schmidt D, Motz R, et al. Outcome of patients with classical infantile pompe disease receiving enzyme replacement therapy in Germany. JIMD Rep. 2015;20:65–75.
54. Chakrapani A, Vellodi A, Robinson P, Jones S, Wraith JE. Treatment of infantile Pompe disease with alglucosidase alpha: the UK experience. J Inherit Metab Dis. 2010;33:747–50.
55. Broomfield A, Sweeney MG, Woodward CE, Fratter C, Morris AM, Leonard JV, et al. Paediatric single mitochondrial DNA deletion disorders: an overlapping spectrum of disease. J Inherit Metab Dis. 2015;38:445–57.
56. Kishnani PS, Corzo D, Leslie ND, Gruskin D, van der Ploeg A, Clancy JP, et al. Early treatment with alglucosidase alpha prolongs long-term survival of infants with Pompe disease. Pediatr Res. 2009;66:329–35.
57. Richard E, Douillard-Guilloux G, Caillaud C. New insights into therapeutic options for Pompe disease. Life. 2011;63:979–86.
58. Safdar A, Nilsson M, Akhtar M, Tarnopolsky M. Exosome-mRNA (EXERNA) therapy for Pompe disease. Mol Genet Metab. 2016;117:S100.
59. Bergsma AJ, Van Der Wal E, Pijnappel WWM, der Pleog AT, Reuser AV. Antisense oligonucleotides useful in treatment of Pompe disease. Patent Application. WO 2015190922 A1. 17 December 2015. Available from https://www.google.com/patents/WO2015190922A1. Accessed 05 June 2017.
60. Bergsma AJ, In't Groen SL, Verheijen FW, van der Ploeg AT, Pijnappel WP. From cryptic toward canonical pre-mRNA splicing in Pompe disease: a pipeline for the development of antisense oligonucleotides. Mol Ther Nucleic Acids. 2016;5:e361.
61. Global Information, Inc. Pompe Disease – Pipeline Review, H2 2016. Available from https://www.giiresearch.com/report/labd200991-pompe-disease-pipeline-review-h2.html. Accessed 05 June 2017.
62. Xu F, Ding E, Migone F, Serra D, Schneider A, Chen YT, et al. Glycogen storage in multiple muscles of old GSD-II mice can be rapidly cleared after a single intravenous injection with a modified adenoviral vector expressing hGAA. J Gene Med. 2005;7:171–8.
63. So K, Iizuka S, Kobayashi H, Kimura T, Fukuda T, Shen J, et al. neonatal gene transfer using lentiviral vector for murine Pompe disease: long-term expression and glycogen reduction. Gene Ther. 2010;17:521–30.
64. van Til NP, Stok M, Aerts Kaya FS, de Waard MC, Farahbakhshian E, Visser TP, et al. Lentiviral gene therapy of murine hematopoietic stem cells ameliorates the Pompe disease phenotype. Blood. 2010;115:5329–37.
65. US Food and Drug Administration Guidance for Industry. Patient-reported outcome measures: Use in medical product development to support labeling claims. 2009. Available from https://www.fda.gov/downloads/drugs/guidances/ucm193282.pdf. Accessed 05 June 2017.
66. US Food and Drug Administration Prescription Drug User Fee Act (PDUFA). Enhancing benefit-risk assessment in regulatory decision-making. 2013. Available from https://www.fda.gov/ForIndustry/UserFees/PrescriptionDrugUserFee/ucm326192.htm. Accessed 05 June 2017.
67. US Food and Drug Administration. The voice of the patient: a series of reports from FDAs patient-focused drug development initiative. Updated 2/16/2017. Available from https://www.fda.gov/forindustry/userfees/prescriptiondruguserfee/ucm368342.htm. Accessed 05 June 2017.
68. European Medicines Agency. The patient's voice in the evaluation of medicines. How patients can contribute to assessment of benefit and risk. 18 October 2013. Available from http://www.ema.europa.eu/docs/en_GB/document_library/Report/2013/10/WC500153276.pdf. Accessed 05 June 2017.

15

Glutathione S-transferase M1 and T1 polymorphisms and the risk of mild hepatotoxicity induced by carbamazepine in a tunisian population study

Chahra Chbili[1*], Anis Hassine[1,2], Neila Fathallah[1], Manel Nouira[1], Salma Naija[2], Sofiene Ben Ammou[2] and Saad Saguem[1]

Abstract

Background: The aim of this study was to evaluate whether the glutathione S-transferase M1 (GSTM1) and T1 (GSTT1) null alleles may contribute to carbamazepine-induced hepatotoxicity.

Methods: A cross-sectional prospective study was conducted to identify the frequency distribution of GSTM1 and GSTT1 alleles in 129 Tunisian epileptic patients treated with carbamazepine. Null alleles were determined using a Polymerase Chain Reaction. Serum alanine aminotransferase (ALT) and aspartate aminotransferase (AST) were measured by standard methods.

Results: Our results showed that the frequencies of GSTM1 (–) null allele and GSTT1 null (–) allele were 74.4 and 17.8% respectively. The ALT and AST levels were elevated in 46 (35.7%) and 33 (25.6%) cases. The mean values of ALT and AST were approximately 1.32 and 3.61 times higher than the upper limit of normal levels, respectively. The values of ALT and AST were significantly higher in GSTM1 (–) allele than in GSTM1 (+) ($p = 10^{-3}$.and 0.004, respectively).
The level of ALT was significantly higher in combination of GSTM1 (–)/T1(–) than in combined GSTM1(–)/T1(+) and combined GSTM1(+)/T1(+) ($p = 0.2$ and 0.03, respectively), and that of AST was significantly higher in combination of GSTM1(–)/T1(–) and in combination of GSTM1(+)/T1(–) than in combination of GSTM1(+)/T1(+) ($p = 10^{-3}$ and 10^{-3}, respectively).

Conclusions: Our findings suggest that the GSTM1 (–) allele may be considered as a key factor for the development of carbamazepine-induced hepatotoxicity. Results related to GSTT (–) allele and elevation in AST levels should be considered with caution as AST may be elevated in other pathophysiological conditions.

Keywords: Glutathione-S-transferase M1, Glutathione-S-transferase T1, Epilepsy, Genetic polymorphisms, Carbamazepine

Background

Carbamazepine (CBZ) is an effective drug used for epilepsy, trigeminal neuralgia and many psychiatric disorders [1]. Although considered as a well tolerated anti-epileptic drug, several adverse drug reactions to CBZ may occur including hypersensitivity syndrome, hematotoxicity and hepatotoxicity [2, 3]. Severe CBZ-induced hepatotoxicity is exceptional. Elevation in hepatic enzymes is reported in almost 22% of CBZ-treated patients [4]. Adverse effects to CBZ have been attributed to reactive metabolites of the drug [3, 5]. In fact, in the liver, CBZ is oxidized to its major metabolite, the 10,11-epoxy-carbamazepine (CBZ-E) [6, 7] and to additional metabolites CBZ-arene oxide and CBZ iminoquinone by the cytochrome P450 enzymes [3]. Glutathione S-transferases (GST) are enzymes involved in phase II reactions and playing a key role in detoxifying drugs and xenobiotics. The implication of the metabolites of

* Correspondence: chahra.chbili@yahoo.com
[1]Metabolic Biophysics, Professional Toxicology and Applied Environmental Laboratory, Department of Biophysics, Medicine Faculty of Sousse, Sousse University, Avenue Mohamed Karoui, 4002 Sousse, Tunisia
Full list of author information is available at the end of the article

CBZ has been suggested to induce adverse-drug reactions, cytotoxicity, and also genotoxicity [3, 5].

Both Glutathione S-transferase class mu (GSTM1) and class thêta (GSTT1) are involved in reactions of gluco-conjugation of the main metabolite and also in the detoxification of toxic metabolites of CBZ [3, 7–9]. Null alleles of the GSTM1 and GSTT1 resulting on a deletion of the entire genes, lack any functional enzyme activity and fail to express the protein.. Therefore, functional polymorphisms in the genes of GSTM1 and GSTT1 enzymes may lead to an increased risk for CBZ-induced adverse effects, including hepatotoxicity. Among ethnic groups, GSTM1 and GSTT1 null allele frequencies are varying from 23 to 62% respectively [10–13]. Drug-induced hepatotoxicity is often unpredictable and may result in a transient elevation in transaminase enzymes, but may be fatal leading to acute liver injury. Many reports have investigated the involvment of GSTs null allele in the occurrence of hepatotoxicity with anti-tubercular drugs, in alzheimer's disease and with troglitazone therapy [14]. In CBZ-induced hepatotoxicity, very few reports have investigated the influence of GSTs alleles in the detoxification of toxic metabolites [14].

To the best of our information, no previous reports in tunisian population nor in subsaharian African population have focused on the effects of GSTM1 and GSTT1 null alleles in elevations of liver enzymes in CBZ-treated patients.

Therefore, in our study, the influence of GSTM1 and GSTT1 null alleles in elevation of transaminase enzyme levels among Tunisian epileptic patients treated with CBZ has been investigated.

Methods

Subjects

Study design

A cross-sectional prospective study has been conducted in the Department of Neurology "Sahloul Hospital of Sousse Tunisia", from September 2010 to July 2015 (Fig. 1).

Inclusion criteria

- Epileptic patients aged between 14 and 80 years old on monotherapy by CBZ.
- At least 1 month of obtaining the maintenance dose of CBZ.
- Pretherapeutic liver function tests in normal ranges.
- Hepatotoxicity was defined as raised levels of transaminase above the upper limit of normal range (ULN) at least once during the period of study. Before initiation of CBZ therapy, a complete cell count and hepatic function test were performed. Then, in the first month, two tests were performed once a week and periodically (every 3 months) as

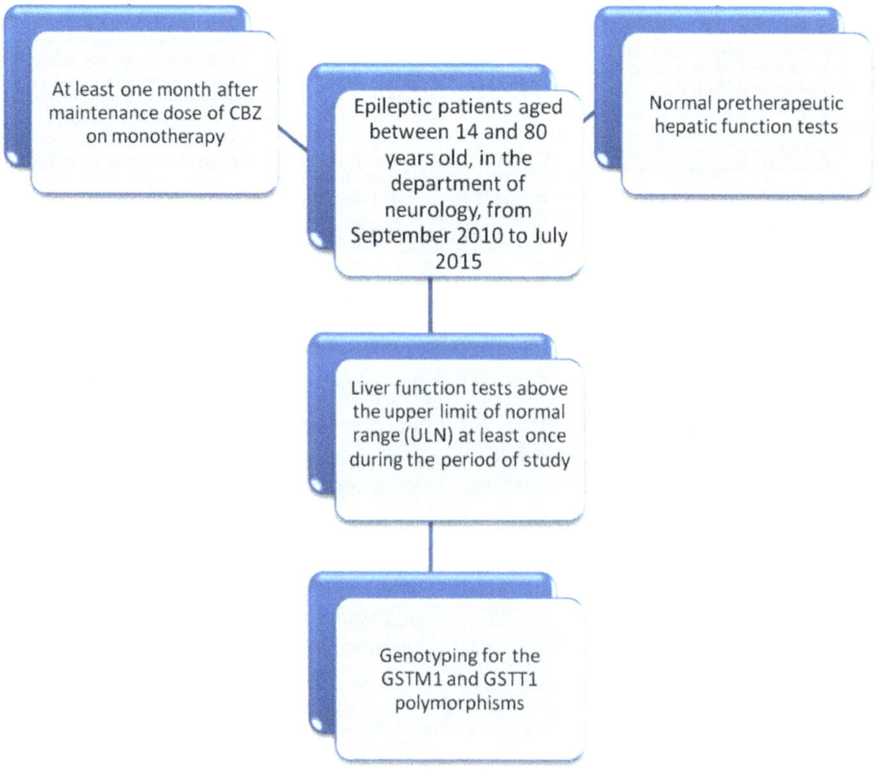

Fig. 1 Flow-diagram of the study

recommended [15]. The ULN for aspartate aminotransferase (AST) and alanine aminotransferase (ALT) were 31 UI/L and 34 IU/L respectively.

Non-inclusion criteria

- Previous chronic or acute liver disease,
- Presence of serological evidence of infection with hepatitis viruses.
- Chronic renal disease.
- History of chronic alcohol intake and/or herbal consumption.
- Drug consumption interfering with the metabolism of CBZ or with liver function tests.

Genotyping

Extraction of genomic DNA was performed from blood samples using the Wizard Genomic DNA Purification Kit (cat. *A1120) (Promega, Madison, USA).

The genotyping of GSTM1 and GSTT1 was performed using a previously described Polymerase Chain Reaction (PCR) [16].

In our study, the deleted gene of GSTM1 is termed GSTM1 null allele or GSTM1 (–). Heterozygotes [GSTM1(+/–) and the homozygous wild type, GSTM1(+/+)] are designed GSTM1 (+). As for the GSTT class, deletion of the entire gene is termed GSTT1(–). While heterozygotes [GSTT1(+/–) and the homozygous wild type GSTT1(+/+)] are designed GSTT1 (+).

Phenotype analysis

An analysis of plasma samples were performed in the Laboratory of Metabolic Biophysics, Professional Toxicology and Applied Environnemental, Department of Biophysics, Medicine Faculty of Sousse, Sousse, Tunisia. Dosage of CBZ and CBZ-E was conducted using previously described high performance liquid chromatography [17].

Serum alanine aminotransferase and aspartate aminotransferase were measured by standard methods adopted by Biochemical Laboratory of University Hospital Sahloul.

Statistical analysis

The mean values of the ALT and AST in epileptic patients were compared according to the different types of genetic polymorphisms of GST by applying the test U Mann–Whitney. Using the Kolmogorov–Smirnov test to a sample, the variables studied follow a non-normal distribution where recourse to the use of non-parametric test (U-test Mann–Whitney).

The correlation between levels of transaminases and the doses per mg/kg/day or the plasma concentration of carbamazepine were studied by Pearson's correlation test.

Association between genotype frequencies of GSTM1/T1 allele distribution and carbamazepine-induced mild hepatotoxicity was analyzed by calculating odds ratios (OR) and 95% confidence intervals (CLs). Statistical analysis was performed using the SPSS software package. A probability of $p < 0.05$ was considered statistically significant.

Ethical considerations

Ethics committee approval and patient consent was obtained for our study.

The local ethical committee of Sahloul University hospital has approved this study. Informations were made anonymous after the collection of the data and blood samples.

Results

Our study included 129 epileptic Tunisian patients (55 males and 74 females). Almost 54.68% suffered from focal seizures with or without secondary generalization (71 patients), 37.5% had generalized tonic-clonic seizures (48 patients) (Table 1). Patients were on CBZ therapy for 28.16 months (range: 18–36 months). Monitoring for epilepsy was performed for 3 years on average.

In our study, frequency distribution of the null allele of GSTM1 (GSTM1-) and the null allele of GSTT1 (GSTT-) were 74.4 and 17.8%, respectively.

The ALT and AST were elevated in 35.7% (46 cases: 30 males /16 females) and 25.6% (33cases: 22 males / 11 females). The mean levels of ALT and AST was 49 ± 6.44 and 112 ± 10.74, respectively.

A 1 mg/body weight/day increase of CBZ maintenance dosages (mg/kg/day) conferred OR of 1.004 (95% CI: 0.89.-1.12; $p = 0.95$) and 0.99 (95% CI: 0.88–1.12; $p = 0.91$) on the elevation in ALT and AST levels respectively; while a 1 µg/mL increase of plasma carbamazepine concentration conferred OR of 1.062 (95% CI: 0.92–1.22; $p = 0.40$) and 1.14 (95% CI: 0.97–1.33; $p = 0.11$) on the elevation in ALT and AST levels, respectively (Table 2). Neither the dosage of CBZ per body weight nor the plasma CBZ concentrations were associated with the ALT and AST

Table 1 Clinical detail in epileptic patients

Total number of patients studied	129
Seizure type (partial/generalized)	71/48
Epilepsy type N (%) (Symptomatic/Cryptogenic)	48/81
Sex (M/F)	55/74
Age (years)	38.26 ± 17
Weight (kg)	63.3 ± 7.6

Table 2 Relationship between mean dosage of CBZ per body weight, mean plasma CBZ concentrations and ALT/AST levels

	ALT		p-value	OR* (95% CI)	AST		p-value	OR* (95% CI)
	Normal (n) 83	Elevated (n) 46			Normal (n) 96	Elevated (n) 33		
Mean dosage (mg/kg/day)	7.92 ± 3.80	7.96 ± 2.06	0.94	1.004 (0.89–1.12)	7.96 ± 3.57	7.88 ± 2.26	0.91	0.99 (0.88–1.12)
Mean plasma carbamazepine concentrations (μg/mL)	6.25 ± 2.70	6.65 ± 2.38	0.40	1.062 (0.92–1.22)	6.18 ± 2.77	7.01 ± 1.88	0.11	1.14 (0.97–1.33)

H0: no difference between mean dosage of CBZ per body weight, mean plasma CBZ concentrations and ALT/AST levels
$p<0.05$ is significant

levels. Levels of ALT and AST seem to not be affected by genders and age.

ALT and AST values were significantly higher in GSTM1 null allele (–) than in GSTM1 (+) ($p = 10^{-3}$ and 0.004, respectively) (Table 3). Concerning GSTT1, these values were not influenced by GSTT1(–).The results concerning the effects of the combinations of GST genotypes on the corresponding values of transaminases was significantly different (Table 2). The level of ALT was significantly elevated in GSTM1(–)/T1(–) and GSTM1(–)/T1(+) than in GSTM1(+)/T1(+) ($p = 0.03$ and 0.2, respectively). The level of AST was significantly higher in GSTM1 (–)/T1(–) and GSTM1(+)/T1(–) than in GSTM1(–)/T1(+) ($p = 10^{-3}$ and 10^{-3}, respectively).

The distribution of GST alleles and the increase of transaminases are shown in Table 4.

The GSTM1 null genotype frequency was 65.1 and 91.3% in patients with normal and elevated levels of ALT, respectively (OR: 5.64; 95% CI: 1.70–20.60; $p = 0.0022$), and was 66.7 and 97% in cases with normal and elevated levels of AST, respectively (OR: 11; 95% CI: 1.56–77.37; $p = 0.0013$). On the contrary, no difference between the frequency of the GSTT1 (–) in the cases with normal or elevated ALT and AST, respectively was found (OR: 0.95; 95% CI: 0.33–2.68; $p = 0.88$) and (OR: 1.73; 95% CI: 0.59–5.01; $p = 0.39$). So, levels of transaminases were influenced by the genotype GSTM1 (–) and seem to not be affected by GSTT1 (–).

The frequency of GSTM1 (–)/T1 (–) (16.41%) was significantly higher than that of the GSTM1(+)/T1(+) (3.13%) in cases with elevated ALT (OR: 0.18; 95% CI: 0.04–0.75; $p = 0.014$). The frequency of GSTM1 (–)/T1 (–) (16.41%) was also significantly higher than that of the GSTM1(+)/T1(+) (1.56%) in cases with elevated AST (OR: 0.08; 95% CI: 0.01–0.45; $p = 0.0012$).

Table 3 Mean values of ALT and AST in each genotype

	ALT (IU/l)	p-value*	AST (IU/l)	p-value*
GSTM1 genotype (n)				
Null (96)	37.5 ± 5,716	**10^{-3}**	35.03 ± 11,8	**0.004**
Present (33)	30.93 ± 6,025		28.81 ± 4,35	
GSTT1 genotype (n)				
Null (23)	34.47 ± 8,36	0.27	35.26 ± 8,20	0.37
Present (106)	36.11 ± 5,96		33.05 ± 11,21	
Combination of GSTM1/GSTT1 (n)				
M1+/T1+ (19)	32.74 ± 6,87		28.42 ± 5,57	
M1+/T1- (8)	33.87 ± 10,66		53.62 ± 23,91	**10^{-3}**[a]
M1–/T1+ (66)	35.86 ± 3,88	**0.02**[a]	29.31 ± 4,57	
M1–/T1- (35)	37.88 ± 8,28	**0.03**[a]	39.71 ± 8,47	**10^{-3}**[a]

Null hypothese H0: no differences between the mean values of ALT and AST in each GSTM1(–) and GSTT1(–), combined GSTM1(–) and GSTT(–) and mean values of ALT and AST
p-value* by Mann-Whitney U test
[a]Compared with M1+/T1+
Bold entries indicate significance

Discussion

We performed a study of association between null alleles of GSTM1 and GSTT1 and risk of mild elevation of liver enzymes in Tunisian epileptic patients treated with CBZ on monotherapy. The GSTM1 and GSTT1 null alleles (GSTM1(–) and GSTT1(–)) consisting on a deletion of the complete genes and resulting in a lack of active enzymes are the most common polymorphisms in these genes. The frequencies of GSTM1 and GSTT1 deficiency vary from 23 to 62% respectively [10–12]. In Tunisian population, GSTM1 null allele frequency was of 34.6% and GSTT1 null allele frequency was of 16.6%. The frequency of double deletion of both GSTM1 and GSTT1 was of 4.82% [18].

In another genetic study of the association of GSTM1 and GSTT1 polymorphisms reported in three Arab populations (Bahraini, Lebanese and Tunisian), including 186 Tunisian healthy subjects, the prevalence of GSTT1 null allele was of 37.1%, GSTM1 null allele was of 63.4% and deleted allele of both genes was found in 21.0% of Tunisians [19].

In our population study, the frequency of patients carrying null alleles of GSTM1 and GSTT1 were consistent with these results.

The GSTM1 (–)allele was associated with elevated levels of both ALT and AST. It seems to affect the levels of transaminases in our population study and to be a risk factor for mild hepatotoxicity induced by CBZ. As for the GSTT1 (–) allele, it seems not to influence the ALT and AST levels. Whereas the combination of GSTM1 (+)/GSTT1 (–) alleles seems to affect the levels

Table 4 Distribution of GSTM1 and GSTT1 alleles in patients with elevated or normal levels of ALT and AST

	ALT		*p*-value	OR* (95% CI)	AST		*p*-value	OR* (95% CI)
	Normal	Elevated			Normal	Elevated		
GSTM1 genotype (n)								
Null	54	42	**0.0022**	5.64 (1.70–20.60)	64	32	**0.0013**	11 (1.56–77.37)
Present	29	4			32	1		
GSTT1 genotype (n)								
Null	15	8	0.88	0.95 (0.33–2.68)	15	8	0.39	1.73 (0.59–5.01)
Present	68	38			81	25		
Combination of GSTM1/GSTT1								
M1+/T1+	15	4		1.0	17	2		1.0
M1+/T1-	5	3	0.68	0.44 (0.05–3.74)	0	8	0.99	4(Undefined)
M1−/T1+	48	18	0.80	0.71 (0.17–2.73)	64	2	0.45	3.76 (0.34–41.37)
M1−/T1-	14	21	**0.014**	**0.18** (0.04–0.75)	14	21	**0.0012**	**0.08** (0.01–0.45)

Null hypothese (H0): no differences between GSTM1 and GSTT1 alleles in patients with elevated or normal levels of ALT and AST
$p<0.05$ is significant
Bold entries indicate significance

of AST. In fact, the GSTM1 (−) allele is rather significantly associated with an increase in ALT levels and in AST levels respectively than the GSTT1 (−) allele. Our results are consistent with those of Ueda et al. [20] who reported that GSTM1 (−) allele was related with the risk of mild hepatotoxicity induced by CBZ in Japanese population. As far as we know, this is the first study reporting an association between the GSTM1 (−) allele and the increasing values of transaminases in Tunisian and subsaharian population.

Many reports have associated the GST null alleles, leading to a lack of functional protein, with an increase susceptibility to several diseases, such as cancer, cardiovascular, epilepsy, schizophrenia and hepatotoxicity [16, 21–24]. The reactive metabolites of drugs causing drug toxicity are detoxified by GST enzymes. So, an inherited weakness of drug eliminating capacity related to a null GST alleles may enhance toxic drug-induced adverse events [3, 5, 7, 10, 25]. A 2-fold ULN increased risk of elevation levels of ALT has been reported in individuals exhibiting the GSTM1 (−) allele among patients treated with isoniazid, rifampicin and pyrazinamide for pulmonary tuberculosis [26, 27]. Simon and colleagues [28] showed that 72% of patients carriers of GSTM1(−)/T1(−) alleles have at least three times elevated ALT levels among Alzheimer's disease. Watanabe and colleagues [27] found higher risk of hepatotoxicity-induced by troglitazone in patients with GSTM1 (−)/T1(−) alleles.

Our study found that the GSTM1 (−) allele, especially when combined with GSTT1 (−) allele, may be a genetic factor associated with the increased risk of hepatotoxicity. In many reports, toxic effects of drugs have been attributed to the formation of chemically reactive metabolites [3, 5]. The metabolites of CBZ, such as 10,11- epoxy-carbamazepine (CBZ-E), arene oxide (s) and iminoquinone (s), may be associated with drug hypersensitivity reactions, cytotoxicity and genotoxicity [3, 5, 7, 25]. The CBZ-E is a chemically reactive metabolite and may be converted into electrophilic reactive intermediate with glutathione (GSH) [26]. So, GST may play a role in the overall covalent binding potential of CBZ-E with liver microsomes and polymorphisms may be responsible for liver-toxicities [29].

In our study, neither the dosage of CBZ per body weight nor the plasma CBZ concentrations were associated with transaminase levels. It is evidence that CBZ-induced hepatotoxicity is dose-independent and carbamazepine toxicity seems to not be correlated with CBZ plasma concentration. It may be rather induced by allergic reactions [3].

GSTM1 seem to affect ALT levels whereas GSTT1 seem to be related to AST levels. These results can be explained, almost partly, by the distribution of transaminases and the GST enzymes. While ALT is mainly distributed in the liver, AST is present in the liver, red blood cells and muscle. Consequently, ALT is therefore considered to be a more accurate sign of liver damage than AST. In addition, GSTM1 is widely expressed in the liver, and GSTT1 is principally expressed in erythrocytes [10, 13]. Consequently, the ALT levels may be more affected by GSTM1 (−) allele while AST may be more susceptible to GSTT1 (−) allele. Thus, our findings suggest that the GSTM1 (−) allele may be considered as a key factor for the development of carbamazepine-induced hepatotoxicity.

However, our findings should be considered with caution. Many limits of our study should be mentioned. First, our population study number is small. Although we tried to be exhaustive and to include all the patients responding to our inclusion criteria, our small sample size just suggests a trend to possible correlation between GSTM1 (–) allele and elevation in ALT and AST levels, additional reports would be indispensable for proving our results in a larger scale.

Second, investigations in patients with elevated AST levels were not performed to rule out other susceptible causes. Moreover, Single laboratory liver test may be of little value.

Conclusions

An association between GST genotyping and a possible effect in transaminases in an epileptic population study on CBZ in monotherapy was attempted. Our results showed a possible correlation between GSTM1 (–) genotype and elevation in ALT and AST levels. GST null allele may be a risk factor for mild hepatotoxicity in Tunisian epileptic patients. Further studies including a larger sample sizes would be necessary for proving our results.

Abbreviations

ALT: Alanine aminotransferase; AST: Aspartate aminotransferase; CBZ: Carbamazepine; CBZ-E: 10,11-epoxy-carbamazepine; CLs: Confidence intervals; GSH: Glutathione; GSTM1 (–): Null allele of the GSTM1; GSTM1: Glutathione S-transferase M1; GSTT1 (–): Null allele of the GSTT1; GSTT1: Glutathione S-transferase T1; HPLC: High-performance liquid chromatography; ORs: Odds ratios; PCR: Polymerase Chain Reaction; SD: Standard deviation; ULN: Upper limit of normal range

Acknowledgements

We thank all the staff of the Laboratory of Metabolic Biophysics, Professional Toxicology and Applied Environmental Laboratory (LR12ES02), Medicine Faculty of Sousse, Tunisia for their help and assistance.

Funding

This study was supported by the "Higher Education and Scientific Research Ministry" in Tunisia.

Authors' contributions

CC performed the experiments analytical studies and wrote the manuscript; FN wrote the manuscript; HA conducted and performed the periodic clinical monitoring; SS planned the study, NM checked the final form of the manuscript, NS improved the English of the manuscript and BAS read and approved the final manuscript. All authors read and approved the final manuscript.

Competing interests

The authors declare that they have no competing interests.

Author details

[1]Metabolic Biophysics, Professional Toxicology and Applied Environmental Laboratory, Department of Biophysics, Medicine Faculty of Sousse, Sousse University, Avenue Mohamed Karoui, 4002 Sousse, Tunisia. [2]Neurology Department of Central Hospital University (CHU), Sousse University, 4002 Sousse, Tunisia.

References

1. Ek O, Ban E, Woo JS, Kim CK. Analysis of carbamazepine and its active metabolite, carbamazepine-10,11-epoxide, in human plasma using high-performance liquid chromatography. Anal Bioanal Chem. 2006;386(6):1931–6.
2. Brodie MJ, Dichter M. Antiepileptic drugs. N Engl J Med. 1996;334(3):168–75.
3. Kalapos MP. Carbamazepine-provoked hepatotoxicity and possible aetiopathological role of glutathione in the events. Retrospective review of old data and call for new investigation. Adverse Drug React Toxicol Rev. 2002;21(3):123–41.
4. Harden CL. Therapeutic safety monitoring: what to look for and when to look for it. Epilepsia. 2000;41:37–44.
5. Pearce RE, Vakkalagadda GR, Leeder JS. Pathways of carbamazepine bioactivation in vitro I. Characterization of human cytochromes P450 responsible for the formation of 2- and 3-hydroxylated metabolites. Drug Metab Dispos. 2002;30(11):1170–9.
6. Breton H, Cociglio M, Bressolle F, Peyriere H, Blayac JP, Hillaire-Buys D. Liquid chromatography-electrospray mass spectrometry determination of carbamazepine, oxcarbazepine and eight of their metabolites in human plasma. J Chromatogr B Analyt Technol Biomed Life Sci. 2005;828:80–90.
7. Bu HZ, Kang P, Deese AJ, Zhao P, Pool WF. Human in vitro glutathionyl and protein adducts of carbamazepine-10,11-epoxide, a stable and pharmacologically active metabolite of carbamazepine. Drug Metab Dispos. 2005;33:1920–4.
8. Bertilsson L, Tomson T. Clinical pharmacokinetics and pharmacological effects of carbamazepine and carbamazepine-10,11-epoxide. An update. Clin Pharmacokinet. 1986;11:177–98.
9. DeBethizy JD, Hayes JR. Metabolism. A determinant of toxicity. In: Hayes AW, editor. Principles and methods of toxicology. 2nd ed. New York: Raven Press; 1988. p. 29–66.
10. Hayes JD, Flanagan JU, Jowsey IR. Glutathione transferases. Annu Rev Pharmacol Toxicol. 2005;45:51–88.
11. Munaka M, Kohshi K, Kawamoto T, Takasawa S, Nagata N, Itoh H, Oda S, Katoh T. Genetic polymorphisms of tobacco- and alcohol-related metabolizing enzymes and the risk of hepatocellular carcinoma. J Cancer Res Clin Oncol. 2003;129:355–60.
12. Lin HJ, Han CY, Bernstein DA, Hsiao W, Lin BK, Hardy S. Ethnic distribution of the glutathione transferase Mu 1-1 (GSTM1) null genotype in 1473 individuals and application to bladder cancer susceptibility. Carcinogenesis. 1994;15:1077–81.
13. Eaton DL, Bammler TK. Concise review of the glutathione S-transferases and their significance to toxicology. Toxicol Sci. 1999;49(2):156–64.
14. Levy M, Goodman MW, Van Dyne BJ, Sumner HW. Granulomatous hepatitis secondary to carbamazepine. Ann Intern Med. 1981;95(1):64–5.
15. Lévy-Chavagnat D. Stratégies de traitement des syndromes épileptiques. Actual Pharm. 2008;475:10–6.
16. Chbili C, B'chir F, Ben Fredj M, Saguem BN, Ben Amor S, Ben Ammou S, Saguem S. Effects of glutathione S-transferase M1 and T1 deletions on epilepsy risk among a Tunisian population. Epilepsy Res. 2014a;108:1168–73.
17. Chbili C, Bannour S, Khlifi S, Ben Hadj Ali B, Saguem S. Relationships between pharmacokinetic parameters of carbamazepine and therapeutic response in patients with bipolar disease. Ann Biol Clin (Paris). 2014b;72:453–9.
18. Gara S, Abessi M, Bendjemena K, Abdennebi M, Guemira F. Deletion polymorphism of glutathione S-transferases M1 and T1 in the Tunisian population. Tunis Med. 2010;88(10):700–2.
19. Salem AH, Yaqoob A, Ali M, Handu S, Fadel R, Abu-Hijleh M, Almawi W. Genetic polymorphism of the glutathione S-transferase M1 and T1 genes in three distinct Arab populations. Dis Markers. 2011;31(5):311–6.
20. Ueda K, Ishitsu T, Seo T, Ueda N, Murata T, Hori M, Nakagawa K. Glutathione S-transferase M1 null genotype as a risk factor for carbamazepine-induced mild hepatotoxicity. Pharmacogenomics. 2007;8:435–842.
21. Gravina P, Spoletini I, Masini S, Valentini A, Vanni D, Paladini E, Bossù P, Caltagirone C, Federici G, Spalletta G, Bernardini S. Genetic polymorphisms of glutathione S-transferases GSTM1, GSTT1, GSTP1and GSTA1 as risk factors for schizophrenia. Psychiatry Res. 2011;187(3):454–6.
22. Cotton SC, Sharp L, Little J, Brockton N. GlutathioneS-transferase polymorphisms and colorectal cancer: a HuGE review. Am J Epidemiol. 2000;151:7–32.
23. Habdous M, Siest G, Herbeth B, Vincent-Viry M, Visvikis S. Polymorphismes des glutathion S-transférases et pathologies humaines: bilan des études épidémiologiques. Ann Biol Clin. 2004;62:15–24.

24. Martin NJ, Collier AC, Bowen LD, Pritsos KL, Goodrich GG, Arger K, Cutter G, Pritsos CA. Polymorphisms in the NQO1, GSTT and GSTM genes are associated with coronary heart disease and biomarkers of oxidative stress. Mutat Res. 2009;674(1–2):93–100.
25. Pirmohamed M, Kitteringham NR, Guenthner TM, Breckenridge AM, Park BK. An investigation of the formation of cytotoxic, protein-reactive and stable metabolites from carbamazepine in vitro. Biochem Pharmacol. 1992;43:1675–82.
26. Roy B, Chowdhury A, Kundu S, Santra A, Dey B, Chakraborty M, Majumder PP. Increased risk of antituberculosis drug –induced hepatotoxicity in individuals with glutathione S-transferase M1 null mutation. J Gastroenterol Hepatol. 2001;16(9):1033–7.
27. Watanabe I, Tomita A, Shimizu M, Sugawara M, Yasumo H, Koishi R, Takahashi T, Miyoshi K, Nakamura K, Izumi T, Matsushita Y, Furukawa H, Haruyama H, Koga T. A study to survey susceptible genetic factors responsible for troglitazone- associated hepatotoxicity in Japanes patients with type 2 diabetes mellitus. Clin Pharmaco Ther. 2003;73(5):435–55.
28. Simon T, Becquemont L, Mary-Krause M, de Waziers I, Beaune P, Funck-Brentano C, Jaillon P. Combined glutathione s-transferases M1 and T1 genetic polymorphism and tacrine hepatotoxicity. Clin Pharmacol Ther. 2000;67(4):432–7.
29. Chbili C, Fathallah N, Nouira M, Laouani A, Hassine A, Ben Amor S, Ben Ammou S, Saguem S. Effects of glutathione S-transferase M1 and T1 deletions on carbamazepine metabolism among a Tunisian population. Genes Genomics. 2015;37(12):991–7.

Severe localised granulomatosis with polyangiitis (Wegener's granulomatosis) manifesting with extensive cranial nerve palsies and cranial diabetes insipidus

James E. Peters[1,2*], Vivek Gupta[2], Ibtisam T. Saeed[3], Curtis Offiah[4] and Ali S. M. Jawad[2]

Abstract

Background: Granulomatosis with polyangiitis (GPA, formerly Wegener's granulomatosis) is a multisystem vasculitis of small- to medium-sized blood vessels. Cranial involvement can result in cranial nerve palsies and, rarely, pituitary infiltration.

Case presentation: We describe the case of a 32 year-old woman with limited but severe GPA manifesting as progressive cranial nerve palsies and pituitary dysfunction. Our patient initially presented with localised ENT involvement, but despite treatment with methotrexate, she deteriorated. Granulomatous inflammatory tissue around the skull base resulted in cavernous sinus syndrome, facial nerve palsy, palsies of cranial nerves IX-XII (Collet-Sicard syndrome), and the rare complication of cranial diabetes insipidus due to pituitary infiltration. The glossopharyngeal, vagus and accessory nerve palsies resulted in severe dysphagia and she required nasogastric tube feeding. Her neurological deficits substantially improved with treatment including high dose corticosteroid, cyclophosphamide and rituximab.

Conclusions: This case emphasises that serious morbidity can arise from localised cranial Wegener's granulomatosis in the absence of systemic disease. In such cases intensive induction immunosuppression is required. Analysis of previously reported cases of pituitary involvement in GPA reveals that this rare complication predominantly affects female patients.

Keywords: Granulomatosis with polyangiitis, Wegener's granulomatosis, Vasculitis, Diabetes insipidus, Pituitary, Collet-Sicard syndrome, Cavernous sinus syndrome, ANCA, Rituximab, Cyclophosphamide

Background

Granulomatosis with polyangiitis (GPA, formerly Wegener's granulomatosis) is an autoimmune vasculitis of small- to medium-sized blood vessels. The Chapel Hill 2012 Consensus Criteria define GPA as "necrotizing granulomatous inflammation usually involving the upper and lower respiratory tract and necrotizing vasculitis affecting predominantly small to medium vessels" [1]. In their seminal 1954 review, Godman and Churg recognized that Wegener's granulomatosis, microscopic polyangiitis, and Churg-Strauss syndrome shared certain clinico-pathological features, and comprised a subset of vasculitides distinct from 'periarteritis nodosa' (now polyarteritis nodosa) [2]. The discovery that anti-neutrophil cytoplasmic antibodies (ANCA) are present in over 90% of patients with GPA and microscopic polyangiitis, and approximately 30% of those with Churg-Strauss syndrome has led to these three clinical syndromes being classified under the umbrella term 'ANCA-associated vasculitis'. Patients with GPA typically show a cytoplasmic pattern of ANCA staining on indirect immunofluorescence ('cANCA pattern'), with antibodies directed against proteinase-3 (PR3), a neutrophil protease.

The generalised form of GPA described by Wegener is characterized histopathologically by the triad of necrotizing

* Correspondence: jp549@cam.ac.uk
[1]Cardiovascular Epidemiology Unit, Department of Public Health and Primary Care, Worts Causeway, University of Cambridge, Cambridge CB1 8RN, UK
[2]Department of Rheumatology, The Royal London and Mile End Hospitals, Barts Health NHS Trust, Bancroft Road, London E1 4DG, UK
Full list of author information is available at the end of the article

vasculitis, pauci-immune focal necrotizing glomerulonephritis and necrotizing granulomatous inflammation of the respiratory tract. This systemic form of the disease can be life-threatening, particularly in the presence of pulmonary haemorrhage or rapidly progressive crescenteric glomerulonephritis. Prior to the introduction of cyclophosphamide [3], mortality was over 80% [4]. Modern treatment involves intensive immunosuppressive therapy with high dose corticosteroids and cyclophosphamide or rituximab to induce remission [5, 6]. Once remission is achieved, patients are switched to less toxic maintenance immunosuppression, such as azathioprine and low dose glucocorticosteroid.

A limited form of Wegener's granulomatosis, with lesions localised to the lung, was later identified [7]. Patients with limited (now generally referred to as 'localised') disease are more likely to be young, female and ANCA negative than those with generalised GPA [8]. Localised GPA typically manifests with middle ear and respiratory tract features such as otitis media, sinusitis, nasal collapse and airway stenosis [8, 9].

Here we describe a patient with localised but severe granulomatosis with polyangiitis (Wegener's granulomatosis) manifesting with progressive cranial nerve palsies and pituitary dysfunction. This case emphasises that localised cranial Wegener's granulomatosis can result in serious morbidity in the absence of systemic disease. In such cases intensive induction immunosuppression is required.

Case presentation

Our patient, a white British female, presented at the age of 32 years with epistaxis, nasal congestion, recurrent bilateral otitis media and progressive hearing loss to an Ear, Nose and Throat (ENT) clinic at her local hospital. A year prior to this she had been fitted with bilateral hearing aids for hearing loss of unknown cause. She subsequently developed a left lower motor neurone facial palsy. A computed tomography (CT) scan showed a left nasopharyngeal mass and inflammatory changes in the middle ear and mastoid air cells. Nasolaryngoscopy revealed inflammation and ulceration of the left nasal turbinate, septum and posterior pharyngeal wall. She had never used cocaine. She underwent an exploratory mastoidectomy with grommet insertion.

Biopsies of the right and left nasopharynx, left middle meatus and septum revealed florid acute and chronic inflammation with mucosal ulceration and extensive necrosis of stroma and cartilage. The inflammatory infiltrate consisted of neutrophils, lymphocytes, and plasma cells, with zones of histiocytes representing granulomata (Fig. 1). Large numbers of multinucleated giant cells were present. Eosinophils were inconspicuous. Histological assessment of vasculitis was difficult due to the extensive necrosis and marked tissue inflammation, but necrotizing vasculitis of small vessels was evident. There was no evidence of malignancy, and stains for fungi and mycobacteria were negative.

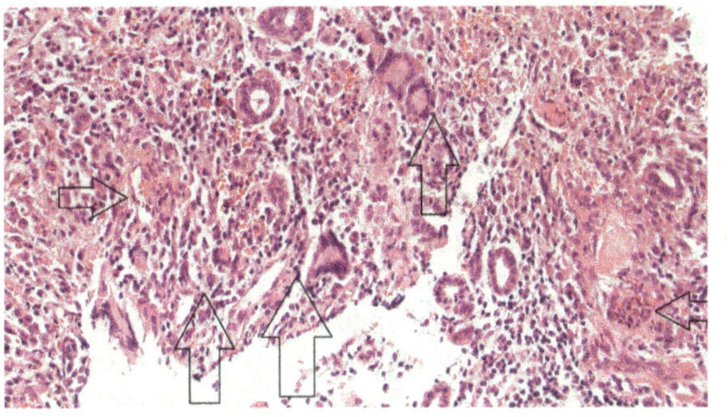

Fig. 1 Histopathology. Nasal biopsy. H&E stain, magnification X100. Vertical arrows show granuloma. Horizontal left facing arrow: necrosis. Horizontal right facing arrow: angiitis with necrosis in vessel wall.

Anti-neutrophil cytoplasmic antibody (ANCA) testing was positive by immunofluorescence with a cytoplasmic staining pattern. Anti-proteinase-3 (PR3) antibodies measured by enzyme-linked immunosorbent assay (ELISA) were mildly elevated (5.8, normal range < 2). Anti-myeloperoxidase (MPO) antibodies were not detected. CT thorax revealed no pulmonary abnormality and no lymphadenopathy. Serum calcium and angiotensin-converting enzyme (ACE) were normal.

On the basis of the clinico-pathological findings, she was diagnosed with localised granulomatosis with polyangiitis (GPA, formerly known as Wegener's granulomatosis). Detailed work-up revealed no evidence of pulmonary, renal or other systemic features. She was treated with methotrexate 25 mg weekly and prednisolone 60 mg daily. The prednisolone was weaned to 10 mg over a period of 6 months. As the steroid dose was reduced she deteriorated. She developed headaches, nausea, diplopia, dysphonia and progressive dysphagia to both solids and liquids, resulting in weight loss of 3 stone.

She was referred to our institution by her general practitioner approximately 1 year after her initial presentation. Physical examination revealed left ptosis, a dilated and unreactive left pupil, paresis of left eye movements consistent with palsies of cranial nerves III, IV and VI, a left lower motor neurone facial palsy, and deviation of the tongue to the right. There was wasting of the right sternocleidomastoid. Laryngoscopy revealed a right-sided vocal cord palsy. Blood tests showed mild elevation of the inflammatory markers; the erythrocyte sedimentation rate (ESR) was 34 mm/hour, and the C-reactive protein (CRP) was 26 mg/L. Renal function, urinalysis and urine microscopy were normal. Repeat ANCA testing revealed cytoplasmic pattern ANCA staining, but antibodies to PR3 and MPO were negative.

A contrast-enhanced CT scan of her head and neck (Fig. 2) demonstrated predominantly dural-based enhancing soft tissue abnormality affecting the central skull base. This chronic inflammatory tissue involved the sella turcica (with resultant erosion of the floor of the sella turcica) and both cavernous sinuses. There was associated abnormality involving the pituitary parenchyma, the pituitary stalk and the hypothalamus. Contiguous chronic inflammatory infiltrative changes were also evident in the orbital apices, the petrous temporal bones encasing the carotid canals and the extra-cranial infratemporal fossae including the pterygopalatine fossae. As a result of the cavernous sinus, petrous temporal bone and infratemporal fossae involvement, both internal carotid arteries were occluded in their skull base carotid canal segments, with the anterior circulation sustained through collateral vessels. The sinonasal region demonstrated chronic inflammatory features, with mucosal and submucosal fibrosis and ulceration. Bilateral chronic middle ear and mastoid inflammatory changes were evident. Radiological features of right Collet-Sicard syndrome (palsy of cranial nerves IX-XII) were also present. The appearances, particularly in relation to the skull base infiltration, had progressed significantly compared to 6 months earlier. Her pituitary hormone profile showed elevated prolactin (1353 munit/L; upper limit of normal range = 496) and reduced thyroid-stimulating hormone (TSH) (0.23 munit/L) with normal free thyroxine. On further enquiry, she reported amenorrhoea for the past year.

She had not yet had any children and was keen to do this in the future. We therefore initially opted for treatment with rituximab over cyclophosphamide. She received Rituximab 1 g, with a plan for a second dose two weeks later. Methotrexate was replaced with Azathioprine. She

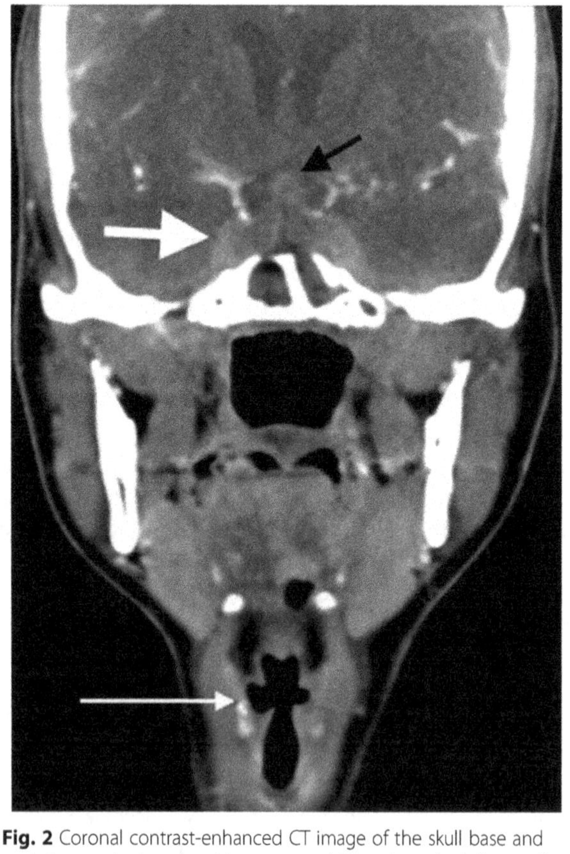

Fig. 2 Coronal contrast-enhanced CT image of the skull base and neck (pre-cyclophosphamide treatment). There is marked abnormal chronic inflammatory infiltration of the cavernous sinuses bilaterally (bold white arrow) and hypophyseal involvement (black arrow). Multiple lower cranial nerve palsies (Collet-Sicard syndrome) as a result of the skull base inflammatory involvement were evident on imaging, including right vocal cord palsy indicated by adducted right true vocal cord and enlarged right laryngeal ventricle (long white arrow)

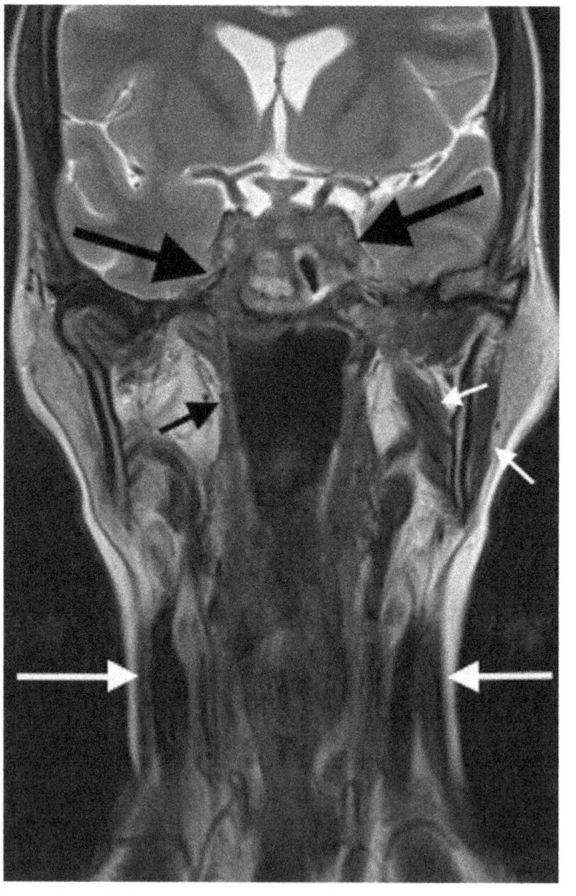

Fig. 3 Coronal T2-weighted MRI image of the skull base and neck (pre-cyclophosphamide treatment). There is severe chronic inflammatory soft tissue abnormality affecting the cavernous sinuses and central and lateral skull base, including the left cavernous sinus and right sphenoid bone and foramen rotundum (large black arrows). Secondary cranial nerve palsies are present. Palsy of the mandibular division of the right trigeminal nerve has resulted in atrophy of the right masticator space muscle, in comparison to the more normal muscle volume on the left (short white arrows). Lower cranial nerve palsies are demonstrated by atrophy of the right superior pharyngeal constrictor muscle (short black arrow) and sternocleidomastoid muscles (long white arrows)

also received one pulse of intravenous (i.v.) methyl prednisolone 500 mg, and her oral prednisolone was increased from 10 mg to 30 mg. Given her modest baseline immunosuppressive treatment, and because of the insidious presentation and lack of systemic features, at the time we felt this mid-range prednisolone dose rather than 1 mg/kg was reasonable. Her CRP fell to 6 mg/L and she was discharged from hospital.

She was seen as an emergency 10 days later. She had developed complete dysphagia to solids and liquids and was unable to manage even small sips of water. Both pupils were now dilated and reacted sluggishly to light, and she had a new right-sided ptosis, indicating a new right-sided third nerve palsy. She also had a new right-sided sixth nerve palsy. Assessment of her swallowing showed that she was aspirating and had an ineffective cough reflex. She was kept nil-by-mouth, and fed through a nasogastric tube. The safety of her airway was assessed by the anaesthetic and ENT teams because of concern that she was at high risk of life-threatening airway obstruction or aspiration should the vocal cord palsies become bilateral. Her CRP had risen to 33 mg/L.

A cranial magnetic resonance imaging (MRI) scan (Figs. 3 and 4a) confirmed the CT findings, and provided greater imaging sensitivity and specificity regarding the extent and severity of the osseus skull base infiltrative changes, the intracranial dural-based disease burden, and the cranial nerve palsies. Muscle atrophy due to denervation as a result of the latter was particularly well demonstrated. In addition, the MRI provided greater detail on the degree of hypothalamic-pituitary axis involvement, and allowed for subsequent imaging assessment of response to treatment.

She was treated with three pulses of i.v. methyl prednisolone 500 mg, with rapid improvement in her diplopia and normalization of the CRP. The right pupillary abnormality improved but the left pupil remained dilated (Fig. 5). Her oral prednisolone was increased to 60 mg, and she received three fortnightly doses of i.v. cyclophosphamide 750 mg (15 mg/kg) followed by three further doses at three-weekly intervals. Azathioprine was stopped. She also was given the second rituximab dose. She received topical mupirocin to reduce nasal *Staphylococcus* carriage and was started on oral co-trimoxazole both to reduce the risk of opportunistic infections and because this may reduce relapses in GPA [10]. Her swallowing remained compromised and she remained an inpatient for ongoing feeding via the nasogastric tube. Subsequently a percutaneous gastrostomy tube was inserted.

Her admission was complicated by hypernatraemia with serum sodium rising to 157 mmol/L. She required 4–5 L of fluid per day to maintain her sodium level in the normal range. She had two episodes of syncope due to postural hypotension. Her fluid balance chart revealed polyuria. Blood glucose and calcium were normal. Repeat dedicated pituitary MRI showed pathological enhancement and diffuse thickening of the pituitary (Fig. 4 b&c). She was diagnosed with cranial diabetes insipidus and treated with desmopressin, with normalization of her serum sodium. She was discharged home with feeding via the gastrostomy tube.

After six pulses of cyclophosphamide, she showed marked clinical improvement. Her diplopia had resolved and eye movements had returned to normal. She was able to eat and drink normally. Her right-sided third nerve palsy had entirely resolved. Her left pupil remained dilated and reacted sluggishly to light, and a mild left facial weakness persisted. A further cranial MRI showed marked regression of the inflammatory changes in the skull base (Fig. 6). She was switched to maintenance therapy with azathioprine, and the prednisolone dose was slowly weaned to 5 mg daily. She remained clinically well on this treatment, with no progression of cranial disease on MRI, for 20 months following completion of cyclophosphamide. At this point, she had a relapse of ENT disease with nasal blockage and epistaxis requiring a tapering course of prednisolone 30 mg daily.

Discussion

Our patient first presented with localised GPA confined to the nasopharynx and ear. Despite initial treatment with full-dose methotrexate and steroids, her disease progressed. She developed the unusual complications of extensive cranial nerve palsies (involvement of nerves II-IV, V_3, and VI-XII) and diabetes insipidus due to granulomatous infiltration of the skull base.

Our report highlights several learning points. First, it demonstrates that localised GPA can be aggressive and result in serious morbidity. Assessment of disease severity is a key aspect of the management of AAV since it guides treatment decisions [5, 6]. Disease severity can be classified as life-threatening, organ-threatening (i.e. disease that will result in permanent tissue damage and/or loss of function unless appropriately treated), or non-organ threatening. Although our patient had anatomically localised cranial GPA, she developed organ-threatening disease with severe progressive cranial nerve involvement as a result of compression by inflammatory tissue. This included a vocal cord palsy, which resulted in dysphonia. If she had not been treated promptly, this could have become bilateral which can lead to life-threatening airway obstruction [11]. Glossopharyngeal, vagus and accessory nerve palsies resulted in severe dysphagia necessitating nasogastric feeding.

Second, this case illustrates central nervous system (CNS) manifestations of GPA, including the rare complication of cranial diabetes insipidus due to pituitary infiltration and compression. In contrast to peripheral nerve

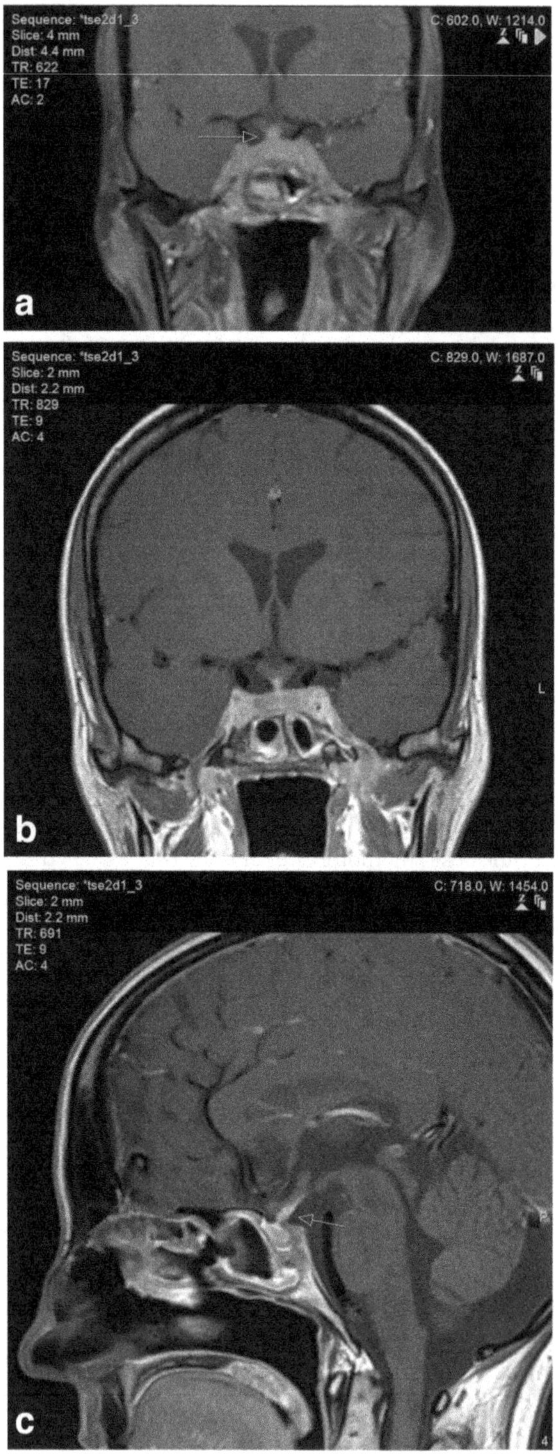

Fig. 4 MR images of the brainstem, skull base and pituitary gland. (a) Coronal contrast-enhanced fat-saturated T1-weighted image of the central skull base demonstrates pathological enhancement of the cavernous sinus, pituitary gland and pituitary stalk (arrow). The abnormalities are non-discrete and radiologically inconsistent with a microadenoma or invasive macro adenoma of the pituitary gland. (b) Dedicated thin-section coronal contrast-enhanced T1-weighted image of the pituitary demonstrates the abnormal enhancement and thickening of the pituitary stalk as well as the cavernous sinus and pituitary parenchyma in more detail. (c) Dedicated thin-section sagittal contrast-enhanced T1-weighted image of the pituitary demonstrates the abnormal generalised thickening and enhancement of the pituitary stalk (arrow) consistent with granulomatous infundibulitis

involvement, CNS disease in GPA is uncommon. In a European cohort of 128 GPA patients, 56 patients (44%) had peripheral neuropathy (either symmetrical polyneuropathy or mononeuritis multiplex), whilst only 9 patients (7%) had CNS involvement, of whom 6 had cranial nerve palsies [12]. CNS involvement occurred in 8% of cases in a cohort from the National Institutes of Health (NIH) [13], and cranial nerve palsies occurred in 21 of 324 patients (6%) attending the Mayo Clinic [14]. CNS disease in GPA is proposed to develop by three distinct but sometimes co-existing mechanisms [15]: by contiguous spread of granulomatous tissue from adjacent sites in the middle ear and sinuses (as in our patient), by primary granuloma formation within the CNS, or from vasculitis affecting the CNS. Seror et al. described three patterns of GPA-related CNS disease: chronic hypertrophic pachymeningitis, pituitary gland involvement, and cerebral vasculitis [16].

Yokoseki et al. reported a series of 36 patients with hypertrophic pachymengitis, of whom 17 had ANCA against MPO and 4 against PR3 [17]. Although the number of PR3 positive patients was small, this study found a higher frequency of pulmonary and renal disease in PR3 positive cases than in MPO+ cases, and that leptomeningeal and parenchymal involvement in the brain were more common in PR3 positive hypertrophic pachymeningitis compared with MPO positive and idiopathic hypertrophic pachymeningitis. In the presence of leptomengingeal AAV,

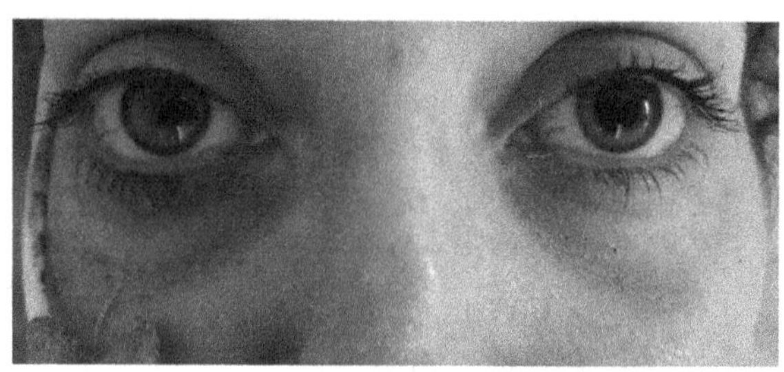

Fig. 5 Photograph demonstrating dilated left pupil and nasal deformity. This was taken after 3 pulses of i.v. methyl prednisolone

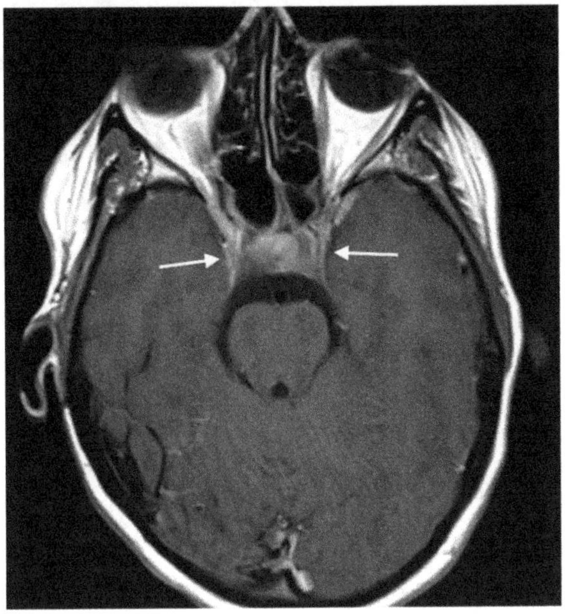

Fig. 6 Axial intracranial contrast-enhanced T1-weighted MR image after six pulses of cyclophosphamide. There is reduction in the volume of abnormal cavernous sinus enhancing chronic inflammatory tissue (arrows) compared with pre-treatment imaging

cerebrospinal fluid analysis may reveal elevated protein and pleiocytosis, but these findings are non-specific. Other causes of hypertrophic pachymeningitis include other immune-mediated diseases (e.g. sarcoidosis and IgG4-related disease), infections, and neoplasms (particularly lymphoma) [17]. Lymphoma mimicking GPA with positive PR3 antibodies has been described [18]. However, in our patient, the radiological picture and the clinical course were not consistent with lymphoma.

Our patient had both chronic pachymeningitis and pituitary gland involvement, with meningeal thickening and pituitary infiltration evident on cranial imaging, and clinical and biochemical evidence of pituitary disease. Pituitary dysfunction due to GPA is rare, occurring in 9 of 819 patients (1.1%) in the French Vasculitis Study Group database [19], and 8 of 637 patients (1.3%) in a series from the Mayo Clinic [20]. We identified 58 previously reported cases of GPA with sellar involvement in the literature (Table 1), and analysed their clinical and demographic features. There was a significant female preponderance; 40 (69%) of the patients were female. Patients with pituitary involvement tended to be younger than GPA patients in general (median age at time of pituitary involvement 39. 5 years, interquartile range 29–50 years). Pituitary involvement generally occurred early in the disease course. Of 46 cases where we were able to identify the age of onset of both GPA and pituitary involvement, in 28 (61%), pituitary disease was either the presenting feature or was diagnosed within a year of GPA onset. ENT involvement was the most common additional clinical GPA manifestation, occurring in 39 patients (67%). Other extra-CNS manifestations were, in order of decreasing frequency, pulmonary ($n = 25$), renal ($n = 16$), musculoskeletal ($n = 15$), ocular ($n = 14$), mucocutaneous ($n = 12$), peripheral neuropathy ($n = 4$), cardiac ($n = 1$), digital infarcts ($n = 1$), gastro-intestinal ($n = 1$). Diabetes insipidus was the most common endocrine abnormality, occurring in 47 patients (81%). In 4 of these, diabetes insipidus occurred following sellar surgery. Anterior pituitary hormone abnormalities occurred less frequently: hypogonadism was present in 32 patients, secondary hypothyroidism in 20, hyperprolactinaemia in 19, and growth hormone deficiency in 5. Reliable estimation of the frequency of adrenocorticotropic hormone (ACTH) deficiency was difficult due to therapeutic administration of exogenous corticosteroids in many cases. Typical MRI appearances include a sellar mass, sometimes with suprasellar extension, diffuse enlargement of the pituitary, thickening of the infundibulum (pituitary stalk), and enhancement with gadolinium contrast. Loss of the normal posterior pituitary hyperintensity on T1 weighted images was reported in 17 cases, and correlated with the presence of diabetes insipidus. In a few cases, hyperprolactinaemia and the presence of a pituitary lesion on imaging caused diagnostic confusion with a prolactinoma [21, 22]. However, diabetes insipidus and the loss of the normal high signal in the posterior pituitary on T1 weighted MRI are unusual in small pituitary adenomas. Our patient had diffuse pituitary and infundibular changes radiologically inconsistent with a pituitary adenoma.

The third issue raised by this case is the wisdom of methotrexate treatment at the time of her initial presentation. The NORAM trial compared methotrexate with cyclophosphamide for the treatment of early, non-organ threatening systemic disease [23]. Whilst there was no significant difference in the primary endpoint of overall remission rates at 6 months, relapse rate at 18 months was higher in the methotrexate group, and there was delayed remission in the methotrexate group in patients with more extensive disease or pulmonary involvement. The lack of a difference between methotrexate and cyclophosphamide at 6 months might reflect the fact that patients in both treatment groups were still receiving steroids at this timepoint. Post-trial follow-up has revealed that patients in the methotrexate arm of the trial received more corticosteroids, cyclophosphamide, and other immunosuppressive agents than those in the cyclophosphamide group [24], indicating less effective disease control with methotrexate compared to cyclophosphamide induction therapy. In light of these data and our clinical experience, it is the authors' personal view that methotrexate should be used for only the mildest cases of GPA, and we have a low threshold for switching to stronger immunosuppressive therapy in the face of active

Table 1 Previous reports of sellar involvement in GPA

1st Author & year	PMID	No. of cases	Age at GPA diagnosis	Age at time of sellar involvement	Sex	Pituitary Imaging (MRI unless stated)	Endocrinological abnormalities	Non-CNS features	ANCA
Haynes 1978 [29]	692550	1	26*	25	M	NA	DI Hyperprolactinaemia Normal TSH Normal LH & FSH	Lung, renal	N/A
Hurst 1983 [30]	6625709	1	47*	47	F	CT normal	DI Normal prolactin Normal TSH Post-menopausal LH/FSH	Polyarthritis, ENT, ocular, mucocutaneous, pulmonary	N/A
Lohr 1988 [31]	3172100	1	19*	19	F	Intrasellar mass	N/A	ENT, pulmonary	N/A
Rosete 1991 [32]	1865428	1	51*	51	F	CT: pituitary enlargement	DI	N/A	N/A
Czarnecki 1995 [33]	7611087	1	31	34	F	Sellar mass with suprasellar extension. Enhancement of the stalk and hypothalamus. Loss of PS.	DI Hyperprolactinaemia	ENT, arthralgia	N/A
Roberts 1995 [34]	7758239	2	71*	71	F	Intrasellar mass with suprasellar extension	DI (post-surgery) ↓ TSH ↓ LH & FSH ↓ cortisol Normal prolactin	None	cANCA +ve
			28*	28	F	Intrasellar mass with low-density centre	DI (post-surgery) Normal prolactin Normal TSH Normal LH & FSH Normal cortisol	Ocular, arthralgia, cutaneous, renal	cANCA +ve
Bertken 1997 [35]	9265867	1	36*	36	F	Macrocystic pituitary mass with suprasellar extension. Hydrocephalus	DI (post surgery) ↓ TSH response ↓ LH & FSH responses	ENT, pulmonary, ocular	ANCA -ve
Hajj-Ali 1999 [36]	10461488	1	N/A	21	F	Normal	DI	N/A	N/A
Katzman 1999 [21]	10219422	2	41*	41	F	Pituitary enlargement. Loss of PS	DI Hyperprolactinaemia Normal TSH Normal LH & FSH	Constitutional, arthralgia, ENT, ocular, cutaneous	cANCA +ve
			18*	18	F	Pituitary enlargement with contrast-enhancement. Loss of PS	DI Hyperprolactinaemia Normal TSH Normal LH & FSH	ENT, pulmonary	cANCA +ve
Miesen 1999 [37]	10069203	1	46*	45	M	Stalk thickening, contrast-enhancement. Loss of PS	DI Hyperprolactinaemia Hypogonadism Normal TSH Normal LH & FSH Normal cortisol & ACTH	ENT, renal, pulmonary	ANCA +ve
Goyal 2000 [38]	11003280	1	N/A (many years before pituitary involvement)	48	F	Sellar mass with suprasellar extension. Contrast-enhancement	DI ↓ TSH	Renal, pulmonary	cANCA +ve
Tappouni 2000 [39]	11096156	1	58*	57	F	Pituitary mass	DI	Constitutional, ENT, cutaneous, renal, pulmonary	PR3 +ve
Woywodt 2000 [40]	11028850	1	30*	30	M	N/A (diagnosed at autopsy)	N/A	N/A	N/A
Garovic 2001 [41]	11136194	1	47*	47	F	Cystic enlargement of the pituitary. Non-enhancing with gadolinium	DI ↓ prolactin ↓ TSH ↓ gonadotropins	Constitutional, cutaneous, pulmonary	cANCA +ve
Tao 2003 [42]	14642162	1	N/A	19	F	Pituitary and stalk enlargement with heterogenous enhancement	DI ↓ TSH Hypogonadism	N/A	N/A

Table 1 Previous reports of sellar involvement in GPA *(Continued)*

1st Author & year	PMID	No. of cases	Age at GPA diagnosis	Age at time of sellar involvement	Sex	Pituitary Imaging (MRI unless stated)	Endocrinological abnormalities	Non-CNS features	ANCA
Muir 2004 [43]	15150009	1	13*	13	M	Diffuse pituitary enlargement. Foci of ↑ T1 signal. More extensive ↑ T2 signal. Central contrast-enhancement. Loss of PS.	DI	ENT, pulmonary	ANCA +ve
Vittaz 2004 [44]	15687906	2	45	47	M	Pituitary mass, with contrast-enhancement. Pituitary stalk thickened & infiltrated. Loss of PS	Hyperprolactinaemia ↓ testosterone ↓ LH, normal FSH ↓ cortisol & ACTH Normal TSH	Constitutional, polyarthritis, peripheral neuropathy, pulmonary	PR3 +ve
			46	50	F	Pituitary enlargement	DI Hyperprolactinaemia Hypogonadism	Polyarthritis, ocular, mucocutaneous, ENT	ANCA +ve
Duzgun 2005 [45]	15864593	1	47*	47	F	Loss of PS	DI Anterior pituitary hormones normal	Polyarthritis, pulmonary, ENT, renal	PR3 +ve
Seror 2006 [16]	16523054	3	45	50	F	Nodular pituitary enlargement. Homogenous contrast-enhancement. Loss of PS	DI Hyperprolactinaemia Thyrotropic deficiency Hypogonadism Corticotropic deficiency	ENT, ocular, mucocutaneous	PR3 +ve
			26	41	F	Nodular pituitary enlargement. Contrast-enhancement	DI Normal anterior pituitary hormones	ENT, arthralgia, ocular, renal	PR3 +ve
			55	57	M	Pituitary enlargement & central necrosis. Heterogenous enhancement.	DI Hyperprolactinaemia Panhypopituitarism	Peripheral neuropathy, pulmonary, retinal vasculitis, digital, cerebral and renal infarcts	PR3 +ve
Spisek 2006 [46]	16322901	1	30*	29	M	Sellar cystic lesion	DI ↓ TSH ↓ LH & FSH ↓ ACTH ↓ IGF-1	ENT	PR3 +ve
McIntyre 2007 [47]	17318440	1	22*	22	F	Heterogeneous enhancing pituitary mass	DI Hypogonadism	Cutaneous, ocular, renal	PR3 +ve
Thiryayi 2007 [48]	17188492	1	21*	21	F	Sellar mass with central hypo-intensity	DI (post-surgery) Hypogonadism (post-surgery)	Constitutional, arthralgia	cANCA +ve
Yong 2008 [49]	17492510	1	33*	33	M	Pituitary stalk thickening. Contrast-enhancing nodule at the superior aspect of the stalk. Loss of PS.	DI Hypogonadism ↓ ACTH Normal prolactin Normal TSH Normal IGF-1	ENT	PR3 +ve
Cunnington 2009 [50]	20107566	3	19	24	M	Pituitary enlargement	DI Anterior pituitary hormones normal	Constitutional, ENT, pulmonary, ocular, cutaneous	PR3 +ve
			33	34	F	Diffusely enlarged gland containing a poorly enhancing lesion with supra-sellar extension. Loss of PS.	DI Normal prolactin Normal TSH	Constitutional, ENT	cANCA+ve
			26	35	M		DI ↓ TSH	Constitutional, ENT, pulmonary	cANCA +ve

Table 1 Previous reports of sellar involvement in GPA *(Continued)*

1st Author & year	PMID	No. of cases	Age at GPA diagnosis	Age at time of sellar involvement	Sex	Pituitary Imaging (MRI unless stated)	Endocrinological abnormalities	Non-CNS features	ANCA
						Diffusely enlarged pituitary and thickened stalk.			
Xue 2009 [51]	19172275	1	63*	63	F	Normal	DI TSH normal LH & FSH normal	Constitutional, pulmonary, peripheral neuropathy	PR3 +ve
Barlas 2011 [52]	21116602	1	35	37	F	Anterior enlargement. Central area with low signal on T1 and high signal on T2. Post contrast enhancement of pituitary and stalk. Loss of PS.	DI Hyperprolactinaemia	ENT, pulmonary, polyarthritis	cANCA +ve
Santoro 2011 [53]	22147097	1	53*	53	F	Hypointensity of adenohypophysis on T1. Hyperintense sectors on R side on T2. Peripheral contrast-enhancement. Stalk-thickening. Loss of PS.	DI ↓ TSH Hypogonadism Normal prolactin	Polyarthritis, cutaneous, pulmonary, renal	cANCA +ve
Tenorio-Jimenez 2011 [54]	22673710	1	23	38	F	MRI: marked infundibular thickening, sellar mass with hypointensity on T1. Loss of PS	Hyperprolactinaemia ↓ TSH Hypogonadism Post pituitary hormones unaffected	ENT, pulmonary, renal	cANCA +ve (−ve by the time of sellar manifestations)
Hughes 2013 [55]	23186961	1	N/A	30	F	Sellar mass	Panhypopituitarism	Ocular	N/A
Pereira 2013 [56]	22898089	1	48*	48	F	Appearances of pituitary microadenoma, but histopathlogy revealed necrotizing granulomatous inflammation	Hyperprolactinaemia ↓ TSH Post pituitary hormones unaffected	ENT	N/A
Kapoor 2014 [20]	25077899	8	N/A	67	F	Peripherally enhancing cystic sellar mass compressing the stalk	Hyperprolactinaemia Hypogonadism Normal TSH	ENT, renal	7/8 cases PR3 +ve
			N/A	48	F	Multiple non-enhancing cystic areas in the pituitary, convexity of superior margin of pituitary	DI ↓ prolactin ↓ TSH Hypogonadism Corticotropic deficiency	ENT, pulmonary, cutaneous	
			N/A	28	F	Sellar mass with large zone of central non-enhancement and peripheral enhancement. Stalk displacement	DI Hypogonadism Normal prolactin Normal TSH Normal IGF-1 Normal cortisol	ENT, pulmonary, renal	
			N/A	55	M	Sellar mass with suprasellar extension	DI Hypogonadism Normal prolactin Normal TSH Normal cortisol Normal IGF-1	ENT, pulmonary, renal, cutaneous, joints	
			N/A	35	M	Necrotic sellar mass with peripheral enhancement & suprasellar extension. Thickened contrast-enhancing stalk	DI ↓ TSH Hypogonadism Normal prolactin Normal cortisol Normal IGF-1	ENT	

Table 1 Previous reports of sellar involvement in GPA *(Continued)*

1st Author & year	PMID	No. of cases	Age at GPA diagnosis	Age at time of sellar involvement	Sex	Pituitary Imaging (MRI unless stated)	Endocrinological abnormalities	Non-CNS features	ANCA
			N/A	54	M	Enlarged pituitary measuring 12 mm, with heterogeneous enhancement. Slight diffuse thickening of the stalk	DI ↓ TSH Hypogonadism Normal prolactin Normal IGF-1	ENT, pulmonary, renal, cardiac	
			N/A	68	M	Homogeneously enhancing sellar mass, extending into the cavernous sinus bilaterally. Stalk preserved.	↓ prolactin ↓ TSH Hypogonadism ↓ IGF-1	ENT, joints	
			N/A	28	F	Sellar mass extending into the suprasellar cistern, with low T2 signal in the periphery and a bright centre. Peripheral enhancement with central cystic change. Thickening of pituitary stalk	DI Normal prolactin Normal TSH Normal cortisol Normal IGF-1	ENT	
De Parisot 2015 [19]	25906106	9	46*	46	F	Enlarged posterior pituitary. Infiltration of posterior pituitary. Loss of PS	DI	ENT, ocular	
			60	70	M	Normal	↓ TSH Hypogonadism ↓ IGF-1 Normal prolactin	ENT, peripheral neuropathy	
			23	24	F	Enlarged pituitary. Irregularity of infundibulum. Heterogeneous enhancement of anterior pituitary. Loss of PS	DI ↓ TSH Hypogonadism Normal prolactin Normal IGF-1	ENT	
			24*	24	M	Enlarged infundibulum	DI Hyperprolactinaemia ↓ TSH Hypogonadism Normal IGF-1	Renal, ocular, joints, gastro-intestinal	
			66	77	M	Enlarged pituitary. Stalk infiltration. Loss of PS.	↓ TSH Hypogonadism ↓ IGF-1 Normal prolactin	None	
			67	68	F	Normal	DI Hyperprolactinaemia Normal TSH Normal LH & FSH Normal IGF-1	ENT	
			28	42	F	Heterogeneous enhancement of pituitary	DI Hyperprolactinaemia Hypogonadism ↓ ACTH	ENT, lung	
			55	57	M	Sellar mass, heterogeneous. Enhancement. Enlargement and infiltration of stalk. Loss of PS	DI Hyperprolactinaemia ↓ TSH Hypogonadism ↓ ACTH	Pulmonary	
			46	50	F	Enlargement and infiltration of pituitary. Heterogeneous enhancement, contact with optic chiasm	DI Hyperprolactinaemia Hypogonadism Normal TSH Normal IGF-1	ENT, ocular	
Eli 2016 [22]	27521731	1	32*	29	F		Hyperprolactinaemia	ENT, pulmonary	MPO +ve

Table 1 Previous reports of sellar involvement in GPA *(Continued)*

1st Author & year	PMID	No. of cases	Age at GPA diagnosis	Age at time of sellar involvement	Sex	Pituitary Imaging (MRI unless stated)	Endocrinological abnormalities	Non-CNS features	ANCA
						Homogenously enhancing sellar mass. Thickened stalk.			
Esposito 2017 [57]	28540625	3	37*	37	F	Sellar mass extending into the suprasellar cistern with peripheral enhancement and central cystic lesion. Stalk deviation.	DI Hypogonadism GH deficiency	Constitutional, ENT	PR3 +ve
			36*	36	F	Cystic pituitary mass	DI Anterior pituitary function normal	Constitutional, myalgia, ENT, pulmonary	PR3 +ve
			32*	32	F	Sellar mass with homogeneous. Thickening of the pituitary stalk	DI Anterior pituitary function normal	ENT	PR3 +ve

Abbreviations: *ACTH* adrenocorticotropic hormone, *cANCA* cytoplasmic pattern ANCA staining, *DI* diabetes insipidus, *GH* growth hormone, *IGF-1* insulin-like growth factor 1, *LH* luteinising hormone, *FSH* follicular stimulating hormone, *MPO* myeloperoxidase, *N/A* data not available, *PMID* PubMed ID, *PR3* proteinase-3, *PS* posterior signal.
*indicates cases where pituitary involvement was diagnosed prior to or at the time of GPA diagnosis
For the purposes of the Table, a TSH within the reference range but inappropriately low for the T4 has been included in the category "↓ TSH"

disease. This view is supported by the 2015 EULAR guidelines which reserve methotrexate for the treatment of non-organ threatening disease [6]. The EULAR guidelines specifically spell out that methotrexate is not suitable therapy for meningeal disease, or for nasal/paranasal disease with bony involvement, cartilage collapse or deafness, and thus do not support the use of methotrexate in this patient, even at the time of her initial presentation. The absence of pulmonary or renal disease and the perception that localised disease is benign may have contributed to her initial under-treatment, and the failure to escalate immunosuppression at her local hospital.

The final issue is the choice of rituximab versus cyclophosphamide. We initially opted for rituximab over cyclophosphamide to reduce the risk of infertility. However, in view of rapid clinical deterioration we commenced cyclophosphamide. The RAVE and RITUXIVAS studies both showed non-inferiority of rituximab compared to cyclophosphamide in AAV [25, 26]. However, the results from these trials cannot necessarily be extrapolated to our patient. In the RITUXIVAS trial all patients had glomerulonephritis. The RAVE study was not restricted to patients with renal involvement, but did not have any patients with cranial nerve palsies in the rituximab treatment arm. Nevertheless, case series suggest that rituximab can be effective in cranial GPA [27, 28]. It should be highlighted that rituximab has a relatively slow onset of action, and in retrospect our initial "bridging" steroid therapy (one pulse of 500 mg iv methyl prednisolone and 30 mg oral prednisolone) was insufficient. The patient improved markedly after we commenced high-dose corticosteroids and cyclophosphamide. For severe cases where rapid control of disease is necessary, this combination of cyclophosphamide and rituximab may be preferable to either drug alone. Indeed, in the RITUXIVAS trial i.v. cyclophosphamide 15 mg/kg was given alongside the rituximab doses in weeks 1 and 3 [26].

Conclusions

Pituitary involvement is a rare complication of GPA. It disproportionately affects female patients and tends to occur early in the disease course. Diabetes insipidus is the most commonly associated endocrinological abnormality. Our case report highlights that localised GPA is not necessarily indolent and that methotrexate may be inadequate treatment for localised disease. The presence of adverse features such as neurological involvement requires prompt recognition and aggressive therapy. Organ- or even life-threatening disease can occur in the absence of pulmonary or renal involvement. In this case a good outcome was achieved with high-dose steroid and dual treatment with cyclophosphamide and rituximab with minimal adverse events. In cases of severe neurological compromise due to GPA where a rapid therapeutic effect is required, such combination therapy may be a useful strategy. Finally, such cases should be managed by a multi-disciplinary team in a tertiary referral centre.

Abbreviations

ACE: Angiotensin-converting enzyme; ACTH: Adrenocorticotropic hormone; CNS: central nervous system; CRP: C reactive protein; CT: Computed tomography; ELISA: Enzyme-linked immunosorbent assay; ENT: Ear, nose and throat; ESR: Erythrocyte sedimentation rate; EULAR: European League Against Rheumatism; GPA: Granulomatosis with polyangiitis; MPO: Myeloperoxidase; MRI: Magnetic resonance imaging; NIH: National Institutes of Health; PR3: Proteinase-3; TSH: Thyroid-stimulating hormone

Acknowledgements

We thank Prof. David Jayne for his comments on the manuscript.

Funding
Dr. Peters was supported by a Career Development Award from the Cambridge British Heart Foundation Centre for Research Excellence (RE/13/6/30180) and a UK Research Institutes Innovation Fellowship at HDR UK (MR/S004068/1).

Authors' contributions
JP, VG and AJ synthesised and interpreted the clinical data. JP performed the literature search and analysed the data. JP wrote the manuscript with assistance from VG, CO and AJ. IS analysed and interpreted the histopathology. CO analysed and interpreted the radiology. All authors provided critical input to the manuscript, and read and approved the final version.

Competing interests
The authors declare that they have no competing interests.

Author details
[1]Cardiovascular Epidemiology Unit, Department of Public Health and Primary Care, Worts Causeway, University of Cambridge, Cambridge CB1 8RN, UK. [2]Department of Rheumatology, The Royal London and Mile End Hospitals, Barts Health NHS Trust, Bancroft Road, London E1 4DG, UK. [3]Department of Histopathology, Queen's Hospital, Rom Valley Road, Romford RM7 0AG, UK. [4]Department of Radiology, The Royal London Hospital, Barts Health NHS Trust, Whitechapel Road, London E1 1BB, UK.

References
1. Jennette JC, Falk RJ, Bacon PA, Basu N, Cid MC, Ferrario F, et al. 2012 revised international Chapel Hill consensus conference nomenclature of Vasculitides. Arthritis Rheum. 2013;65(1):1–11.
2. Godman GC, Churg J. Wegener's granulomatosis: pathology and review of the literature. AMA Arch Pathol. 1954;58(6):533–53.
3. Fauci AS, Wolff SM. Wegener's granulomatosis: studies in eighteen patients and a review of the literature. Medicine (Baltimore). 1973;52(6):535–61.
4. Walton EW. Giant-cell granuloma of the respiratory tract (Wegener's granulomatosis). Br Med J. 1958;2(5091):265–70.
5. Ntatsaki E, Carruthers D, Chakravarty K, D'Cruz D, Harper L, Jayne D, et al. BSR and BHPR guideline for the management of adults with ANCA-associated vasculitis. Rheumatology (Oxford). 2014;53(12):2306–9.
6. Yates M, Watts RA, Bajema IM, Cid MC, Crestani B, Hauser T, et al. EULAR/ERA-EDTA recommendations for the management of ANCA-associated vasculitis. Ann Rheum Dis. 2016;75(9):1583–94.
7. Carrington CB, Liebow A. Limited forms of angiitis and granulomatosis of Wegener's type. Am J Med. 1966;41(4):497–527.
8. Stone JH, Wegener's Granulomatosis Etanercept Trial Research G. Limited versus severe Wegener's granulomatosis: baseline data on patients in the Wegener's granulomatosis etanercept trial. Arthritis Rheum. 2003;48(8):2299–309.
9. Peters JE, Salama AD, Ind PW. Wegener's granulomatosis presenting as acute systemic vasculitis following 20 years of limited tracheobronchial disease. J Laryngol Otol. 2009;123(12):1375–7.
10. Stegeman CA, Tervaert JW, de Jong PE, Kallenberg CG. Trimethoprim-sulfamethoxazole (co-trimoxazole) for the prevention of relapses of Wegener's granulomatosis. Dutch Co-Trimoxazole Wegener study group. N Engl J Med. 1996;335(1):16–20.
11. Peters JE, Burke CJ, Morris VH. Three cases of rheumatoid arthritis with laryngeal stridor. Clin Rheumatol. 2011;30(5):723–7.
12. de Groot K, Schmidt DK, Arlt AC, Gross WL, Reinhold-Keller E. Standardized neurologic evaluations of 128 patients with Wegener granulomatosis. Arch Neurol. 2001;58(8):1215–21.
13. Hoffman GS, Kerr GS, Leavitt RY, Hallahan CW, Lebovics RS, Travis WD, et al. Wegener granulomatosis: an analysis of 158 patients. Ann Intern Med. 1992; 116(6):488–98.
14. Nishino H, Rubino FA, DeRemee RA, Swanson JW, Parisi JE. Neurological involvement in Wegener's granulomatosis: an analysis of 324 consecutive patients at the Mayo Clinic. Ann Neurol. 1993;33(1):4–9.
15. Drachman DA. Neurological complications of Wegener's granulomatosis. Arch Neurol. 1963;8(2):145–55.
16. Seror R, Mahr A, Ramanoelina J, Pagnoux C, Cohen P, Guillevin L. Central nervous system involvement in Wegener granulomatosis. Medicine (Baltimore). 2006;85(1):54–65.
17. Yokoseki A, Saji E, Arakawa M, Kosaka T, Hokari M, Toyoshima Y, et al. Hypertrophic pachymeningitis: significance of myeloperoxidase anti-neutrophil cytoplasmic antibody. Brain. 2014;137(Pt 2):520–36.
18. Shinkawa Y, Hatachi S, Yagita M. Intravascular large B-cell lymphoma with a high titer of proteinase-3-anti-neutrophil cytoplasmic antibody mimicking granulomatosis with polyangiitis. Mod Rheumatol. 2016:1–3.
19. De Parisot A, Puechal X, Langrand C, Raverot G, Gil H, Perard L, et al. Pituitary involvement in granulomatosis with polyangiitis: report of 9 patients and review of the literature. Medicine (Baltimore). 2015;94(16):e748.
20. Kapoor E, Cartin-Ceba R, Specks U, Leavitt J, Erickson B, Erickson D. Pituitary dysfunction in granulomatosis with polyangiitis: the Mayo Clinic experience. J Clin Endocrinol Metab. 2014;99(11):3988–94.
21. Katzman GL, Langford CA, Sneller MC, Koby M, Patronas NJ. Pituitary involvement by Wegener's granulomatosis: a report of two cases. AJNR Am J Neuroradiol. 1999;20(3):519–23.
22. Eli IM, Raheja A, Corn HJ, Simmons DL, Palmer CA, Couldwell WT. Sellar Wegener granulomatosis masquerading as Cabergoline-resistant Prolactinoma. World Neurosurg. 2016;95:622. e621-622 e625
23. De Groot K, Rasmussen N, Bacon PA, Tervaert JW, Feighery C, Gregorini G, et al. Randomized trial of cyclophosphamide versus methotrexate for induction of remission in early systemic antineutrophil cytoplasmic antibody-associated vasculitis. Arthritis Rheum. 2005;52(8):2461–9.
24. Faurschou M, Westman K, Rasmussen N, de Groot K, Flossmann O, Hoglund P, et al. Brief report: long-term outcome of a randomized clinical trial comparing methotrexate to cyclophosphamide for remission induction in early systemic antineutrophil cytoplasmic antibody-associated vasculitis. Arthritis Rheum. 2012;64(10):3472–7.
25. Stone JH, Merkel PA, Spiera R, Seo P, Langford CA, Hoffman GS, et al. Rituximab versus cyclophosphamide for ANCA-associated vasculitis. N Engl J Med. 2010;363(3):221–32.
26. Jones RB, Tervaert JW, Hauser T, Luqmani R, Morgan MD, Peh CA, et al. Rituximab versus cyclophosphamide in ANCA-associated renal vasculitis. N Engl J Med. 2010;363(3):211–20.
27. Martinez Del Pero M, Chaudhry A, Jones RB, Sivasothy P, Jani P, Jayne D. B-cell depletion with rituximab for refractory head and neck Wegener's granulomatosis: a cohort study. Clin Otolaryngol. 2009;34(4):328–35.
28. Guerry MJ, Brogan P, Bruce IN, D'Cruz DP, Harper L, Luqmani R, et al. Recommendations for the use of rituximab in anti-neutrophil cytoplasm antibody-associated vasculitis. Rheumatology (Oxford). 2012;51(4):634–43.
29. Haynes BF, Fauci AS. Diabetes insipidus associated with Wegener's granulomatosis successfully treated with cyclophosphamide. N Engl J Med. 1978;299(14):764.
30. Hurst NP, Dunn NA, Chalmers TM. Wegener's granulomatosis complicated by diabetes insipidus. Ann Rheum Dis. 1983;42(5):600–1.
31. Lohr KM, Ryan LM, Toohill RJ, Anderson T. Anterior pituitary involvement in Wegener's granulomatosis. J Rheumatol. 1988;15(5):855–7.
32. Rosete A, Cabral AR, Kraus A, Alarcon-Segovia D. Diabetes insipidus secondary to Wegener's granulomatosis: report and review of the literature. J Rheumatol. 1991;18(5):761–5.
33. Czarnecki EJ, Spickler EM. MR demonstration of Wegener granulomatosis of the infundibulum, a cause of diabetes insipidus. AJNR Am J Neuroradiol. 1995;16(4 Suppl):968–70.
34. Roberts GA, Eren E, Sinclair H, Pelling M, Burns A, Bradford R, et al. Two cases of Wegener's granulomatosis involving the pituitary. Clin Endocrinol. 1995;42(3):323–8.
35. Bertken RD, Cooper VR. Wegener granulomatosis causing sellar mass, hydrocephalus, and global pituitary failure. West J Med. 1997;167(1):44–7.
36. Hajj-Ali RA, Uthman IW, Salti IA, Zaatari GS, Haddad MC, Nasr FW. Wegener's granulomatosis and diabetes insipidus. Rheumatology (Oxford). 1999;38(7):684–5.
37. Miesen WM, Janssens EN, van Bommel EF. Diabetes insipidus as the presenting symptom of Wegener's granulomatosis. Nephrol Dial Transplant. 1999;14(2):426–9.
38. Goyal M, Kucharczyk W, Keystone E. Granulomatous hypophysitis due to Wegener's granulomatosis. AJNR Am J Neuroradiol. 2000;21(8):1466–9.
39. Tappouni R, Burns A. Pituitary involvement in Wegener's granulomatosis. Nephrol Dial Transplant. 2000;15(12):2057–8.
40. Woywodt A, Knoblauch H, Kettritz R, Schneider W, Gobel U. Sudden death and Wegener's granulomatosis of the pituitary. Scand J Rheumatol. 2000; 29(4):264–6.

41. Garovic VD, Clarke BL, Chilson TS, Specks U. Diabetes insipidus and anterior pituitary insufficiency as presenting features of Wegener's granulomatosis. Am J Kidney Dis. 2001;37(1):E5.
42. Tao J, Dong Y. Pituitary involvement in Wegener's granulomatosis: a case report and review of the literature. Chin Med J. 2003;116(11):1785–8.
43. Muir BM, Hulett RL, Zorn JG. Wegener's granulomatosis complicated by central diabetes insipidus in a pediatric patient. AJR Am J Roentgenol. 2004; 182(6):1560–2.
44. Vittaz L, Ramanoelina J, Mahr A, Cohen R, Cohen P, Reach G, et al. Pituitary involvement in Wegener's granulomatosis. Two cases. Presse Med. 2004; 33(22):1585–90.
45. Duzgun N, Morris Y, Gullu S, Gursoy A, Ensari A, Kumbasar OO, et al. Diabetes insipidus presentation before renal and pulmonary features in a patient with Wegener's granulomatosis. Rheumatol Int. 2005;26(1):80–2.
46. Spisek R, Kolouchova E, Jensovsky J, Rusina R, Fendrych P, Plas J, et al. Combined CNS and pituitary involvement as a primary manifestation of Wegener granulomatosis. Clin Rheumatol. 2006;25(5):739–42.
47. McIntyre EA, Perros P. Fatal inflammatory hypophysitis. Pituitary. 2007; 10(1):107–11.
48. Thiryayi W, Donaldson MH, Border D, Tyagi A. An enhancing pituitary lesion in a young woman: a diagnostic dilemma. J Clin Neurosci. 2007;14(3):286–8.
49. Yong TY, Li JY, Amato L, Mahadevan K, Phillips PJ, Coates PS, et al. Pituitary involvement in Wegener's granulomatosis. Pituitary. 2008;11(1):77–84.
50. Cunnington JR, Jois R, Zammit I, Scott D, Isaacs J. Diabetes insipidus as a complication of Wegener's granulomatosis and its treatment with biologic agents. Int J Rheumatol. 2009;2009:346136.
51. Xue J, Wang H, Wu H, Jin Q. Wegener's granulomatosis complicated by central diabetes insipidus and peripheral neutrophy with normal pituitary in a patient. Rheumatol Int. 2009;29(10):1213–7.
52. Barlas NB, Hassan HH, Al Badr FB, Bilal A. Structural and functional involvement of pituitary gland in Wegener's granulomatosis. Clin Neuroradiol. 2011;21(1):31–3.
53. Santoro SG, Guida AH, Furioso AE, Glikman P, Rogozinski AS. Panhypopituitarism due to Wegener's granulomatosis. Arq Bras Endocrinol Metabol. 2011;55(7):481–5.
54. Tenorio Jimenez C, Montalvo Valdivieso A, Lopez Gallardo G, McGowan B. Pituitary involvement in Wegener's granulomatosis: unusual biochemical findings and severe malnutrition. BMJ Case Rep. 2011;2011
55. Hughes J, Barkhoudarian G, Ciarlini P, Laws ER, Mody E, Inzucchi SE, et al. Refractory pituitary granulomatosis with polyangiitis (Wegener's) treated with rituximab. Endocr Pract. 2013;19(1):e1–7.
56. Pereira EA, Plaha P, Hofer M, Karavitaki N, Cudlip SA. Hypophyseal Wegener's granulomatosis presenting by visual field constriction without hypopituitarism. Clin Neurol Neurosurg. 2013;115(6):762–4.
57. Esposito D, Trimpou P, Giugliano D, Dehlin M, Ragnarsson O. Pituitary dysfunction in granulomatosis with polyangiitis. Pituitary. 2017;20(5):594–601.

17

Personalized objects can optimize the diagnosis of EMCS in the assessment of functional object use in the CRS-R

Yuxiao Sun[1], Jianan Wang[1], Lizette Heine[2,3], Wangshan Huang[1], Jing Wang[1], Nantu Hu[1], Xiaohua Hu[4], Xiaohui Fang[1], Supeng Huang[1], Steven Laureys[2] and Haibo Di[1*]

Abstract

Background: Behavioral assessment has been acted as the gold standard for the diagnosis of disorders of consciousness (DOC) patients. The item "Functional Object Use" in the motor function sub-scale in the Coma Recovery Scale-Revised (CRS-R) is a key item in differentiating between minimally conscious state (MCS) and emergence from MCS (EMCS). However, previous studies suggested that certain specific stimuli, especially something self-relevant can affect DOC patients' scores of behavioral assessment scale. So, we attempted to find out if personalized objects can improve the diagnosis of EMCS in the assessment of Functional Object Use by comparing the use of patients' favorite objects and other common objects in MCS patients.

Methods: Twenty-one post-comatose patients diagnosed as MCS were prospectively included. The item "Functional Object Use" was assessed by using personalized objects (e.g., cigarette, paper) and non-personalized objects, which were presented in a random order. The rest assessments were performed following the standard protocol of the CRS-R. The differences between functional uses of the two types of objects were analyzed by the McNemar test.

Results: The incidence of Functional Object Use was significantly higher using personalized objects than non-personalized objects in the CRS-R. Five out of the 21 MCS studied patients, who were assessed with non-personalized objects, were re-diagnosed as EMCS with personalized objects ($\chi^2 = 5$, df = 1, $p < 0.05$).

Conclusions: Personalized objects employed here seem to be more effective to elicit patients' responses as compared to non-personalized objects during the assessment of Functional Object Use in DOC patients.

Keywords: Coma recovery scale-revised, Functional object use, Personalized objects, Non-personalized objects

Background

Behavioral assessment is the gold standard for diagnosis in patients with disorders of consciousness (DOC) [1, 2], and the Coma Recovery Scale-Revised (CRS-R) is an important tool for the assessment of DOC such as the "vegetative state" (now also coined unresponsive wakefulness syndrome; VS/UWS) [3] and the minimally conscious state (MCS) [4]. Differential diagnosis of the level of consciousness in patients with DOC is of great importance, for instance in the decisions on treatment, care, and end-of-life [5]. Clinical diagnosis is based on reliable behavioral responsiveness to the stimuli suggested by the CRS-R. The lower scores for each sub--scale represent reflexive behavior and the higher scores represent relatively conscious behavior. Several items from different sub-scales identify consciously mediated behaviors, and final diagnosis is based on the best behavior over all sub-scales (and multiple assessments).

When the patient shows Functional Object Use (score 6 in the motor function sub-scale) or Accurate Functional

* Correspondence: dihaibo19@aliyun.com
[1]International Vegetative State and Consciousness Science Institute, Hangzhou Normal University, Hangzhou, China
Full list of author information is available at the end of the article

Communication (score 2 in the communication sub-scale) , he/she is diagnosed as an EMCS, which is no longer a DOC. Difference between EMCS and MCS coincide with an increase in functional connectivity collaboration between anti-correlated brain networks [6]. The difference between MCS and EMCS can clinically be based on responses to presented stimuli (e.g., Functional Object Use). Previous research has shown that self-referential stimuli are more effective to elicit patient's responses than non-self-referential stimuli [5, 7]. Laureys et al. found that patients with MCS had a broader range of brain activation using their own names than using any other sound stimuli when patients were scaned with PET [8]. Perrin et al. found that preserved semantic processing could be observed in non-communicative brain-damaged patients, particularly for the subject's own name [9]. In addition, a study with functional magnetic resonance imaging (fMRI) found that 7 patients with VS/UWS who responded to their own names became MCS after 3 months and showed the value of using patient's own name [10]. Other self-referential stimuli such as familiar faces result in a higher number of responses [11]; a preferred music (i.e., a self-referential, autobiographical and emotional stimulus) [12], or a familiar voice of a relative has an effect on behavioral and cognitive processes of patients with DOC [12].

It is thus hypothesized that self-referential stimuli might improve diagnostic assessment, and subsequently decrease the level of misdiagnosis.

To our knowledge, different stimuli indeed have different effects on the behavioral response of patients. The aim of the present study is to compare the frequency of Functional Object Use elicited by the stimuli suggested by the CRS-Rand the personalized stimuli in order to optimize the behavioral assessment of the motor function sub-scale.

Methods

Twenty-one patients diagnosed as MCS were recruited (standard diagnosis procedure using the CRS-R for 4 times within 2 weeks; 11 patients were diagnosed as MCS+ and 10 patients as MCS-; mean age 54.67 ± 13. 58 years old; 15 male, 6 female); mean time since injury was 6 ± 3.81 months). Each patient had the motor ability to move their hands and arms (i.e., motor sub-scale scores ≥1 by using noxious stimuli to upper limbs) [13]. Etiology was traumatic in 11 (52%) patients and non-traumatic in 10 (48%) patients. Table 1 shows the clinical data for each of the 21 patients diagnosed as MCS using the CRS-R. The study was approved by the Ethics Committee of Hangzhou Normal University and Wujing Hospital which complies with the Code of Ethics of the World Medical Association (Declaration of Helsinki). Written informed consents were obtained by the patient's legal surrogates.

This study has been designed in line with the CONSORT recommendations for reporting randomized trials (see Additional file 1).

Patients using a central nervous system stimulant, neuro-muscular blocking agents, or sedative for 24 h, with unstable status, concurrent disease (e.g., pyrexia, pneumonia, diarrhea), or dyskinesia of the upper limbs (i.e., motor sub-scale scores < 1 by using noxious stimuli to upper limbs), or receiving hyperbaric oxygen treatments within 2 h were excluded.

CRS-R assessment tools suggested by the CRS-R (cup and comb) and personalized stimulants (cigarette, paper, pen, mobile phone, tooth brush, fan, and lipstick) were used as assessment instruments. All personalized objects used were collected from patients' bedsides in the hospital, or from their previous daily life.

Each patient was assessed at least twice by assessor "A" on different days within 1 week, with the CRS-R including the sub-item Functional Object Use as suggested by the CRS-R protocol. Patients were tested 2 more times using the CRS-R including Functional Object Use with personalized objects by a second experienced assessor "B" on the same day as by assessor "A". The order of all the assessments was randomized and the time elapse between standard and 'personalized' assessments was set as short as possible (within 2 h). Personalized objects were chosen by family members, or nurses in cases where the patient lacked frequent company of family members. Objects were those be highly appreciated and/or used by patients in their previous daily live. Functional Object Use was evaluated by assessor "A" through standardized methodology as described in the CRS-R. In brief, the assessor placed one of the objects in the patient's hand and instructed the patient that "Show me how to use a [name object]." Then, she placed the second object in the patient's hand and restated the same instruction (see Additional file 2). All the objects were presented in a random order [2, 4].

During the assessment, patients were all subject to a standardized arousal facilitation protocol (i.e., deep pressure stimulation from the facial musculature to the toes was employed if needed, in order to prolong the length of time the patients maintained aroused, and this protocol was re-administered if patients showed sustained eye closure again or behavioral responsiveness ceased despite sustained eye opening [2, 4].)

Differences between Functional Object Use assessed by non-personalized and personalized stimulants were analyzed using the McNemar test. Results were considered significant at $p < 0.05$.

Six months after completion of the protocol, family members and/or nursing staff were asked to perform the

Table 1 Function Object Use with personalized objects

Patient	Aetiology /Time since injury (month)	CRS-R[1]			CRS-R Personalized Objects		
		Diagnosis	Functional Object Use[2]		Re-Diagnosis	Functional Object Use	
			comb	cup		Object 1	Object 2
1	Traumatic/8	MCS-(2-1-3-2-0-3)	0/2	0/2	EMCS (2-2-6-1-0-3)	Paper (2/2)	Pen (2/2)
2	Non-traumatic/6	MCS+(2-1-2-2-1-2)	0/2	0/2	MCS+(2-1-2-2-1-2)	0/2	0/2
3	Non-traumatic/3	MCS+(3-5-3-2-1-3)	0/2	0/2	EMCS (3-5-6-2-1-3)	Paper (2/2)	Pen (2/2)
4	Traumatic/7	MCS+(2-1-2-2-1-2)	0/2	0/2	MCS+(2-1-2-2-1-2)	0/2	0/2
5	Traumatic/3	MCS+(1-3-3-2-0-2)	0/2	0/2	MCS+(3-3-3-3-1-2)	0/2	0/2
6	Non-traumatic/5	MCS+(3-1-4-1-0-2)	0/2	0/2	MCS+(3-1-4-1-0-2)	0/2	0/2
7	Traumatic/10	MCS-(0-2-2-1-0-2)	0/2	0/2	MCS-(0-2-2-1-0-2)	0/2	0/2
8	Traumatic/3	MCS-(1-3-1-1-0-2)	0/2	0/2	EMCS (1-3-6-1-0-2)	Phone (2/2)	Tooth Brush (2/2)
9	Non-traumatic/18	MCS-(2-1-2-1-1-2)	2/2	0/2	EMCS (1-2-6-1-0-3)	Comb (2/2)	Phone (2/2)
10	Non-traumatic/10	MCS-(2-0-1-2-0-2)	0/2	0/2	EMCS (3-5-6-2-1-3)	Phone (2/2)	Fan (2/2)
11	Non-traumatic/6	MCS+(3-5-1-2-1-2)	0/2	0/2	MCS+(3-5-1-2-1-2)	0/2	0/2
12	Traumatic/6	MCS+(2-3-2-2-1-2)	0/2	0/2	MCS+(2-2-2-2-1-2)	0/2	0/2
13	Non-traumatic/3	MCS+(4-5-2-3-1-3)	0/2	0/2	MCS+(4-5-2-3-1-3)	0/2	0/2
14	Traumatic/3	MCS+(4-5-4-2-1-2)	0/2	0/2	MCS+(4-5-4-2-1-2)	0/2	0/2
15	Non-traumatic/2	MCS+(4-5-4-2-0-2)	0/2	0/2	MCS+(4-5-4-2-0-2)	0/2	0/2
16	Non-traumatic/5	MCS-(2-3-3-1-0-2)	0/2	0/2	MCS-(2-3-3-1-0-2)	0/2	0/2
17	Traumatic/9	MCS-(2-3-2-1-0-2)	0/2	0/2	MCS-(2-3-2-1-0-2)	0/2	0/2
18	Traumatic/1	MCS-(1-1-4-1-0-2)	0/2	0/2	MCS-(2-1-4-1-0-2)	0/2	0/2
19	Non-traumatic/9	MCS+(4-5-2-2-0-2)	0/2	0/2	MCS+(4-5-2-2-0-2)	0/2	0/2
20	Traumatic/4	MCS-(2-3-3-1-0-2)	0/2	0/2	MCS-(2-3-3-1-0-2)	0/2	0/2
21	Traumatic/6	MCS-(2-3-2-2-0-2)	0/2	0/2	MCS-(2-3-2-2-1-2)	0/2	0/2

Notes: [1] CRS-R includes 6 sub-scales: Auditory Function Scale, Visual Function Scale, Motor Function Scale, Oromotor/Verbal Function Scale, Communication Scale, Arousal Scale

[2] Functional Object Use is included in Motor Function Scale, and patients will be diagnosed as EMCS if get score in this item

CRS-R including the personalized objects used for each patient.

Results

Reaction to different objects

The incidence of Functional Object Use was significantly higher using personalized objects than non-personalized objects in the CRS-R ($\chi^2 = 5$, df = 1, $p < 0.05$, Fig. 1).] Five out of 21patients who were diagnosed as MCS (1 MCS+, 4 MCS-) without using personalized objects, were however re-diagnosed as EMCS with personalized objects, making a 23.8% diagnosis improvement (see details in Table 1). Four of the 5 patients (1 MCS+, 3 MCS-) only responded to personalized objects, but had no response to the non-personalized objects. The other patient previously diagnosed as MCS- was able to functionally use both one personalized object (mobile phone) and one non-personalized object (comb). Patients made an action of paper folding when investigators showed them a piece of paper (i.e., patient 1 and patient 3); they drew lines on the paper when given the pen (i.e., patient 1 and patient 3); they took the phone and shifted it closer to their ears like answering the phone when displayed a phone (i.e., patient 8 and patient 9); they moved the tooth brush around the mouth when given a tooth brush (i.e., patient 8); and they moved the comb to their heads when given a comb (i.e., patient 9).

Moreover, at 6 months follow-up all of the 5 EMCS patients were reportedly able to use the same personalized objects as tested before in a manner score-able as functional object use.

Discussion

The aim of the study was to determine whether the assessment of Functional Object Use in DOC patients was influenced by the choice of objects. In this study, diagnosis of 5 patients changed when personalized objects were employed instead of the two the standard CRS-R protocol suggests.

Our results are in line with a large amount of research showing that the elicitation of patients' behavioral response can be improved when their personal experience and personal preferences are taken into consideration. Several previous studies found that using the patient's

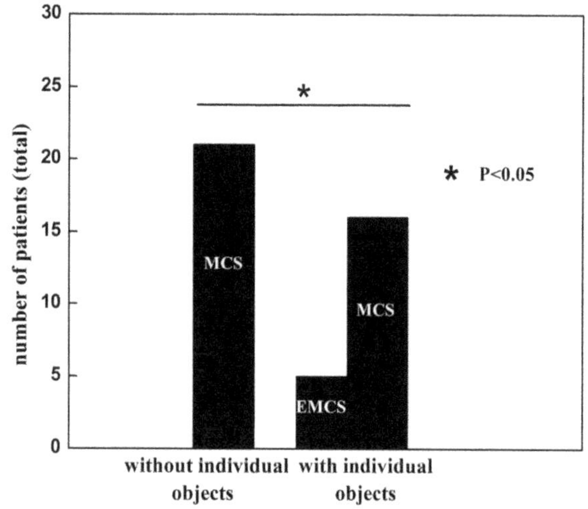

Fig. 1 Functional Object Use with personalized objects. Number of patients diagnosed as MCS and EMCS as a function of the employed assessment (with/without personalized objects)

own name is more suitable to elicit a behavioral response as compared to a standard sound [14, 15]. Di et al.'s study proved that using a mirror (auto-referential stimuli) during the assessment of visual fixation in patients with DOC can elicit higher positive response rate compared to other neutral stimuli [16]. Furthermore, our results are in accordance with a recent study by Stenberg et al. [17], demonstrating improved behavioral responses with personalized stimuli in the visual subscale during the CRS-R assessment in 3 DOC patients. The emotional richness and complexity of personally relevant stimuli are considered to be crucial in promoting active responses of covert behaviors during assessment for DOC patients [7, 11, 12, 18].

Notably, we used a cigarette, paper, pen, mobile phone, tooth brush, fan and the standard comb and cup (as recommended in the CRS-R) and compared the frequency of behavioral response elicited by the different stimuli in 21 patients diagnosed as MCS. Patients for example made the action of origami shipshape when investigators showed the paper (i.e., patient 1 and patient 3); they drew lines on the paper when given the pen (i.e., patient 1 and patient 3); they took the phone and shift closer to their ears like answering the phone when displaying the phone (i.e., patient 8 and patient 9); they moved the tooth brush to around the mouth when given the tooth brush (i.e., patient 8); and they moved the comb to the head when given the comb (i.e., patient 9). Reaction of non-personalized objects included any movement that was not related to the item. The choice of objects was based on reports from family and clinicians from observations of affective behaviors like smiling, laughing, frowning, crying that occur spontaneously in response to the personal objects (cigarette, paper, pen, mobile phone, tooth brush, fan). One out of the five patients (i.e., patient 9) showed "Functional Object Use" to both a personalized object and a non-personalized object. When the non-personalized objects (comb and cup) were presented, the patient only showed a motor response to the comb and was diagnosed as MCS-. However, after being given personalized objects, he could use both the comb and a phone and was therefore re-diagnosed as EMCS. This indicates that personally relevant stimuli might specifically be important for those patients on the edge between MCS and EMCS.

In addition, patient 9 and patient 10 showed a parallel improvement on the motor and the arousal sub-scale while using personalized objects. This might be in line with the mood and arousal hypothesis put forward in previous studies [7]. Thus, the choice of personalized objects seems to be crucial to the accurate assessment of DOC patients' conscious state [11, 18]. As the score of the motor sub-scale was stable across the repeated testing of the CRS-R, and the assessments were counterbalanced, it is unlikely that fluctuations in motricity underly differences in responses to personally relevant objects compared to neutral objects.

Outcome information from the family at 6 months after this study showed that all 5 patients were able to use the personalized objects (but not one or both of the neutral objects except for patient 9)) in a similar way as during the study. It indicates that patients were in a stable state and no behavioral improvement was expected to have occurred in the short period of the study. This is corroborated by the information that no improvement in conscious state was observed by the family or nursing staff (behaviors indicative of upper severe disability or higher [19]). However, main outcome measures were performed using interviews with families, and results should obviously be interpreted with care due to possible family bias.

Conclusions

Personalized objects employed here seemed more sensitive to elicit patients' responses as compared to common objects (e.g., comb, cup) during the assessment of Functional Object Use in patients with DOC.

Abbreviations

CRS-R: Coma Recovery Scale-Revised; DOC: Disorders of consciousness; EMCS: emergence from MCS; fMRI: Functional magnetic resonance imaging; MCS: Minimally conscious state; VS/UWS: Vegetative state/unresponsive wakefulness syndrome

Acknowledgements

Not applicable.

Funding
This study was supported by the National Natural Science Foundation of China (81471100, 811247008), the National High Technology Research and Development Program of China (2015AA020514), the Hangzhou Normal University (JTAS2011-01-016), the Belgian Funds for Scientific Research (FNRS), Fonds Léon Fredericq, and the University of Liège. LH is doctoral researcher and SL is research director at FNRS.

Authors' contributions
YS, JAW, XH, XF, SH collected data and managed the patients; YS, JW and WH performed data analyses; SL and HD designed the study; YS, JW and NH wrote the paper. LH, HD and JW revised the manuscript for important intellectual content. All authors discussed the results and commented on the manuscript. All authors read and approved the final manuscript.

Competing interests
The authors declare that they have no competing interests.

Author details
[1]International Vegetative State and Consciousness Science Institute, Hangzhou Normal University, Hangzhou, China. [2]GIGA, GIGA-Consciousness, Coma Science Group, University & Neurology Department, Hospital of Liege, Liege, Belgium. [3]Audition Cognition and Psychoacoustics Team, Lyon Neuroscience Research Center, Lyon, France. [4]Rehabilitation Center for Brain Damage, Wujing Hospital of Hangzhou City, Hangzhou, China.

References
1. Giacino JT, Schnakers C, Rodriguez-Moreno D, Kalmar K, Schiff N, Hirsch J. Behavioral assessment in patients with disorders of consciousness: gold standard or fool's gold? Prog Brain Res. 2009;177:33–48.
2. Di H, He M, Zhang Y, Cheng L, Wang F, Nie Y, Huang W, Laureys S, Schnakers C. Chinese translation of the coma recovery scale-revised. Brain Inj. 2017; https://doi.org/10.1080/02699052.2016.1255780:1-3.
3. Laureys S, Celesia GG, Cohadon F, Lavrijsen J, Leon-Carrion J, Sannita WG, Sazbon L, Schmutzhard E, von Wild KR, Zeman A, et al. Unresponsive wakefulness syndrome: a new name for the vegetative state or apallic syndrome. BMC Med. 2010;8:68.
4. Giacino JT, Kalmar K, Whyte J. The JFK coma recovery scale-revised: measurement characteristics and diagnostic utility. Arch Phys Med Rehabil. 2004;85(12):2020–9.
5. Owen AM, Coleman MR. Detecting awareness in the vegetative state. Ann N Y Acad Sci. 2008;1129:130–8.
6. Di Perri C, Bahri MA, Amico E, Thibaut A, Heine L, Antonopoulos G, Charland-Verville V, Wannez S, Gomez F, Hustinx R, et al. Neural correlates of consciousness in patients who have emerged from a minimally conscious state: a cross-sectional multimodal imaging study. Lancet Neurol. 2016;15(8):830–42.
7. Perrin F, Castro M, Tillmann B, Luaute J. Promoting the use of personally relevant stimuli for investigating patients with disorders of consciousness. Front Psychol. 2015;6:1102.
8. Laureys S, Perrin F, Faymonville ME, Schnakers C, Boly M, Bartsch V, Majerus S, Moonen G, Maquet P. Cerebral processing in the minimally conscious state. Neurology. 2004;63(5):916–8.
9. Perrin F, Schnakers C, Schabus M, Degueldre C, Goldman S, Bredart S, Faymonville ME, Lamy M, Moonen G, Luxen A, et al. Brain response to one's own name in vegetative state, minimally conscious state, and locked-in syndrome. Arch Neurol. 2006;63(4):562–9.
10. Di HB, Yu SM, Weng XC, Laureys S, Yu D, Li JQ, Qin PM, Zhu YH, Zhang SZ, Chen YZ. Cerebral response to patient's own name in the vegetative and minimally conscious states. Neurology. 2007;68(12):895–9.
11. Sharon H, Pasternak Y, Ben Simon E, Gruberger M, Giladi N, Krimchanski BZ, Hassin D, Hendler T. Emotional processing of personally familiar faces in the vegetative state. PLoS One. 2013;8(9):e74711.
12. Heine L, Castro M, Martial C, Tillmann B, Laureys S, Perrin F. Exploration of functional connectivity during preferred music stimulation in patients with disorders of consciousness. Front Psychol. 2015;6:1704.
13. Thompson AK, Wolpaw JR. The simplest motor skill: mechanisms and applications of reflex operant conditioning. Exerc Sport Sci Rev. 2014;42(2):82–90.
14. Cheng L, Gosseries O, Ying L, Hu X, Yu D, Gao H, He M, Schnakers C, Laureys S, Di H. Assessment of localisation to auditory stimulation in post-comatose states: use the patient's own name. BMC Neurol. 2013;13:27.
15. Qin P, Di H, Yan X, Yu S, Yu D, Laureys S, Weng X. Mismatch negativity to the patient's own name in chronic disorders of consciousness. Neurosci Lett. 2008;448(1):24–8.
16. Di H, Nie Y, Hu X, Tong Y, Heine L, Wannez S, Huang W, Yu D, He M, Thibaut A, et al. Assessment of visual fixation in vegetative and minimally conscious states. BMC Neurol. 2014;14:147.
17. Stenberg J, Godbolt AK, Moller MC. The value of incorporating personally relevant stimuli into consciousness assessment with the coma recovery scale - revised: a pilot study. J Rehabil Med. 2018; https://doi.org/10.2340/16501977-2309.
18. Di Stefano C, Cortesi A, Masotti S, Simoncini L, Piperno R. Increased behavioural responsiveness with complex stimulation in VS and MCS: preliminary results. Brain Inj. 2012;26(10):1250–6.
19. Wilson JT, Pettigrew LE, Teasdale GM. Structured interviews for the Glasgow outcome scale and the extended Glasgow outcome scale: guidelines for their use. J Neurotrauma. 1998;15(8):573–85.

18

Anti-ganglioside complex antibody profiles in a recurrent complicated case of GQ1b-seronegative miller fisher syndrome and Bickerstaff brainstem encephalitis

Hiroto Ito[1*], Yuki Hatanaka[3], Yuki Fukami[4], Yumiko Harada[1], Rei Kobayashi[1], Hisashi Okada[1], Ayumi Uchibori[2], Atsuro Chiba[2] and Satoshi Okuda[1]

Abstract

Background: Guillain-Barré syndrome (GBS), Miller Fisher syndrome (MFS) and Bickerstaff brainstem encephalitis (BBE) are a group of autoimmune neurological disorders (GBS spectrum disorder) that rarely recur. Recently, anti-ganglioside complex antibodies (GSC-Abs) were identified in patients with GBS spectrum disorder. However, there has been no case report describing GSC-Abs profiles in a recurrent case showing different phenotypes.

Case presentation: We report the case of a 33-year-old male patient with GQ1b-seronegative BBE-GBS after two prior episodes of MFS-GBS. Our patient showed ophthalmoplegia, ataxia, areflexia and a weakness of the extremities (MFS and GBS symptoms) in all episodes. In the episode reported here, our patient showed disturbed consciousness and an extensor response to cutaneous plantar stimulation was observed (BBE symptoms), with severe disability and requirement for artificial respiration management. GSC-Abs detected in previous episodes were also detected in the subsequent episodes, while new GSC-Abs emerged in each episode. Interestingly, whereas antibodies to GA1/GQ1b and GA1/GT1a, which are commonly identified in patients with GBS, MFS or BBE, appeared in all episodes, antibodies to GD1a/GD1b and GD1b/GT1b, which are predominantly associated with severe disability and the requirement for artificial respiration management in GBS, emerged for the first time in this episode.

Conclusion: This study reports novel phenomena about the GSC-Abs profiles and its relationship with clinical features in a case with recurrent GBS spectrum disorder, showing different phenotypes in different episodes. Further studies are required to reveal the significance of the GSC-Abs profiles in recurrent GBS spectrum disorder.

Keywords: Bickerstaff brainstem encephalitis, Miller fisher syndrome, Guillain-Barré syndrome, Anti-ganglioside complex antibodies, Recurrence, GQ1b-seronegative

* Correspondence: hiroto.ito.nagoya.uni.med@gmail.com
[1]Department of Neurology, National Hospital Organization Nagoya Medical Center, 4-1-1 Sannomaru, Naka-ku, Nagoya, Japan
Full list of author information is available at the end of the article

Background

Guillain-Barré syndrome (GBS), Miller Fisher syndrome (MFS) and Bickerstaff brainstem encephalitis (BBE) are considered to form a continuous clinical spectrum, GBS spectrum disorder with monophasic symptoms [1]. When they recur, symptoms tend to be similar, although most cases exhibit some differences compared with the previous episodes [2–4]. Recently, ganglioside complexes (GSCs) such as GD1a/GD1b were identified as target antigens for serum antibodies in patients with GBS spectrum disorder [5]. However, anti-ganglioside complex antibody (GSC-Abs) profiles and their relationship with clinical features in different episodes of recurrent cases are unknown. Herein, we report the GSC-Abs profiles and clinical features of a patient with BBE-GBS but without antibodies to GQ1b after two prior episodes of MFS-GBS.

Case presentation

A 33-year-old Japanese man presented with disturbed consciousness. He had a medical history of recurrent MFS-GBS. At age 25, in August, he developed diplopia, difficulty in speaking and swallowing, and an unsteady gait two weeks after suffering from diarrhea. On admission, he showed flaccid tetraparesis (Medical Research Council (MRC) scale grade 3 in the lower limbs, 4 in the upper limbs), external ophthalmoplegia and areflexia. His consciousness was alert, and pathological reflexes were not observed. Nerve conduction studies (NCS) on day 7 showed a slight reduction in sensory nerve action potential (SNAP, recorded orthodromically) amplitude in all examined nerves (5.5 μV in the right median nerve; normal range > 7.9 μV) and slightly prolonged distal motor latency (4.3 ms in the right median nerve only; normal range < 3.7 ms). Slightly slowed F-wave conduction velocity (FWCV) was also observed in all examined nerves (58.0 m/s in the median nerve; normal range > 59.0 m/s). Serum IgG antibodies on admission were measured by enzyme-linked immunosorbent assay to gangliosides (GM1, GM2, GM3, GD1a, GD1b, GD2, GD3, GT1a, GT1b, GQ1b, GA1) and combinations of gangliosides (GM1, GD1a, GD1b, GT1b, GQ1b, GA1). Enzyme-linked immunosorbent assay for IgG antibodies against isolated gangliosides and ganglioside complexes were performed as previously reported [6, 7]. Antibodies to GA1 and GSCs were positive, especially GA1/GQ1b and GA1/GT1a, which had high titers (Fig. 1a). After admission, the weakness in all limbs worsened, and the patient became chair-bound on day 7 after admission. He was then treated with intravenous immunoglobulin (IVIG, 0.4 g/kg/day for 5 days) and began to recover. Within a month, he was discharged with a crutch and later fully recovered. Serum reactivities to GSCs on day 30 were reduced (respective optical density (OD) values of GA1, GA1/GQ1b and GA1/GT1a were 0.69, 1.71, and 1.84 on day 1, and 0.29, 0.84 and 0.85 on day 30).

a

First episode	GA1	GM1	GD1b	GD1a	GT1b	GT1a	GQ1b
Single	2+	–	–	–	–	–	–
GA1		–	–	–	2+	3+	3+
GM1			–	–	–	1+	2+
GD1b				–	–	2+	3+
GD1a					–	–	–
GT1b						–	–
GT1a							–
GQ1b							

b

Second episode	GA1	GM1	GD1b	GD1a	GT1b	GT1a	GQ1b
Single	–	–	–	–	–	–	–
GA1		–	2+	2+	2+	2+	3+
GM1			–	–	–	1+	1+
GD1b				–	–	1+	2+
GD1a					–	–	–
GT1b						–	–
GT1a							–
GQ1b							

c

Third episode	GA1	GM1	GD1b	GD1a	GT1b	GT1a	GQ1b
Single	–	–	–	–	–	1+	–
GA1		–	2+	2+	3+	3+	3+
GM1			–	–	1+	2+	2+
GD1b				1+	1+	2+	2+
GD1a					–	–	–
GT1b						–	–
GT1a							–
GQ1b							

Fig. 1 Profiles of anti-ganglioside antibodies and GCS-Abs in each episode (**a**: first episode, **b**: second episode, **c**: third episode). Isolated gangliosides and GSC were grouped into categories based on antibody titer as follows: (1+) 0.1 to < 0.5; (2+) 0.5 to < 1.0; and (3+) 1.0 or more. In all episodes, serum reacted more strongly to specific ganglioside complexes such as GA1/GQ1b and GA1/GT1a, compared with isolated gangliosides. GSC-Abs that were positive in the previous episode were also positive during the subsequent episodes, while some GSC-Abs newly appeared in each episode

At age 28, in May, one week after suffering from a common cold, he developed an unsteady gait, diplopia and difficulty in speaking and swallowing. He was then readmitted to the same hospital. On examination, loss of proprioception was especially notable, in addition to dysarthria, ophthalmoplegia, areflexia and a weakness of the lower extremities. He was normal in mental status and did not show pathological reflexes. NCS on day 7 showed slightly prolonged distal motor latency (4.1 ms in the right median nerve only) and a slight reduction of SNAP (recorded orthodromically) amplitude in all examined nerves except for the sural nerve (4.9 μV in the right median nerve). Anti-ganglioside antibodies were negative, and antibodies to GA1/GD1b and GA1/GD1a were detected for the first time (in addition to the GSC-Abs identified in the first episode) (Fig. 1b). Starting at admission, IVIG was administered for 5 days.

Although he was restricted to a wheelchair at the nadir, he left the hospital without any disability two weeks after admission.

At age 33, in July, four days after an upper respiratory infection, he noticed diplopia and weakness of the lower extremities. The following day his gait became unsteady. He then complained of a difficulty in breathing and finally displayed drowsiness, and was admitted to our hospital. On admission, he had incomplete ophthalmoplegia, slurred speech, bilateral facial weakness, ptosis and flaccid quadriparesis (MRC grade 2 in the lower limbs, 3 in the upper limbs). Intention tremor and paresthesia were observed. Deep tendon reflexes were absent and an extensor response to cutaneous plantar stimulation was observed. NCS on day 7 showed prolonged distal motor latency in almost all nerves (4.6 ms in the right median nerve) and a reduction of SNAP (recorded antidromically) amplitude in all examined nerves (1.9 μV in the right median nerve; normal range > 10.0 μV). Slowed FWCV was also observed only in tibial nerves (37.6 m/s; normal range > 45.5 m/s). Antibodies to isolated GT1a and GD1a/GD1b, GT1b/GD1b and GM1/GT1b were detected for the first time (in addition to the GSC-Abs identified in previous episodes) (Fig. 1c). His cerebrospinal fluid was abnormal, with an increase in protein (73 mg/dl) and evidence of pleocytosis (432/3 μl; polymorphonuclear/mononuclear leukocyte ratio: 45/55). Brain and spinal magnetic resonance imaging were normal. Electroencephalography on day 5 showed a slow α-rhythm and occasional diffuse theta activity. *Haemophilus influenzae* was found in his sputum culture.

On the day of admission, he developed a more severe disturbed consciousness, and intratracheal intubation was required for potential respiratory failure. He was given IVIG and intravenous methylprednisolone (1000 mg/day on days 1–5). On day 5, he fell into a deep coma without sedation. Starting on day 7, his condition gradually improved. First, his consciousness recovered, which revealed complete flaccid paralysis of the four limbs. Thereafter, the pathological reflexes disappeared. As his limb weakness was still severe, a second IVIG regimen was performed on days 14–18. Finally, the weakness of his four limbs gradually disappeared, and sensory ataxia became apparent. Serum reactivities to GT1a and GSCs on day 40 were reduced (respective OD values of GT1a, GA1/GQ1b and GA1/GT1a were 0.28, 1.28, and 1.29 on day 1, and 0.01, 0.24 and 0.27 on day 40). On day 56, he was transferred to a rehabilitation hospital with a wheelchair. At 10 months after the third onset, he had almost fully recovered, except for hyporeflexia and very mild diplopia and ataxia.

Discussion

In the current case, we diagnosed the first and second episodes as MFS-GBS (first episode mainly GBS, second episode mainly MFS), and the third episode as BBE-GBS. In the third episode, in addition to the previous MFS symptoms, he exhibited new symptoms, including disturbed consciousness and extensor plantar responses, and he required artificial respiration management. Antibodies to GQ1b were negative. However, the GSC-Abs detected in previous episodes were also detected in subsequent episodes, as well as new GSC-Abs during each attack, in part reflecting his clinical features. Antibodies with high titers in the first episode, such as GA1/GQ1b and GA1/GT1a antibodies, also had high titers in recurrent episodes. These antibodies were produced and then reduced in parallel with the neurological symptoms.

The frequency of recurrence in GBS and its variants is low (reported as 2–6% in GBS) [1, 2]. In general, patients with recurrent GBS and its variants show symptoms similar to previous episodes at relapse [2–4]. The emergence of different phenotypes in subsequent episodes is rare [1–4]. In previously reported cases where different phenotypes were observed at relapse, most patients (5 out of 6 patients) developed both MFS and BBE (Table 1) [8–12], possibly because MFS and BBE have pathogenetic and clinical similarities [13]. Given that symptoms at relapse are generally similar to those at previous episodes [2–4], these reports and our case also suggest that MFS and BBE are in close proximity in GBS spectrum disorders. In all cases, BBE was followed by MFS or incomplete MFS. Three of these five patients required artificial respiration management in the last episode, suggesting disease had a tendency to be more severe in recurrent episodes, although all patients responded well to treatment and showed complete or near complete responses (Table 1).

The continued presence of some GSC-Abs and the emergence of new antibodies in our case are consistent with the generally similar, but at the same time unique, clinical features. Our patient exhibited ophthalmoplegia, ataxia, areflexia and a weakness of the extremities in each episode. Antibodies to GA1/GT1a and GA1/GQ1b (commonly identified in patients with GBS, MFS or BBE), GM1/GQ1b, and GD1b/GT1a (commonly identified in patients with GBS or MFS) appeared in all episodes [5]. Antibodies to GD1a/GD1b and GD1b/GT1b, which emerged only in the third episode, are predominantly associated with severe disability in GBS and the requirement for artificial respiration management [5]. Recently, complex enhanced or attenuated anti-GQ1b or GT1a antibodies were reported to underlie the different clinical features in anti-GQ1b antibody syndrome [14]. In our case, subtle differences in the specificities of GSC-Abs in each episode may account for the differential clinical features observed.

The profiles of antibodies to isolated gangliosides and GSCs may be related to recurrence. Previous studies

Table 1 Reported cases describing the different phenotypes during various episodes

Case	Age	Sex	Episode	Preceding illness	DOC	Ophthalm oplegia	Ataxia	Areflexia	Hyper reflexia	PR	Limb weakness	GQ1b Ab	GSC Ab	Phenotype	FG at nadir	Treatment	Outcome	Reference
1	38	F	First	URI	–	+	+	+	–	–	–	+	n.e	MFS	1	IAPP	CR	[8]
	38		Second	URI	–	–	–	+	–	–	+	+	n.e	GBS	4	IAPP	CR	
2	10	F	First	URI	–	+	+	+	–	–	–	n.e	n.e	MFS	2	n.d	CR	[9]
	17		Second	n.d	–	–	+	+	–	–	–	n.e	n.e	Incomplete MFS	1	n.d	CR	
	19		Third	Fever	+	+	+	+	–	+	±	+	n.e	BBE	5	IVIG	NCR	
3	48	M	First	n.d	–	+	n.d	n.d	n.d	n.d	+	n.e	n.e	MFS-GBS	5	n.d	CR	[10]
	53		Second	–	+	+	+	+	–	+	+	–	n.e	BBE-GBS	5	IVIG	CR	
4	35	M	First	n.d	–	+	n.d	n.d	n.d	n.d	–	n.e	n.e	Incomplete MFS	1	–	CR	[11]
	38		Second	n.d	+	+	+	–	+	–	–	n.e	n.e	BBE	5	IVIG	CR	
	43		Third	Fever	+	+	+	–	+	–	–	–	n.e	BBE	5	IVIG	CR	
5	46	M	First	n.d	+	+	+	+	–	n.d	–	–	n.e	MFS (BBE)[a]	3	IVIG	NCR	[12]
	46		Second	n.d	+	+	+	+	–	+	±	–	n.e	BBE	2	IVIG	NCR	
6	25	M	First	URI	–	+	+	+	–	–	+	–	+	MFS-GBS	4	IVIG	CR	Our case
	28		Second	URI	–	+	+	+	–	–	+	–	+	MFS-GBS	4	IVIG	CR	
	33		Third	URI	+	+	+	+	–	+	+	–	+	BBE-GBS	5	IVIG	NCR	

F female, *M* male, *GBS* guillain-Barré syndrome, *MFS* miller fisher syndromes, *BBE* bickerstaff brainstem encephalitis, *Incomplete FS* acute ophthalmoparesis, acute ataxic neuropathy, acute ptosis and acute mydriasis, *URI* upper respiratory infection, *DOC* disturbance of consciousness, *PR* pathological reflex, *Limb weakness* + MMT ≤ 3 at least one limb, *Limb weakness* ± MMT ≥ 4, *MFS-GBS* MFS with definite limb weakness (MMT ≤ 3), *BBE-GBS* BBE with definite limb weakness (MMT ≤ 3), *n.e* not examined, *n.d* not documented, *FG* fuctional grade, *IAPP* immunoadsorption plasmapheresis, *IVIG* intravenous immunoglobulin, *CR* complete recovery, *NCR* near complete recovery (Mild diplopia, weakness, and atxia without disability)

[a]Although this case was considered "Fisher-Bickerstaff syndrome" and the first episode was considered MFS in reference [9], we consider the first episode as BBE because of the presence of drowsiness [1]

revealed a high frequency of IgG antibodies to GQ1b in MFS patients (83–95%) [6, 13, 15] and BBE patients (66–68%) [13, 16]. By comparison, GQ1b-seronegative and GSC-seropositive MFS patients represented only 4 (1.9%) of 207 MFS patients [15]. Interestingly, those patients were all male, and one of them relapsed [15], similar to our case. The relapsed patient in that study had antibodies to GM1/GQ1b and GM1/GT1a in the second episode [15], which also continued to be positive in our case. Furthermore, we reviewed the positive rate of antibodies to GQ1b in reported recurrent cases where patients showed both BBE and MFS. During recurrence, among patients who showed both BBE and MFS, only 1 female patient out of 5 (20.0%) was positive for antibodies to GQ1b, and the other GQ1b-seronegative patients were male (Table 1) [8–12]. This rate for antibodies to GQ1b was low compared with 83–95% in patients with monophasic MFS and 66–68% in patients with monophasic BBE [6, 13, 15, 16]. Some of the patients with both BBE and MFS may have had GQ1b-seronegative and GSC-seropositive profiles.

Conclusion

We observed novel phenomena in this recurrent complicated case of GQ1b-seronegative MFS-GBS and BBE-GBS. GSC-Abs that were positive in previous episodes were also detected in subsequent episodes, while new GSC-Abs appeared in each episode, partly reflecting the clinical features. Based on our review of previous reports, GQ1b-seronegative and GSC-seropositive profiles in patients with MFS or BBE might be associated with recurrence, but further studies are needed to identify patients with a risk for recurrence.

Abbreviations

BBE: Bickerstaff brainstem encephalitis; FWCV: F-wave conduction velocity; GBS: Guillain-Barré syndrome; GSC-Abs: Anti-ganglioside complex antibodies; IVIG: Intravenous immunoglobulin; MFS: Miller Fisher syndrome; MRC: Medical Research Council; NCS: Nerve conduction studies; OD: Optical density; SNAP: Sensory nerve action potential

Acknowledgements

The authors are grateful to Dr. Yu Miyazaki (Osaka University) for useful discussions. We thank J. Ludovic Croxford, PhD, from Edanz Group (http://www.edanzediting.com/ac) for editing a draft of this manuscript.

Authors' contributions

HI, YHat, YHar, RK, HO, SO made the clinical diagnosis, made clinical management decisions and supervised the manuscript draft. HI and YF drafted the first manuscript and reviewed the literature. YHat was involved in the direct management of the patient in the first and second episodes, and HI in the third episode. AU and AC measured serum IgG antibodies against isolated gangliosides and GSC for all episodes. All authors have read and approved the final manuscript.

Competing interests

The authors declare that they have no competing interests.

Author details

[1]Department of Neurology, National Hospital Organization Nagoya Medical Center, 4-1-1 Sannomaru, Naka-ku, Nagoya, Japan. [2]Department of Neurology, Kyorin University, 6-20-2 Shinkawa, Mitakai, Tokyo, Japan. [3]Department of Neurology, Teikyo University, 2-11-1 Kaga, Itabashi-ku, Tokyo 173-8605, Japan. [4]Department of Neurology, Nagoya University Hospital, 65 Tsurumai-cho, Showa-ku, Nagoya, Aichi, Japan.

References

1. Wakerley BR, Uncini A, Yuki N. Guillain–Barré and miller fisher syndromes—new diagnostic classification. Nature. Rev Neurol. 2014;10:1–8.
2. Kuitwaard K, van Koningsveld R, Ruts L, Jacobs BC, van Doorn PA. Recurrent Guillain-Barré syndrome. J Neurol Neurosurg Psychiatry. 2009;80:56–9.
3. Heckmann JG, Dütsch M. Recurrent miller fisher syndrome: clinical and laboratory features. Eur J Neurol. 2012;19:944–54.
4. Ishii J, Yuki N, Kawamoto M, Yoshimura H, Kusunoki S, Kohara N. Recurrent Guillain-Barré syndrome, miller fisher syndrome and Bickerstaff brainstem encephalitis. J Neurol Sci. 2016;364:59–64.
5. Kaida K, Kusunoki S. Antibodies to gangliosides and ganglioside complexes in Guillain-Barré syndrome and fisher syndrome: mini-review. J Neuroimmunol. 2010;223:5–12.
6. Chiba A, Kusunoki S, Obata H, Machinami R, Kanazawa I. Serum anti-GQ1b IgG antibody is associated with ophthalmoplegia in miller fisher syndrome and Guillain-Barré syndrome: clinical and immunohistochemical studies. Neurology. 1993;43:1911–7.
7. Uchibori A, Gyohda A, Chiba A. Ca(2+)-dependent anti-GQ1b antibody in GQ1b-seronegative fisher syndrome and related disorders. J Neuroimmunol. 2016;298:172–7.
8. Mochizuki A, Ota K, Iijima M, Yamauchi T, Iwata MA. Case of relapsing Guillain-Barré syndrome following miller fisher syndrome. Rinsho Shinkeigaku. 1996;36:675–9.
9. Hamaguchi T, Yamaguchi K, Komai K, Yamada M, Yokoji H, Satake R, Yoshino H. Recurrent anti-GQ1b IgG antibody syndrome showing different phenotypes in different periods. J Neurol Neurosurg Psychiatry. 2003;74:1350.
10. Sharma V, Chan YC, Ong THL, Bickerstaff W-SEP. S brainstem encephalitis: can it recur? J Clin Neurosci. 2006;13:277–9.
11. Osada T, Ikeda M, Ito D, Takahashi K, Suzuki N. A 43-year-old male case of brainstem encephalitis remitting and relapsing three times. Undo Syogai. 2007;17:7–11.
12. Dong HQ, Liu Z, Tang Y, Lu Y, Wang Q, Jia JP. Recurrent fisher-Bickerstaff syndrome: report of a Chinese case. Chin Med J. 2011;124:2786–8.
13. Ito M, Kuwabara S, Odaka M, Misawa S, Koga M, Hirata K, Yuki N. Bickerstaff's brainstem encephalitis and fisher syndrome form a continuous spectrum. J Neurol. 2008;255:674–82.
14. Fukami Y, Wong AHY, Funakoshi K, Safri AY, Shahrizaila N, Yuki N. Anti-GQ1b antibody syndrome: anti-ganglioside complex reactivity determines clinical spectrum. Eur J Neurol. 2016;23:320–6.
15. Koga M, Gilbert M, Takahashi M, Li J, Hirata K, Kanda T, Yuki N. GQ1b-seronegative fisher syndrome: clinical features and new serological markers. J Neurol. 2012;259:1366–74.
16. Odaka M, Yuki N, Yamada M, Koga M, Takemi T, Hirata K, Bickerstaff KS. S brainstem encephalitis: clinical features of 62 cases and a subgroup associated with Guillain-Barré syndrome. Brain. 2003;126:2279–90.

19

Wilson's disease combined with systemic lupus erythematosus

Yun Zhang[1], Dongmei Wang[2], Wei Wei[3] and Xuejun Zeng[1*]

Abstract

Background: Wilson's disease (WD) is an inherited disorder in which defective biliary excretion of copper leads to its accumulation, particularly in the liver and brain. Systemic lupus erythematosus (SLE) is a multi-system disorder that can manifest in any system. Cases with concomitant WD and SLE, unrelated to treatment with penicillamine, have been rarely reported.

Case presentation: We report a case of a young woman who had typical neuropsychiatric symptoms and laboratory tests results of WD. She also had concomitant massive hematuria and proteinuria, fever, multiple positive autoimmune antibodies, hypocomplementemia, abnormal lumbar puncture findings and evidence of Sjögren syndrome, which are all rare in WD. Hence, we considered the diagnosis of SLE. Tapering of steroid dosage also confirmed the diagnosis.

Conclusion: Wilson's disease and SLE have varied clinical manifestations. Herein, we reported a rare case in which the two conditions concomitantly existed. In clinical practice, differential diagnosis of the two diseases is necessary for patients with hepatic, neurological, and psychiatric manifestations.

Keywords: Wilson's disease, Systemic lupus erythematosus

Background

Wilson's disease (WD) is an inherited disorder with defective biliary excretion of copper that leads to its accumulation, particularly in the liver and brain. Systemic lupus erythematosus (SLE) is a multi-system disorder that can manifest in any system. We report a case of a young woman who had typical neuropsychiatric symptoms of WD as well as other abnormalities unrelated to WD. The diagnosis of SLE gradually emerged, although cases with concomitant WD and SLE, unrelated to treatment with penicillamine, have been rarely reported.

Case presentation

An 18-year-old female was admitted to Peking Union Medical College Hospital in November 2016 with the chief complaints of abnormal limb movements and slurred speech for two years, which worsened 20 days ago. Initially, her movements were slower, her hands were clumsy, and she could not speak clearly. In the past 20 days, she gradually developed dysdipsia, unsteady gait, dyskinesia, significantly increased involuntary movements of limbs and fell > 4 times. Cranial magnetic resonance imaging (MRI) showed abnormal signals in bilateral basal ganglia and thalamus. Electroencephalography (EEG) demonstrated diffused 4–6 Hz theta waves. Slit-lamp examination showed Kayser–Fleischer (KF) ring in both eyes. Her serum ceruloplasmin concentration was 0.033 g/L (Normal range: 0.2–0.6). The symptoms progressively worsened, and she had a fever, with temperature between 37.5 and 38.0 °C, without chills, cough or diarrhea. The patient had difficulty in opening her mouth, could only speak one word at a time, and had occasional torsion spasm at the time of admission.

The patient had xerostomia, keratoconjunctivitis sicca, frequent oral ulcers, with no significant weight loss. There was no history of other diseases, but her mother recalled that she talked less, had behavioral changes, abnormal gait, involuntary smile and involuntary movements of

* Correspondence: zxjpumch@126.com
[1]Department of General Internal Medicine, Peking Union Medical College Hospital (PUMCH), Chinese Academy of Medical Science (CAMS) and Peking Union Medical College (PUMC), Beijing 100730, China
Full list of author information is available at the end of the article

all limbs since five years. The parents and older sister did not have similar symptoms. Physical examination revealed that the patient had normal comprehension, with low-grade fever, hepatomegaly, splenomegaly, dystonia, lack of coordination, slight tremor, dysarthria, dysphagia and right side Babinski sign positive.

After admission, routine tests revealed decreased white blood cell count of 2.87*109/L (Normal range: 4–10). Liver function test showed slightly elevated transaminase level and normal bilirubin level. Albumin level was decreased to 32 g/L (Normal range: > 35). Renal parameters were marginally elevated with proteinuria (1.12 g/24 h) and hematuria (++). Lumbar puncture showed elevated intracranial pressure, normal white blood cell count of 2/ul, elevated protein of 0.69 g/L and elevated immunoglobulin G (IgG) of 58.8 mg/L (Normal range: 0–40). Anti-AQP-4 (Anti-aquaporin 4) IgG and myelin basic protein were negative. MRI revealed symmetric abnormal signals with low signal in T1-weighted image, and high signals in T2-weighted and FLAIR images of bilateral basal ganglia thalamus, midbrain, and pons (Fig. 1). Computed tomography (CT) scans revealed diffused lesions in the liver, uneven density, and hepatosplenomegaly. The patient, her parents and her sister underwent genotype test for

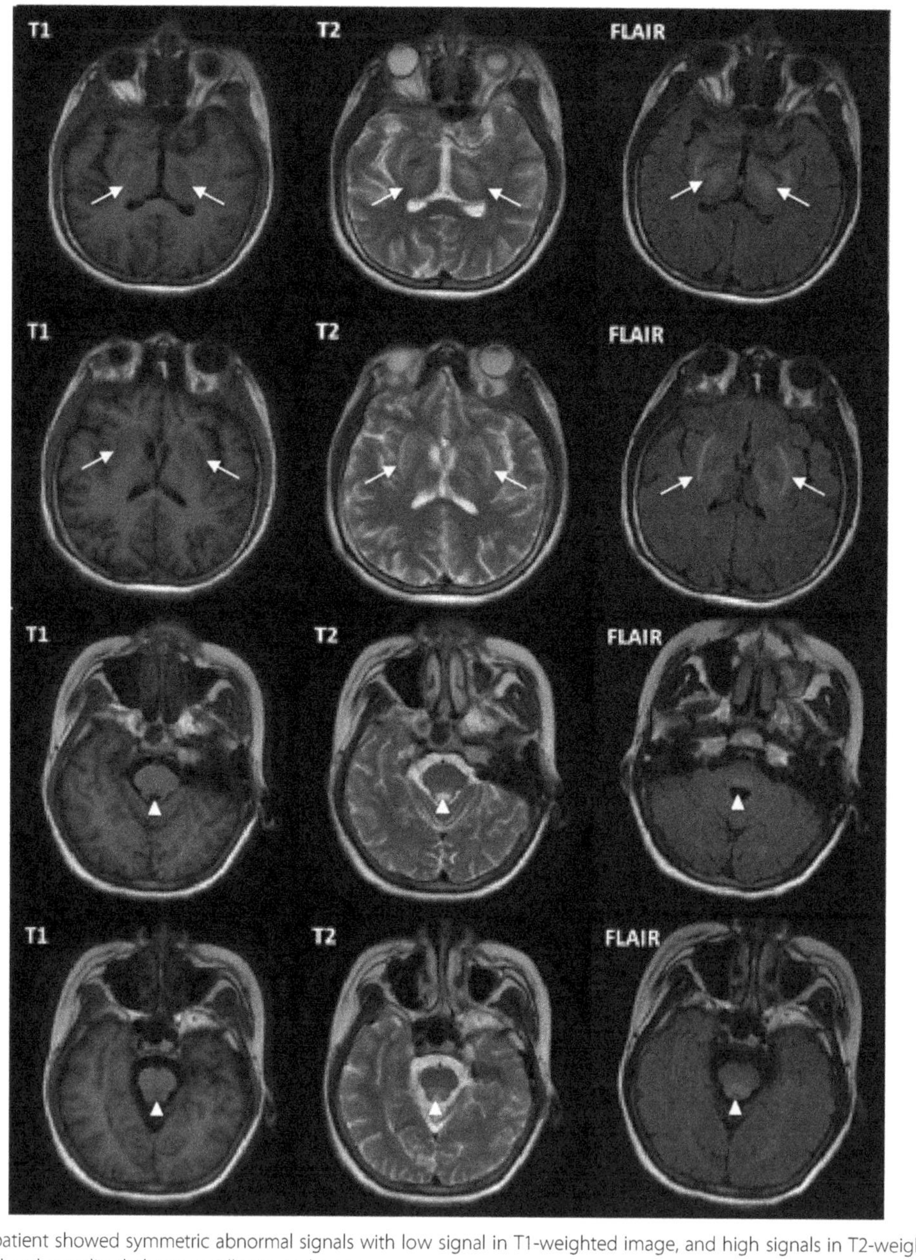

Fig. 1 MRI of the patient showed symmetric abnormal signals with low signal in T1-weighted image, and high signals in T2-weighted and FLAIR images of bilateral basal ganglia, thalamus, midbrain, and pons

WD, which showed that the patient had a compound heterozygous mutation, while her family members did not.

Other laboratory findings included elevated ESR, C-reactive protein, IgG, IgM and hypocomplementemia. The titers of antinuclear antibody (ANA) (S1:640), anti-SSA antibody (+++) and anti-rRNP antibody (+++) were remarkably increased, while anticardiolipin antibodies (ACL), Lupus anticoagulants (LA), and anti-β2-glycoprotein-1 (anti-β2GP1) antibodies were all positive. Stomatological and ophthalmological evaluations provided objective evidence of salivary gland (salivary flow rate and parotid sialography) and ocular (Schirmer's test and ocular dye score) involvement. Salivary gland biopsy showed typical histopathology of Sjögren syndrome. Magnetic resonance angiography (MRA) showed normal arteries, and ultrasound examinations of arteries and veins of bilateral legs, bilateral subclavian, supra-mesenteric, inferior-mesenteric, bilateral renal found no thrombotic evidence.

Based on all the findings, the final diagnosis for this patient was WD, SLE, secondary Sjögren syndrome with anti-phospholipid (aPL) antibodies. Therefore, we started therapy with iv sodium dimercaptopropane sulfonate (DMPS), full dose zinc sulfate for WD, and methylprednisolone (80 mg iv for 7 days, then 40 mg po for 3 weeks), and hydroxychloroquine po for SLE, respectively. Since has three kinds of aPL antibodies were positive, the patient was also treated with anticoagulant therapy (low molecular weight heparin, and then aspirin po). One month later, her neurological symptoms and laboratory tests showed improvement. WBC count, liver function test including transaminase level, bilirubin level and serum albumin level, urine test, ESR, CRP, IgG and complement levels were all normal. Repeat lumbar puncture showed normal parameters. The titer of ANA had declined (S1:160), and aPL (ACL, LA, anti-β2GP1) antibodies were negative. The steroid dosage was gradually tapered and the patient was given oral dimercaptosuccinate (DMSA), zinc sulfate, hydroxychloroquine and aspirin for maintenance.

The patient was followed-up every three months at the outpatient clinic. Six months after discharge, her symptoms recurred, and she developed hyponatremia, hematuria and proteinuria, when the steroid was reduced to 2 mg/day. Hence, methylprednisolone dosage was increased to 16 mg/day, while the other treatment remained unchanged. Symptoms and abnormal laboratory findings were relieved in the next follow-up.

Discussion and conclusions

Wilson's disease (WD) is an inherited disorder caused by mutations of the ATP7B gene on chromosome 13, which encodes a copper-transporting P-type ATPase (ATP7B) residing in the trans-Golgi network of hepatocytes. Our patient had a compound heterozygous mutation of ATP7B (Fig. 2), while her parents and sister did not. The clinical features of WD may include hepatic, neurological, and psychiatric manifestations. More than 90% of patients with neurological manifestations have a KF ring [1–3].

Our patient first showed symptoms of abnormal behavior several years before diagnosis. Literature review indicated that psychiatric problems can be the earliest manifestation in adult patients. In addition to the three main movement disorders including dystonia, lack of coordination, and tremor, our patient also presented some common neurological features of WD, such as dysarthria and dysphagia. MRI and CT scans showed typical findings of WD. However, lumbar puncture revealed increased pressure, increased protein level and immunoglobulin level, which were unrelated to WD. Moreover, our patient had massive hematuria and proteinuria, which are rare in WD. Because of fever, multiple autoimmune antibody

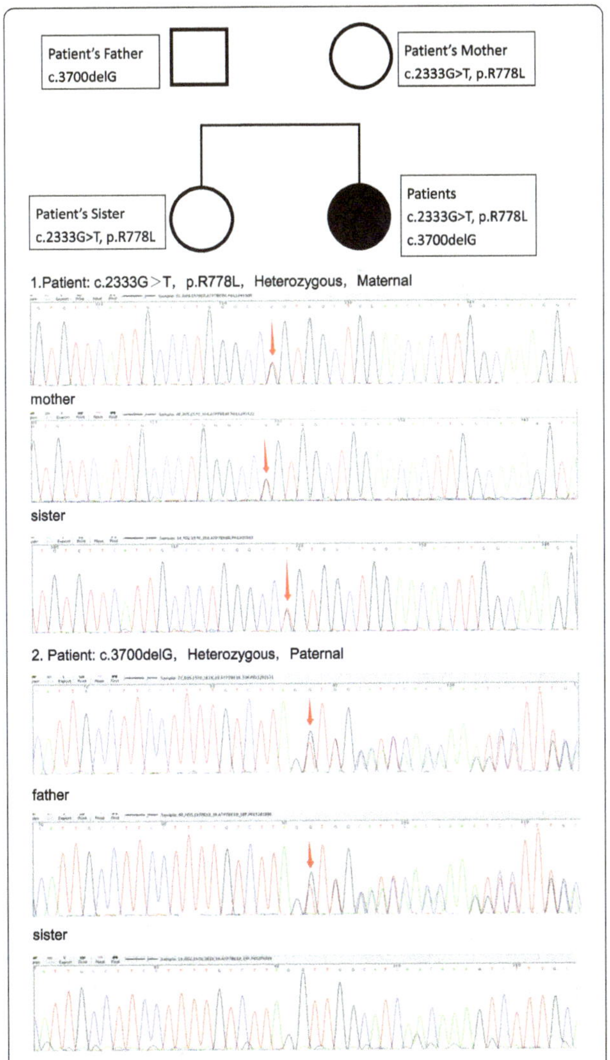

Fig. 2 Sequence analysis of ATP7B in the family

positive, hypocomplementemia, renal involvement, abnormal lumbar puncture findings and evidence of Sjögren syndrome, we considered the diagnosis of SLE. Tapering of steroid dosage also confirmed the diagnosis.

WD can concurrently occur with autoimmune hepatitis and Coomb's positive autoimmune hemolytic anemia [4, 5]. SLE has been reported to be associated with WD in patients treated with penicillamine in the form of drug-induced lupus (DILE). DILE has several different features from SLE [6]. But concomitant SLE and WD without penicillamine treatment is rare [7–9]. A possible pathogenetic mechanism of Fas-mediated apoptosis might play a role in autoimmune disease and WD [10]. In such patients, penicillamines should be avoided. According to the guidelines, we used iv DMPS and oral DMSA for this patient, followed by maintainance zinc monotherapy for WD, and 4 mg methylprednisolone and hydroxychloroquine for SLE. The patient has been following-up for 1.5 years, and her liver function and neurological condition continues to be stable [11].

Wilson's disease and SLE have varied clinical manifestations. Herein, we reported a rare case in which the two conditions concomitantly existed. In clinical practice, differential diagnosis of the two diseases is necessary for patients with hepatic, neurological, and psychiatric manifestations.

Abbreviations
ACL: Anticardiolipin antibodies; Anti-AQP4: Anti-aquaporin 4; Anti-β2GP1: Anti-β2-glycoprotein-1 antibodies; aPL: Anti-phospholipid; APS: Anti-phospholipid antibody syndrome; CT: Computed tomography; DILE: Drug-induced lupus; DMPS: Sodium dimercaptopropane sulfonate; DMSA: Dimercaptosuccinate; EEG: Electroencephalograph; IgG: Immunoglobulin G; KF ring: Kayser–Fleischer ring; LA: Lupus anticoagulants; MRA: Magnetic resonance angiography; MRI: Magnetic resonance imaging; SLE: Systemic lupus erythematosus; WD: Wilson's disease

Acknowledgments
We thank all the physicians from the division of general internal medicine of PUMCH who contributed to the patient care.

Funding
This work was supported by the National Health and Family Planning Commission of People's Republic of China (No. 201502024).

Authors' contributions
YZ drafted the main manuscript. DW collected the clinical data and redrafted the manuscript. WW participated in the care of the patient and paper review. XZ conceptualized and executed the case report. All authors read and approved the final manuscript.

Competing interests
The authors declare that they have no competing interests.

Author details
[1]Department of General Internal Medicine, Peking Union Medical College Hospital (PUMCH), Chinese Academy of Medical Science (CAMS) and Peking Union Medical College (PUMC), Beijing 100730, China. [2]Department of Neurology, Nanfang Hospital, Southern Medical University, Guangzhou 510515, China. [3]Department of Internal Medicine, Peking Union Medical College Hospital (PUMCH), Chinese Academy of Medical Science (CAMS) and Peking Union Medical College (PUMC), Beijing 100730, China.

References
1. Roberts EA, Schilsky ML. A practice guideline on Wilson disease. Hepatology. 2003;38(2):1475–92.
2. Gitlin JD. Wilson disease. Gastroenterology. 2003;125(6):1868–77.
3. Thomas GR, Forbes JR, Roberts EA, et al. The Wilson disease gene: spectrum of mutations and their consequences. Nat Genet. 1995;9(2):210–7.
4. Milkiewicz P, Saksena S, Hubscher SG, et al. Wilson's disease with superimposed autoimmune features: report of two cases and review. J Gastroenterol Hepatol. 2000;15(5):570–4.
5. Guha SK, Modak D, Basu A, et al. Coomb's positive autoimmune Haemolytic Anaemia in a case of Wilson disease: co-incidence or association? JIACM. 2009;10(1 & 2):78–80.
6. Walshe JM. Penicillamine and the SLE syndrome. J Rheumatol Suppl. 1981;7:155.
7. Dell'Era L, Boati E, Nebbia G, et al. Wilson's disease treated with penicillamine and lupus erythematosus: related or distinct entities? Minerva Pediatr. 2012;64(1):55.
8. Kim TY, Lee SH, Kim TJ, et al. A case of fulminant hepatic failure in Wilson's disease combined with systemic lupus erythematosus. Taehan Kan Hakhoe Chi. 2002;8(1):100–4.
9. Santhakumar R, Gayathri K, Ramalingam PK, et al. Wilson's disease with systemic lupus erythematosus. J Assoc Physicians India. 2016;64(4):81.
10. Stassi G, Di FV, Todaro M, et al. Involvement of Fas/FasL system in the pathogenesis of autoimmune diseases and Wilson's disease. Arch Immunol Ther Exp. 1999;47(3):129.
11. Ranucci G, Dato FD, Tufano M, et al. Long term follow-up of Wilson disease patients diagnosed in childhood: reasons for treatment changes. Dig Liver Dis. 2013;45(5444):e273.

20

Marathons and myasthenia gravis

Simone Birnbaum[1,2,3*], Tarek Sharshar[4,5,6], Bruno Eymard[1], Marie Theaudin[7], Pierre Portero[2] and Jean-Yves Hogrel[1]

Abstract

Background: The cardinal symptoms of auto-immune myasthenia gravis are fatigue and weakness. Endurance events such as marathon running would seem incompatible with this chronic disease. Many patients stop sport altogether. There is limited literature of patients with auto-immune myasthenia gravis undergoing regular endurance exercise.

Case presentation: We report the case of a 36-year-old female who began long-distance running whilst experiencing initial symptoms of myasthenia gravis. She was diagnosed with auto-immune myasthenia gravis and whilst advised to stop all sport, her way of fighting and living with this chronic and unpredictable disease was to continue running to maintain a healthy body and mind. Despite suffering from ocular, bulbar and localized limb fatigability, she managed to complete multiple marathons and achieve disease stability with cholinesterase inhibitors.

Conclusions: Marathon and half-marathon running lead to distinct changes in mediators of inflammation in an exercise-dose-dependent manner. Despite symptoms of weakness and fatigue in certain muscles in myasthenia gravis, physical exertion remains possible and may not worsen symptoms as demonstrated in this case and recent studies. The immunomodulatory role of exercise could be considered in this case however this hypothesis remains to be confirmed in future studies with quantitative data.

Keywords: Myasthenia gravis, Marathon, Auto-immune disease, Health, Endurance exercise

Background

Auto-immune myasthenia gravis (MG) is a chronic disease whereby dysfunction at the neuromuscular junction causes symptoms of fatigue and weakness [1]. Endurance events such as marathon running would seem incompatible with MG. Many patients stop sport altogether, finding activities of daily living to be challenging enough in themselves [2]. Even for the general public, marathon running is not practiced by a large majority, one must train regularly and have a high endurance capacity.

There are only three case studies combining sport and MG reported in the literature. Scheer et al. (2012) describe a 52 year old ultra-endurance athlete with mild MG (MGFA IIa), treated with 10 mg of prednisone who completed a 220 km ultra-marathon over 5 days [3]. Fatigue, leg weakness, dysphagia and breathing problems were reported, relieved by rest, shade and 60 mg of pyridostigmine every 90 min (max daily dose 720 mg). He began running 5 years prior to MG diagnosis and maintained a combined weekly running distance of 70 km. Stout et al. (2001) report a 26 year old athletic (baseball and weight lifting) student who suffered from extreme weakness and atrophy due to his MG, he was unable to do a single push-up at diagnosis [4]. Once stabilized he began exercising again at low levels which prevented further weakness but he struggled to regain force until undergoing a 15-wk upper and lower limb resistance training program, with oral creatine supplementation and he was able to make force gains (37% leg extension) and increase training volume (34–40% upper limb). Finally, Leddy et al. (2000) describe a 17 year old college football player with mild generalized MG (antibody-negative, 15% decrement RNS-EMG), treated with 60 mg prednisone every other day and 60 mg pyridostigmine q.i.d [5]. Following an initial period of weakness at the time of diagnosis, his strength returned to normal after

* Correspondence: s.birnbaum@institut-myologie.org
[1]Institute of Myology, GH Pitié-Salpêtrière (AP-HP), Bd de l'Hôpital, 75651 Paris Cedex 13, France
[2]Bioingénierie, Tissus et Neuroplasticité, EA 7377 Université Paris-Est Créteil Faculté de Médecine, 8 rue Jean Sarrail, 94010 Créteil, France
Full list of author information is available at the end of the article

6 weeks and aside from a relapse associated with a period of non-compliance with medication, he became stable without treatment and was able to participate in full football practice.

Three recent uncontrolled trials have demonstrated benefits and tolerance of supervised physical activity (resistance or aerobic) programs for patients with stable MG [6–8]. Additionally, using the contralateral limb as a control, Lohi et al. found improvements in lower limb force following dynamic training and no deterioration nor negative side effects in a group of 11 subjects with mild MG [9]. A review article has suggested that risk factors for exacerbation of MG include prolonged exercise, running uphill and activity with stairs, however no specific data was provided to support these claims [10]. Currently there are no official guidelines regarding participation in sport and MG [11, 12].

Case presentation

Here we report a 36-year-old female nurse, working full-time 12-h night shifts in a busy intensive care service, with generalized (MGFA IIb) auto-immune MG, symptomatic and dependent on cholinesterase inhibitors. Past medical history includes eczema in her teens, she is a carrier for sickle disease (sickle cell trait (SCT)) and she carried two pregnancies to term. Red blood cells have slightly reduced mean corpuscular volume and mean corpuscular hemoglobin concentration, 75.5 fl and 25.7 pg, respectively. She has no clinical symptoms of anemia and no specific treatment or monitoring. Surgical history includes 1 cesarean (2004), linea alba repair (2011) and breast implant (2014). She is a nonsmoker and does not drink alcohol. She is right-handed. She has a normal body mass index, 20.3 kg/m^2, weighing 52 kg for 1.60 m.

Despite already experiencing abnormal weakness, she began running a year before being diagnosed with MG. Prior to running, she played amateur level basketball however this became incompatible with working night-shifts. MG diagnosis was based on clinical signs (right hand weakness - difficulty brushing teeth and hair, carrying light loads, cutting meat, a heavy head, nasal voice, ptosis, diplopia, dysphagia and difficulty masticating and articulating), serum auto-antibodies against nicotinic acetylcholine receptors (AChR) (> 100 nmol/l) and significant decrement on repetitive nerve stimulation (3 Hz) EMG (50% right trapezius, 24% right anconeus, 15% left anconeus, 43% tongue/mouth (CN V/XII)). Myasthenic muscle score (MMS) was 65/100. Initial treatment consisted of intravenous immunoglobulins (2 g/kg over 3 days (100 g)) and 60 mg pyridostigmine (t.i.d). Thoracic CT scan did not show thymoma but was in favour of thymic hyperplasia. Thymectomy was not performed as per the patient's request.

Despite the patient being informed at diagnosis that sport was contra-indicated, she kept running. Training consisted of 1–2 10 km weekly runs with the beginning being the most difficult. MG symptoms persisted including fatigue, dysphagia and episodes of diplopia at the end of pyridostigmine dose thus aziathoprine (100 mg) was introduced. She performed a half marathon 2 months later, followed by a full marathon and another half marathon. No major difficulty was experienced and performances significantly improved: 5h13mins (8.1 km/h) for a marathon pre-diagnosis to 4h51mins (8.7 km/h) post diagnosis (and treatment), Figs. 1 & 2.

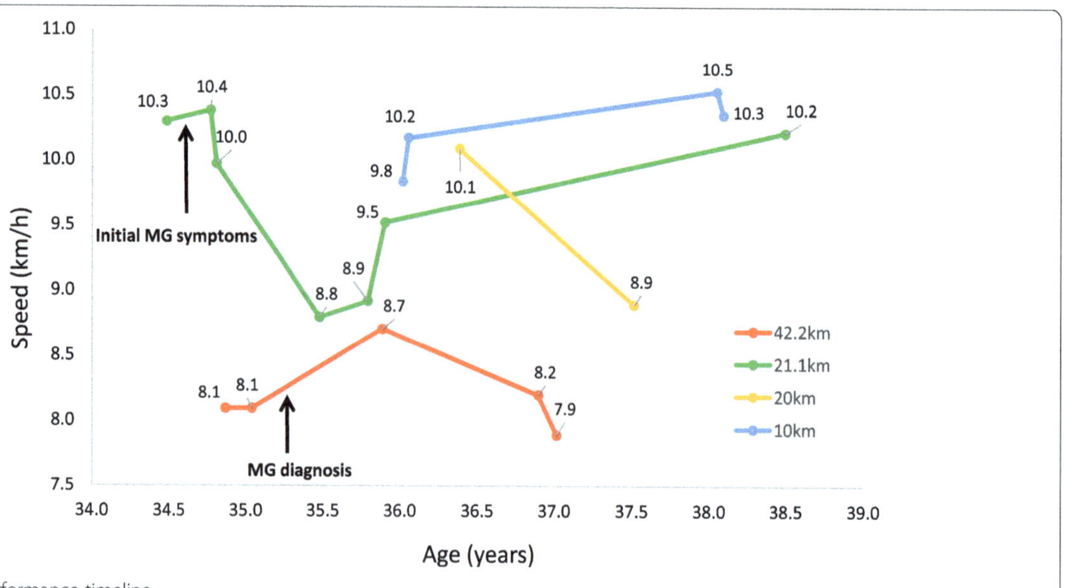

Fig. 1 Running performance timeline

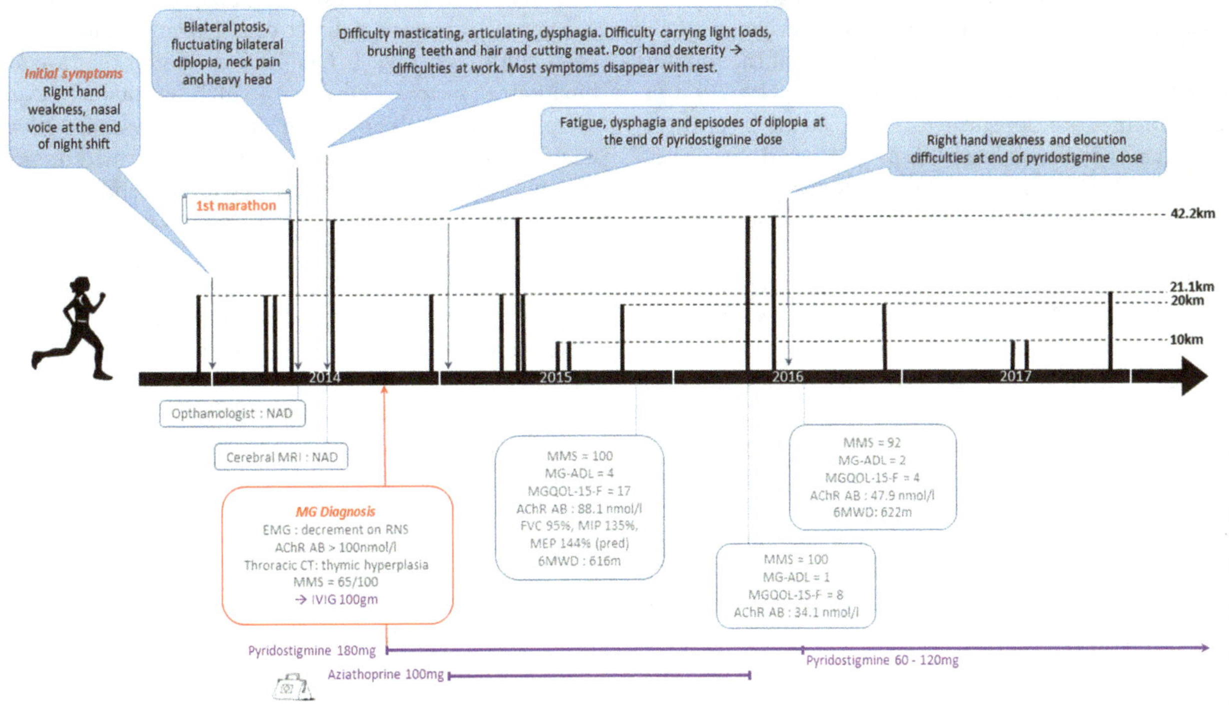

Fig. 2 Diagnosis, clinical evaluation and running timeline

On clinical evaluation 1 year after MG diagnosis, she had above average respiratory strength (MIP and MEP 135% and 144% of theoretical) and normal respiratory function (FVC 95% of theoretical). On maximal voluntary testing, limb strength was normal (knee extensors and elbow flexors: 128% and 101% of theoretical, respectively and right handgrip strength: 88%). Walking endurance was also considered normal (92% of theoretical 6MWD). The MMS suffered from a ceiling effect with the patient achieving the maximal score of 100 and a score of 4 on the MG-ADL due to episodes of dysphagia, dyspnea with effort and UL fatigue with brushing her teeth and hair. She reported recurrent MG symptoms including loss of hand dexterity (difficulty manipulating medication at work), bulbar symptoms such as dysphagia on her own saliva, a nasal voice and ocular symptoms (ptosis and diplopia). MG-specific quality of life (MGQOL-15-F) was reduced (17/60) particularly with regards to professional and social aspects, reflected in the WHO-QOL Bref with the social relationship and physical health domains being reduced, 11/20 and 13/20 respectively [13, 14].

She continued regular running without any particular changes in her MG, recurrent right hand weakness persisted and she experienced occasional ocular and bulbar symptoms primarily at the end of pyrodistigmine dose. Quality of life improved significantly over time (Fig. 2) and strength remained stable (knee extensors and elbow flexors: 128% and 100% of theoretical, respectively, right handgrip strength: 93%). She discontinued aziathoprine (treatment duration 14 months) and remained exclusively treated with cholinesterase inhibitors (60 mg, b.i.d).

Discussion and conclusion

It is well known that MG does not affect all muscles to the same extent and whilst some muscles may clearly be affected, other muscles may function normally and can be trained without adverse effects. Thus, continuing activities and daily life seems important for maintaining "unaffected" muscles and for psychological benefits. With regards to physical activity a close link between endurance running and the immune system activity has been demonstrated [15]. During sustained physical activity, repeated muscle contractions stimulate the production of inflammatory cytokines such as Interleukin-6 (IL-6) by myocytes. IL-6 may act as an inhibitor to pro-inflammatory cytokines such as TNF-α which is a potent mediator of tissue damage [16, 17]. IL-6 also stimulates the production of IL-10 (an anti-inflammatory cytokine) and IL-1ra, generating an anti-inflammatory environment. Whether these effects can modify disease activity in MG currently remains unclear. These exercise-induced mediators of inflammation are susceptible to exercise dose, with greater increases seen following a marathon as compared to a half marathon, for example [16]. A disease-specific response has been suggested for the change in cytokine kinetics in relation to exercise [18].

Whilst evidence of exercise-induced change of cytokines remains sparse in MG, there is growing evidence of the presence of inflammation and modulation of the immune response by cytokines in MG pathogenesis [19, 20]. Certain cytokines are upregulated (IL-17, IL-21, IL-6, IL-10) and others downregulated (IL-4) compared to control subjects [19, 21–23]. A recent study evaluated serum IL-6 before and after a twice-weekly, 3 month training program in subjects with ocular or mild, generalized MG. Serum Il-6 levels remained unchanged [7]. However, circulating microRNAs (miR150-5p and miR21-5p) decreased [7]. These immuno-microRNAs have been suggested as new biomarkers in AChR MG, notably miR150-5p as a marker for disease severity [24, 25].

Another factor which warrants consideration here is the localized role of IL-6 in triggering satellite cells in the myogenic process [26]. Whilst research has demonstrated the role of IL-6 in muscle atrophy, this has predominantly involved pathological situations such as cancer cachexia and ageing [27] where there is chronic inflammation. When released at low concentration into satellite cell niches IL-6 could promote repair and regenerate skeletal muscle tissue [27]. It seems that IL-6 is deregulated in the muscles of MG patients, possibly due to AChR antibodies deregulating the IL-6 pathway [28].

In the case of this patient, weakness induced by MG mechanisms tends to affect the same muscles which were initially affected, regardless of increased exertion. Whether this patient has benefitted from protective effects of exercise or not is difficult to determine, however, this case study demonstrates that an endurance sport such as running marathons and MG are not mutually exclusive. The immunosuppressor treatment likely played an essential role in attenuating the autoimmune attack enabling the patient to improve and optimize her physical capacities. Clinical scores improved and remained stable and running performance improved and remained relatively consistent (Figs. 1 and 2). The level of antibodies against AChR decreased over time (Fig. 2) however this also coincided with immunosuppressor treatment.

In stabilized MG there are no clear arguments to fear adverse effects of physical activity and as well as positive psychological effects, patients will benefit from cardiovascular and muscular adaptions as well as possible immunomodulatory effects. It is important to consider each individual case and weigh up the benefits and risks and possibly put into place a supervised or specific return to sport program where necessary. As can be expected in the absence of disease, inter-individual variation is likely with strenuous physical exercise.

It seems important to discuss the possible consequences of exercise and sickle cell trait which are not currently clear in the literature. Case-control studies have found an increased prevalence of sudden death on exertion, often called "exercise collapse associated with sickle trait" however a direct causal relationship has not been confirmed [29]. It has been suggested that a combination of factors [30] such as high altitude or severe dehydration combined with intense physical activity could cause red blood cells to become deformed or sickled and cause complications such as rhabdomyolysis. This may be due to lower capillary density and tortuosity, reduced small vessels and a higher percentage of broader micro vessels [31]. Microvascular remodeling may be a compensatory mechanism to facilitate normal blood flow [29] which may be present in this patient considering the raised but not excessive elevation of CK following a marathon (data not presented). SCT may not be a completely benign carrier state nor a true disease entity but rather a potential risk factor which could be monitored. Maintaining physical fitness may be a protective agent by decreasing the endothelial activation through improvements in nitric oxide and antioxidant availability [32, 33]. Precautions would be the same as for exercise with MG i.e.; adequate hydration, control heat exposure and monitor exertion intensity [34].

This case report demonstrates that despite being in the first 2 years of MG disease onset in which exacerbations and instability are most common, and despite regular intense endurance running, the MG has remained stable. A growing body of literature suggests that regular physical exercise may lead to anti-inflammatory effects in chronic auto-immune diseases. The immunomodulatory role of exercise could be considered in this case study. However, further studies regarding the specific effects of exercise on disease activity in MG are necessary to confirm these speculations.

Patient perspective

"I am myasthenic and marathonian, running allows me to take time for myself, to evacuate stress and to think. It's a real therapy".

Abbreviations

6MWD: Six-minute walk distance; AChR: Acetycholine receptor; b.i.d: Twice a day; CN: Cranial nerve; EMG: Electromyogram; IL-6: Interleukin-6; MG: Autoimmune myasthenia gravis; MG-ADL: Myasthenia Gravis Activites of Daily Living score; MGFA: Myasthenia Gravis Foundation of America disease classification; MGQOL-15-F: Myasthenia Gravis 15 item French Quality Of Life scale; MIP/MEP: Maximal inspiratory pressure/Maximal expiratory pressure; MMS: Myasthenic Muscle Score; SCT: Sickle cell trait; t.i.d: Three times a day; TNF-α: Tumour Necrosis Factor alpha; UL: Upper limb; WHO-QOL Bref: World Health Organisation Quality Of Life short questionnaire

Acknowledgements

The authors would like to thank the patient for accepting publication of her case. Thank you to Aurelie Canal for her assistance in data collection and presentation.

Funding

No specific funding was provided for this case report.

Authors' contributions

SB contributed to the concept, drafting and reporting of the case. MT, BE and SB acquired clinical data and revised the manuscript. TS, PP, JY, contributed to reporting and revising the manuscript. All authors read and approved the final manuscript.

Competing interests

The authors declare that they have no competing interests.

Author details

[1]Institute of Myology, GH Pitié-Salpêtrière (AP-HP), Bd de l'Hôpital, 75651 Paris Cedex 13, France. [2]Bioingénierie, Tissus et Neuroplasticité, EA 7377 Université Paris-Est Créteil Faculté de Médecine, 8 rue Jean Sarrail, 94010 Créteil, France. [3]Unité de Recherche Clinique Paris Île- de- France Ouest (URC PIFO), Raymond Poincaré Hospital, AP-HP, Garches, France. [4]Medical and Surgical Neurointensive Care Centre, Hospital Sainte Anne, Paris, France. [5]Laboratory of human histopathology and animal models, Institute Pasteur, Paris, France. [6]Université Paris Descartes, Paris, France. [7]Department of Neurology, CHUV, Rue du Bugnon, 46 1011 Lausanne, Switzerland.

References

1. Phillips WD, Vincent A. Pathogenesis of myasthenia gravis: update on disease types, models, and mechanisms. F1000Res. 2016;5(F1000 Faculty Rev):1513.
2. Paul RH, Nash JM, Cohen RA, Gilchrist JM, Goldstein JM. Quality of life and well-being of patients with myasthenia gravis. Muscle Nerve. 2001;24:512–6.
3. Scheer BV, Valero-Burgos E, Costa R. Myasthenia gravis and endurance exercise. Am J Phys Med Rehabil. 2012;91:725–7.
4. Stout JR, Eckerson JM, May E, Coulter C, Bradley-Popovich GE. Effects of resistance exercise and creatine supplementation on myasthenia gravis: a case study. Med Sci Sports Exerc. 2001;33:869–72.
5. Leddy JJ, Chutkow JG. Myasthenia gravis in a collegiate football player. Med Sci Sports Exerc. 2000;32:1975–9.
6. Rahbek MA, Mikkelsen EE, Overgaard K, Vinge L, Andersen H, Dalgas U. Exercise in myasthenia gravis: a feasibility study of aerobic and resistance training. Muscle Nerve. 2017;56:700–9.
7. Westerberg E, Molin CJ, Lindblad I, Emtner M, Punga AR. Physical exercise in myasthenia gravis is safe and improves neuromuscular parameters and physical performance-based measures: a pilot study. Muscle Nerve. 2017;56: 207–14.
8. Westerberg E, Molin CJ, Sporndly Nees S, Widenfalk J, Punga AR. The impact of physical exercise on neuromuscular function in myasthenia gravis patients: a single-subject design study. Medicine. 2018;97:e11510.
9. Lohi EL, Lindberg C, Andersen O. Physical training effects in myasthenia gravis. Arch Phys Med Rehabil. 1993;74:1178–80.
10. Cass S. Myasthenia gravis and sports participation. Curr Sports Med Rep. 2013;12:18–21.
11. Sussman J, Farrugia ME, Maddison P, Hill M, Leite MI, Hilton-Jones D. Myasthenia gravis: Association of British Neurologists' management guidelines. Pract Neurol. 2015;15:199–206.
12. Sanders DB, Wolfe GI, Narayanaswami P. Developing treatment guidelines for myasthenia gravis. Ann N Y Acad Sci. 2018;1412:95–101.
13. Skevington SM, Lotfy M, O'Connell KA. The World Health Organization's WHOQOL-BREF quality of life assessment: psychometric properties and results of the international field trial. A report from the WHOQOL group. Qual Life Res. 2004;13:299–310.
14. Hawtho rne G, Herrman H, Murphy B. Interpreting the WHOQOL-BREF: preliminary population norms and effect sizes. Soc Indic Res. 2006;77:37–59.
15. Barros ES, Nascimento DC, Prestes J, Nobrega OT, Cordova C, Sousa F, Boullosa DA. Acute and chronic effects of endurance running on inflammatory markers: a systematic review. Front Physiol. 2017;8:779.
16. Niemela M, Kangastupa P, Niemela O, Bloigu R, Juvonen T. Acute changes in inflammatory biomarker levels in recreational runners participating in a Marathon or half-Marathon. Sports Med Open. 2016;2:21.
17. Pedersen BK. Muscle as a secretory organ. Compr Physiol. 2013;3:1337–62.
18. Perandini LA, Sales-de-Oliveira D, Mello S, Camara NO, Benatti FB, Lima FR, Borba E, Bonfa E, Roschel H, Sa-Pinto AL, Gualano B. Inflammatory cytokine kinetics to single bouts of acute moderate and intense aerobic exercise in women with active and inactive systemic lupus erythematosus. Exerc Immunol Rev. 2015;21:174–85.
19. Uzawa A, Kawaguchi N, Himuro K, Kanai T, Kuwabara S. Serum cytokine and chemokine profiles in patients with myasthenia gravis. Clin Exp Immunol. 2014;176:232–7.
20. Uzawa A, Kanai T, Kawaguchi N, Oda F, Himuro K, Kuwabara S. Changes in inflammatory cytokine networks in myasthenia gravis. Sci Rep. 2016;6:25886.
21. Roche JC, Capablo JL, Larrad L, Gervas-Arruga J, Ara JR, Sanchez A, Alarcia R. Increased serum interleukin-17 levels in patients with myasthenia gravis. Muscle Nerve. 2011;44:278–80.
22. Li Y, Rauniyar VK, Yin WF, Hu B, Ouyang S, Xiao B, Yang H. Serum IL-21 levels decrease with glucocorticoid treatment in myasthenia gravis. Neurol Sci. 2014;35:29–34.
23. Molin CJ, Westerberg E, Punga AR. Profile of upregulated inflammatory proteins in sera of myasthenia gravis patients. Sci Rep. 2017;7:39716.
24. Punga T, Le Panse R, Andersson M, Truffault F, Berrih-Aknin S, Punga AR. Circulating miRNAs in myasthenia gravis: miR-150-5p as a new potential biomarker. Ann Clin Transl Neurol. 2014;1:49–58.
25. Punga AR, Punga T. Circulating microRNAs as potential biomarkers in myasthenia gravis patients. Ann N Y Acad Sci. 2018;1412:33–40.
26. Munoz-Canoves P, Scheele C, Pedersen BK, Serrano AL. Interleukin-6 myokine signaling in skeletal muscle: a double-edged sword? FEBS J. 2013; 280:4131–48.
27. Belizario JE, Fontes-Oliveira CC, Borges JP, Kashiabara JA, Vannier E. Skeletal muscle wasting and renewal: a pivotal role of myokine IL-6. Springerplus. 2016;5:619.
28. Maurer M, Bougoin S, Feferman T, Frenkian M, Bismuth J, Mouly V, Clairac G, Tzartos S, Fadel E, Eymard B, et al. IL-6 and Akt are involved in muscular pathogenesis in myasthenia gravis. Acta Neuropathol Commun. 2015;3:1.
29. O'Connor FG, Bergeron MF, Cantrell J, Connes P, Harmon KG, Ivy E, Kark J, Klossner D, Lisman P, Meyers BK, et al. ACSM and CHAMP summit on sickle cell trait: mitigating risks for warfighters and athletes. Med Sci Sports Exerc. 2012;44:2045–56.
30. Quattrone RD, Eichner ER, Beutler A, Adams WB, O'Connor FG. Exercise collapse associated with sickle cell trait (ECAST): case report and literature review. Curr Sports Med Rep. 2015;14:110–6.
31. Vincent L, Feasson L, Oyono-Enguelle S, Banimbek V, Denis C, Guarneri C, Aufradet E, Monchanin G, Martin C, Gozal D, et al. Remodeling of skeletal muscle microvasculature in sickle cell trait and alpha-thalassemia. Am J Physiol Heart Circ Physiol. 2010;298:H375–84.
32. Chirico EN, Faes C, Connes P, Canet-Soulas E, Martin C, Pialoux V. Role of exercise-induced oxidative stress in sickle cell trait and disease. Sports Med. 2016;46:629–39.
33. Aufradet E, Monchanin G, Oyonno-Engelle S, Feasson L, Messonnier L, Francina A, Bezin L, Serpero LD, Gozal D, Dodogba M, et al. Habitual physical activity and endothelial activation in sickle cell trait carriers. Med Sci Sports Exerc. 2010;42:1987–94.
34. Eichner ER. Sickle cell considerations in athletes. Clin Sports Med. 2011;30: 537–49.

21

Autosomal recessive Myotonia congenita caused by a novel splice mutation (c.1401 + 1G > A) in *CLCN1* gene of a Chinese Han patient

Jing Miao, Xiao-jing Wei, Xue-mei Liu, Zhi-xia Kang, Yan-lu Gao and Xue-fan Yu*

Abstract

Background: Autosomal recessive Myotonia congenita (Becker's disease) is caused by mutations in the *CLCN1* gene. The condition is characterized by muscle stiffness during sustained muscle contraction and variable degree of muscle weakness that tends to improve with repeated contractions.

Case presentation: A 21-year-old man presented with transient muscle stiffness since the last 10 years. He had difficulty in initiating movement and experienced muscle weakness after rest, which typically improved after repeated contraction (warm-up phenomenon). There was no significant family history. Medical examination showed generalized muscle hypertrophy. Serum creatine kinase level was 2-fold higher than the normal value. Electromyogram showed myotonic discharges. DNA sequence analysis identified a novel splice mutation (c.1401 + 1G > A) and a known mutation (c.1657A > T,p.Ile553Phe). He rapidly responded to treatment with mexiletine 100 mg three times a day for 6 months.

Conclusions: This case report of autosomal recessive Myotonia congenita caused by a novel compound heterozygous mutation expands the genotypic spectrum of *CLCN1* gene.

Keywords: Myotonia congenita, Autosomal recessive, Case report, *CLCN1* gene

Background

Autosomal recessive Myotonia congenita (Becker's disease) is caused by mutations in *CLCN1* gene, which is located on the 7q35 chromosomal region and contains 23 coding exons. The condition is characterized by muscle stiffness during sustained muscle contraction and a variable degree of muscle weakness, which tends to improve with repeated contraction. The *CLCN1* gene is responsible for chloride (Cl^-) conductance in skeletal muscles, which contributes significantly to the repolarization of action potential.

Till date, several mutations of the CLCN1 gene such as missense and nonsense mutations have been reported in different populations across the world. To the best of our knowledge, only a few splicing mutations of the CLCN1 gene have been reported. These mutations may induce depolarisation of the skeletal muscle cell membrane which leads to hyperexcitablity (myotonia), which may improve on treatment with sodium (Na^+) blocking agents such as mexiletine [1–5]. In this study, we report a Chinese patient suffering from recessive Myotonia congenita caused by compound heterozygous mutations which includes a novel splicing mutation.

Case presentation

A 21-year-old man complained of transient muscle stiffness since 10 years. He experienced difficulty in initiating movement and felt muscle weakness after rest. However the symptoms typically improved after repeated contraction (warm-up phenomenon). The symptoms tended to aggravate during cold weather. He was unable to open his eyes immediately after washing his face with cold water.

* Correspondence: dr_yuxuefan@126.com
Department of Neurology and Neuroscience Center, the First Affiliated Hospital of Jilin University, Changchun 130021, Jilin, People's Republic of China

He had non-consanguineous parents and there was no significant family history. Further, the patient showed normal growth and development. Medical examination showed generalized muscle hypertrophy and normal muscle strength as assessed with the Medical Research Council (MRC) sum score. Deep tendon reflexes were attenuated. No nerve dysfunction or sensory deficit was noted. The serum creatine kinase level was 2-fold higher than the upper limit of the normal reference level. Electromyogram showed myotonic discharges. Biceps muscle biopsy specimen was obtained after written informed consent of the patient. The specimen was precooled with isopentane and frozen in liquid nitrogen. A section of muscle biopsy specimen was stained with hematoxylin-eosin (HE) and modified Gomori's trichrome (MGT). Activity of oxidative enzymes such as succinate dehydrogenase (SDH), NADH-tetrazolium reductase (NADH-TR), and cytochrome c oxidase (COX) were normal. Next generation sequencing of the DNA sample of this patient identified a novel splice mutation (c.1401 + 1G > A) (which was inherited from his father) and a known mutation (c.1657A > T, p.Ile553Phe) (which was inherited from his mother) (Fig. 1). The novel splice mutation was not detected in Human Gene Mutation Database or any of the 200 healthy controls. The splicing site, analyzed by Human Splicing Finder, is implicated in the alteration of the wild-type donor site and most probably have an impact on splicing. Mutation Taster software predicted the effects of the mutation to be 'disease causing'. The patient was prescribed mexiletine 100 mg three times per day for about 6 months. The patient responded well to the treatment and was completely relieved of his symptoms.

Discussion and conclusions

Our patient showed transient muscle stiffness and weakness after rest which improved with repeated contractions. The symptoms were aggravated by cold weather and stress. EMG revealed myotonic discharges and gene sequencing analysis identified novel compound heterozygous mutations in *CLCN1* gene. Finally, a diagnosis of recessive myotonia congenita was established.

The *CLCN1* gene encodes the major skeletal muscle chloride channel CLCN-1. CLCN-1 plays an important part in the maintenance of resting potential, which is activated during the course of depolarization. The mutations of *CLCN1* gene were scattered throughout the entire sequence of the channel protein. The mutations included insertion/deletion, missense, nonsense, and splicing mutations. To the best of our knowledge, very few studies have reported splicing mutations of *CLCN1* gene [1, 2, 4, 5]. The sequences associated with splicing mutation contains two splice sites: one is a donor site, which is an invariant GU at the 5′ end of the intron and another is an acceptor site, which is an invariant AG at the 3′ end of the intron. Meyer-Kleine et al... reported a 5′ splice-donor mutation (c.1471 + 1G > A) in three GM family, which can change the highly conserved consensus sequence [4]. Gianna et al reported four cases that harbored splicing mutations(c.563G > T, c.1169-5 T > G, c.1251 + 1G > A and c.1931-2A > G), which led to skipping exons in a frameshift change during RNA translation or premature termination [5]. In our case, the novel splicing mutation c.1401 + 1G > A in intron 12 affected the 5′ splice-donor sequences resulting in exons skipping and generation of out-of-frame mRNA. However, the specific mechanism is yet to be elucidated. Another mutation (c.1657A > T,p.Ile553Phe) has been reported in Chinese GM patients [6], which may induce small changes in channel properties. This indicates that the mutation may be associated with certain ethnic populations. CLCN-1 is a voltage-dependent ion channel that mediates chloride conductance in the skeletal muscle cell membrane. The mutations of CLCN1 gene may result in a decrease in channel opening probability and render the membrane hyperexcitable, which is manifested as myotonia. This can be improved by administration of Na^+ blocking agents, such as mexiletine [7].

In conclusion, this case report of autosomal recessive myotonia congenita caused by a novel compound heterozygous mutation expands the genotypic spectrum of *CLCN1* gene.

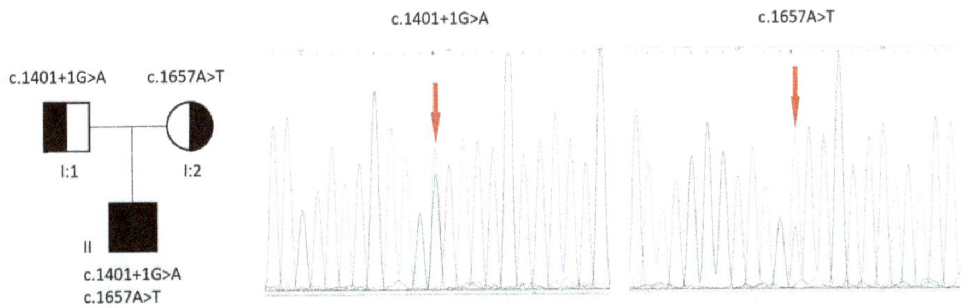

Fig. 1 Pedigree and mutation analysis of the patient. The c.1401 + 1 G > A mutation (red arrow) and c.1657 A > T mutation (red arrow), inherited from his father (I:1) and mother (I:2) respectively, were found in the patient (II)

Abbreviations

COX: cytochrome c oxidase; GM: generalized myotonia; HE: hematoxylin-eosin; MGT: modified Gomori's trichrome; MRC: Medical Research Council; NADH-TR: NADH-tetrazolium reductase; SDH: succinate dehydrogenase

Acknowledgements

The authors thank Medjaden Bioscience Limited for proofreading the manuscript.

Funding

This work was supported by the National Natural Science Foundation of China (No, 81601088), Natural Science Foundation of Jilin Province (No, 20160520164JH) and the 7th Youth Foundation of the First Hospital of Jilin University (No, JDYY72016028).

Authors' contributions

JM drafted the manuscript and figures; XW and XL designed and analyzed the study; ZK and YG analyzed and interpreted histological data; XY revised the manuscript and gave the final approval of the version to be published. All authors read and approved the contents of the case report.

Authors' information

All of authors are from the Department of Neurology and the Neuroscience Center of the First Affiliated Hospital of Jilin University.

Competing interests

The authors declare that they have no competing interests.

References

1. McKay OM, Krishnan AV, Davis M, Kiernan MC. Activity-induced weakness in recessive myotonia congenita with a novel (696+1G>a) mutation. Clin Neurophysiol. 2006;117:2064–8.
2. Ulzi G, Lecchi M, Sansone V, Redaelli E, Corti E, Saccomanno D, et al. Myotonia congenita: novel mutations in CLCN1 gene and functional characterizations in Italian patients. J Neurol Sci. 2012;318:65–71.
3. Cheng W, Tian J, Burgunder JM, Hunziker W, Eng HL. Myotonia congenita-associated mutations in chloride channel-1 affect zebrafish body wave swimming kinematics. PLoS One. 2014;9:e103445.
4. Meyer-Kleine C, Steinmeyer K, Ricker K, Jentsch TJ, Koch MC. Spectrum of mutations in the major human skeletal muscle chloride channel gene (CLCN1) leading to myotonia. Am J Hum Genet. 1995;57:1325–34.
5. Ulzi G, Sansone VA, Magri F, Corti S, Bresolin N, Comi GP, et al. In vitro analysis of splice site mutations in the CLCN1 gene using the minigene assay. Mol Biol Rep. 2014;41:2865–74.
6. Burgunder JM, Huifang S, Beguin P, Baur R, Eng CS, Seet RC, et al. Novel chloride channel mutations leading to mild myotonia among ChineseNeuromuscul Disord. 2008;18:633–40.
7. Andersen G, Hedermann G, Witting N, Duno M, Andersen H, Vissing J. The antimyotonic effect of lamotrigine in non-dystrophic myotonias: a double-blind randomized study. Brain. 2017;140:2295–305.

22

Epileptic spasms in *PPP1CB*-associated Noonan-like syndrome: a case report with clinical and therapeutic implications

Chien-Heng Lin[1†], Wei-De Lin[2†], I-Ching Chou[3,4], Inn-Chi Lee[5], Hueng-Chuen Fan[6,7] and Syuan-Yu Hong[3,8*]

Abstract

Background: Noonan syndrome-like disorder with loose anagen hair-2 (NSLH2) is an extremely rare disease caused by a heterozygous mutation in the PPP1CB gene on chromosome 2p23. The syndrome causes not only numerous dysmorphic features but also hypotonia, developmental delay, and even intellectual disability. We report the first case of NSLH2 in Asia and the 16th in the world. Moreover, the first case of PPP1CB-related infantile spasms. The clinical and therapeutic significance is outlined in this paper.

Case presentation: We found a male infant presented with severe intractable epileptic spasms. Although certain clinical features of somatic dysmorphism were noted, numerous laboratory and neuroimaging studies failed to identify the cause. To determine the underlying etiology, whole-exome sequencing was conducted. We identified a de novo heterozygous mutation, NM_206876.1: c.548A > C (p.Glu183Ala), in the PPP1CB gene. His seizures were almost refractory to conventional antiepileptic drugs but relative seizure control was eventually achieved with a ketogenic diet.

Conclusion: This result expands the clinical spectrum of NSLH2 and strengthens the association between the PPP1CB gene and epileptic seizures. Furthermore, we suggest that the ketogenic diet can offer seizure reduction in particular drug-resistant epilepsy syndromes. Additional studies are warranted to clarify the pathogenic mechanisms underlying this PPP1CB mutation in epileptic seizures.

Keywords: Epileptic spasms, PPP1CB, Noonan syndrome-like disorder with loose anagen hair-2, NSLH2, Ketogenic diet, KD

Background

PP1-beta (symbolized PPP1CB) is a catalytic subunit of protein phosphatase-1 (PP1). PP1 is one of the four major serine/threonine-specific protein phosphatases involved in the dephosphorylation of numerous proteins. These enzymes work in opposition to protein kinases, which are implicated in the regulation of cell growth, proliferation, survival, differentiation, and cytoskeletal changes, to control the level of phosphorylation [1]. PPP1CB is expressed abundantly in the human brain and spine [2, 3].

In 2014, Hamdan et al. reported a patient with a de novo 1-bp insertion in the PPP1CB gene (c.909dupA: p.Tyr450Ilefs*92), which was predicted to cause a frame-shift mutation and premature termination codon. The patient's clinical features included severe intellectual disability, short stature, relative macrocephaly, large mouth, malar hypoplasia, and mildly increased cerebral spinal fluid spaces [4]. Subsequently, Gripp et al. and Ma et al. have respectively studied four and eight unrelated patients with mutations in the PPP1CB gene. All these patients exhibited relative or absolute macrocephaly, prominent forehead, low-set and posteriorly rotated ears, and developmental delay, as well as slow-growing, sparse, or unruly hair [3, 5]. The PPP1CB gene has been

* Correspondence: dazingdog@hotmail.com
†Chien-Heng Lin and Wei-De Lin contributed equally to this work.
[3]Division of Pediatrics Neurology, China Medical University, Children's Hospital, Taichung, Taiwan
[8]Department of Pediatrics, China Medical University Hospital, 2 Yuh-Der Road, Taichung 404, Taiwan
Full list of author information is available at the end of the article

associated with Noonan syndrome-like disorder with loose anagen hair syndrome (NSLH2).

Herein, we report a male infant with a PPP1CB mutation who presented not only with typical clinical features of NSLH2 but also epileptic spasms that were almost refractory to conventional antiepileptic drugs (AEDs). Eventually, relative seizure control was achieved through administering a ketogenic diet (KD). To the best of our knowledge, this is the first case of NSLH2 in Asia and the first case of PPP1CB-related infantile spasms. The clinical and therapeutic significance is outlined in this paper.

Case presentation

The proband patient was the first child of nonconsanguineous healthy parents. His mother gave birth to him at the age of 35 years without any complication. The proband was born at 39 weeks of gestation. His birth weight was 3100 g (30th percentile), his height was 49 cm (~32nd percentile), and his head circumference (HC) was 36.2 cm (90th percentile). The Apgar score was 8/10/10 at birth. The patient did not exhibit any perinatal brain injury, hypoxia, ischemia, cranial trauma, or infection of the central nervous system. Family history of complications, such as epilepsy, febrile convulsion, intellectual disability, and psychotic disorders, was also negative.

A general physical examination at 4 months revealed macrocephaly (HC: 43.5 cm, 90th percentile), prominent forehead, low-set and posteriorly rotated ears, and sparse and slow-growing hair.

His neurological and developmental examination at 4 months demonstrated poor head control, hypotonia, less eye–object pursuit, and a less pronounced smile, but cooed occasionally. A follow-up at 14 months revealed that the patient was unable to sit stably or crawl even under an intensive early intervention.

Paroxysmal epileptic spasms and occasional erratic myoclonic seizures in clustered episodes were first noticed at the age of 4 months, and their frequency gradually increased with age: at 9 months, the patient experienced more than 20 episodes per day, with each episode lasting 1–2 min. An initial interictal electroencephalogram (EEG) at 4 months revealed multifocal spikes and high-voltage wave discharges predominantly in the posterior region (Fig. 1a). At 9 months, the interictal EEG evolved into a pattern of chaotic, disorganized rhythms with superimposed multifocal spike discharges (Fig. 1b).

Numerous AEDs in different combinations were administered at various time points since the patient was 4 months old, namely phenobarbital (5 mg/kg/day), clonazepam (titrated to 0.1 mg/kg/day), topiramate (titrated to 9 mg/kg/day) and vitamins (pyridoxine, pyridoxal phosphate, biotin, folic acid, and vitamin B12), levetiracetam (titrated to 50 mg/kg/day), valproic acid (titrated to 30–40 mg/kg/day), and vigabatrin (titrated to 150 mg/kg/day). However, none of these treatments were effective in treating his seizures at the age of 10 months, at which time he was placed on a KD.

The following laboratory tests were conducted: urinary organic acids and an acylcarnitine profile; urine toxicology screen; blood gases and electrolytes (calculate anion gap); carbohydrate-deficient transferrin and biotinidase activity; serum chemistry of liver function tests, lactate, pyruvate, ammonia, and amino acids; cerebrospinal fluid (lactate, protein and glucose levels, cell count and microscopic differentiation, gram stain and cultures, bacterial antigens, polymerase chain reaction for herpes simplex virus and varicella-zoster virus). The results were all negative. Brain magnetic resonance imaging did not reveal any marked structural abnormalities. In addition, *cardiac sonography* at 4 months showed an atrial septal defect and peripheral pulmonary stenosis. Therefore, whole-exome sequencing (WES) was conducted to determine the underlying etiology.

Genomic DNA for WES was extracted from blood from affected and unaffected parents. Exome capture

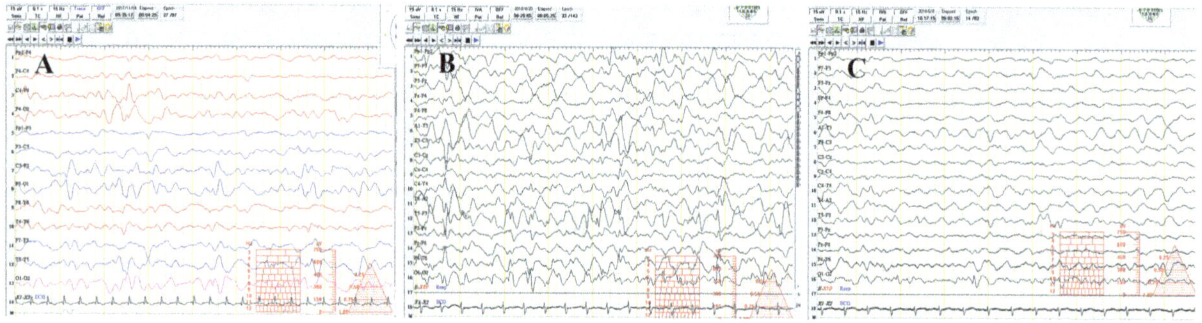

Fig. 1 The interictal electroencephalogram at the age of 4 months consists of multifocal spikes and high-voltage wave discharges appearing mainly in the posterior region (**a**). At 9 months, the interictal electroencephalogram showed a pattern of high-voltage, chaotic, random, and multifocal spikes with or without superimposed in slow waves, and spike and wave activities in almost all cortical areas (**b**). At 13 months, (after 3 months of the KD), his electroencephalogram showed only a few spikes in the posterior region (**c**)

involved the use of the Agilent Human exome V5 (51 Mb) capture kit. Sequencing was performed by 101 bp paired-end sequencing on Hiseq2000 platform (Illumina, San Diego, USA) with an ~150× depth of coverage. Raw reads were aligned to the Human genome (hg19/GRCh37) using the Burrows-Wheeler transform (BWA-MEM; v0.7.8). Variant calling was performed using the recommended best practices of GATK version 1.0.5506 (Broad Institute). Variant annotation and prioritization were performed using a well-developed pipeline, wANNOVAR [6, 7]. Candidate pathogenic variants were defined as missense, nonsense, splice-site and frameshift mutations with a minor allele frequency lower than 0.01, using the 1000 Genomes Project, dbSNP annotations, the Exome Aggregation Consortium (ExAC) and the Genome Aggregation Database (gnomAD). Several prediction programs: PolyPhen-2, Mutation Taster, CADD, and SIFT were used [8].

Only a single heterozygous missense mutation, namely NM_206876.1: c.548A > C (p.Glu183Ala), was identified in the PPP1CB gene. Variant description and *mutation* pathogenicity *prediction* were summarized in Table 1. Sanger sequencing of a DNA sample confirmed that the variant in the patient did not exist in his parents (Fig. 2). Thus, the c.548A > C variant from the proband was confirmed to be de novo. The mutation was not identified in the 1000 Genomes Project, the gnomAD, or in ExAC or dbSNP databases. Additionally, the same variant was ever reported as pathogenic by Ma et al. in 2016 [3].

After administering numerous AEDs in different combinations without a favorable response, we introduced a KD since the patient was 10 months of age. The diet protocol suggested by Neal et al. [9]. was followed. We started by administering medium-chain triglycerides from an infant formula and carefully monitored his blood and urine glucose and ketones, liver and renal functions, triglyceride and cholesterol levels, electrolytes, growth, and body weight gain during the treatment period. Parents, nurses, child nutritionists, and caretakers were enrolled in this treatment plan and educated regarding suitable food items, in addition to the calculation and preparation of ketogenic meals. Subsequently, the spasms gradually decreased to less than 0–2 times per day, and no cluster form was noticed at the follow-up time of 14 months of age, although seizures were occasionally exacerbated during a febrile illness episode. An EEG at 13 months revealed few spikes, mainly in the posterior region (Fig. 1c). However, developmental delay with cognitive and gross motor impairment was still observed.

Discussion and conclusion

A de novo PPP1CB variant (c.548A > C:p.Glu183Ala) was detected through WES. To the best of our knowledge, this is the first reported case of NSLH2 in Taiwan and the 16th in the world [3, 10, 11]. Compared with other rare diseases, a PPP1CB-related disorder is a relative new disease not generally known for its phenotype, genotype, or phenotype–gene relationship.

Since the first case of PPP1CB mutation was reported in 2014,[4] several missense mutations in *PPP1CB* associated with NSLH2 have been identified by GeneDx and numerous studies, namely c.146C > G (p.Pro49Arg), c.166G > C (p.Ala56Pro), c.548A > C (p.Glu183Ala), c.548A > T (p.Glu 183Val), c.658C > T (p.Arg220Cys), c.754G > T (p.Asp 252Tyr), and c.820G > A (p.Glu274Lys) [3, 5, 10, 11].

On the basis of the clinical features of NSLH2 (Phenotype MIM No. 617506) summarized in Online Mendelian Inheritance in Man (OMIM) (https://www.omim.org), its characteristics include intellectual disability, relative or absolute macrocephaly; prominent forehead; low-set and posteriorly rotated ears; congenital heart disease including atrial septal defect, mitral and tricuspid valve insufficiency, hypoplastic left-sided aortic arch, coarctation of the aorta, dilated aortic root, and peripheral pulmonic stenosis; brain abnormalities including septo-optic dysplasia and mild ventriculomegaly; connective tissue abnormalities including high-arched palate, joint hypermobility, and translucent or doughy skin consistency; and epidermal features such as slow-growing, sparse, or unruly hair. Our patient's features exhibited a resemblance to other cases except that this patient experienced epileptic spasms; this was the first observed patient with a *PPP1CB* mutation who had epileptic spasms.

The seizure mechanism and its response to the KD remain unknown. However, Noonan syndrome or Noonan-like syndrome, diseases typified by a disturbance of the transduction signal through the RAS/mitogen-activated protein kinase (MAPK) signal pathway are related to certain genes, such as PTPN11, SOS1, RAF1, KRAS, SHOC2, BRAF, NRAS, MAP2K1, RIT1, SOS2, LZTR1,

Table 1 Method of whole-exome sequencing and the PPP1CB mutation identified in the patient

Patient ID	Variant with NM No.	AF in		*Mutation* pathogenicity *prediction*				
		1KGP	gnomAD	Polyphen HDIV score (pred)	SIFT_score (pred)	LRT score (pred)	Mutation Taster score (pred)	*Reference*
LCY03	PPP1CB: NM_206876.1: c.548A > C (p.Glu183Ala)	–	–	0.014(B)	0.01(D)	0(D)	0.81 (D)	Ma et al. [3].

Pred prediction, *AF* allele frequency, *1KGP* 1000 Genomes Project; *gnomAD* The Genome Aggregation Database; –, not present, *B*, benign *D* deleterious, *SIFT* sorting intolerant from tolerant, *LRT* Likelihood Ratio Test

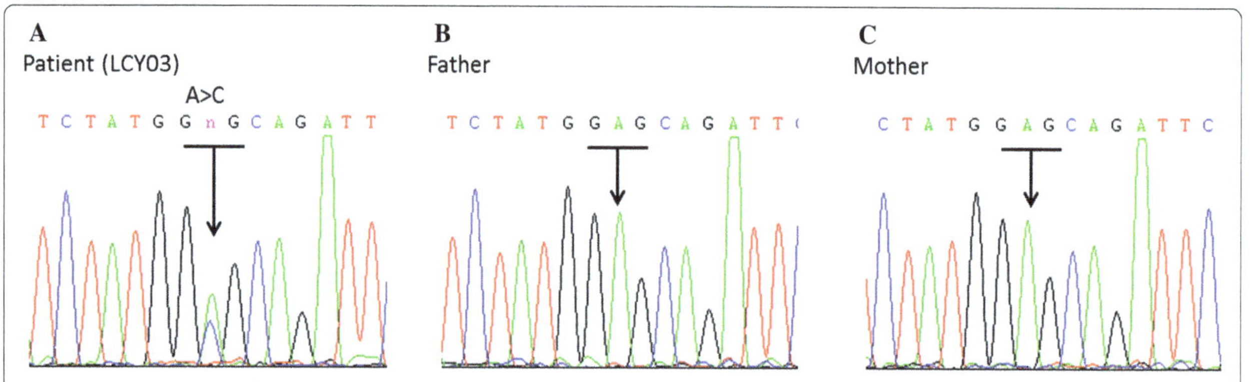

Fig. 2 Sequencing results of the de novo mutation in the *PPP1CB* gene. The arrow indicates an A-to-C substitution at nucleotide 548 (c.548A > C, p.Glu183Ala) in the patient (**a**). This gene was normal in his father (**b**) and mother (**c**)

A2ML1 and PPP1CB [5, 12, 13]. Notably, although seizure disorder (13%) is not uncommon in patients with Noonan syndrome [14], neurological impairment in patients with mutations in the RAS/MAPK pathway could be more severe and linked to certain forms of refractory epilepsy, especially epileptic encephalopathy and infantile spasms [15–17].

Strategies for treating RAS/MAPK-related seizures have not been established. In the aforementioned studies, Adachi et al. [17] reported two individual cases of cardiofaciocutaneous syndrome with severe neurological impairment and infantile spasms caused by heterozygous mutations in KRAS and BRAF genes. None of the AEDs were effective in treating their seizures, but the patient with KRAS mutation (p. D153V) had a partial response to ACTH therapy. The clinical and genetic characteristics of RAS/MAPK-associated epilepsy syndromes are summarized in Table 2 [15–18]. In recent studies, the ketogenic diet has proven to be a safe and effective treatment for children with not only drug-resistant epilepsies but also epileptic encephalopathies [19–23]. However, some adverse effects that can happen in the short-term when using dietary treatment of KD should be kept in mind and closely monitored, e.g. gastrointestinal symptoms; dyslipidemia;

Table 2 Clinical and genetic characteristics of RAS/MAPK-associated epileptic encephalopathies

Clinical manifestation	RAS/MAPK-associated genes			
	BRAF	*MEK1*	*KRAS*	*PPP1CB*
Associated syndrome	CFC	CFC3	Noonan syndrome 3	NSLH2
Reported mutations	L485F; L485S; F468S; Q257R; del E11; F595 L; T599R; G534R; D638E; K499 N	F53F; Y130N	D153V	E183A
Age of onset of epileptic encephalopathies	Birth to 11y	2 reported patients (1y and15y)	3 m with Myo/11 m with IS	4 m
Seizure type	CPS, GTCS or sGTCS, Abs, IS, Tonic spasms, SE	GTCS, Abs, CPS	IS, Myo	IS, Myo
Interictal EEG	Hypsarrhythmia (some patients)	Focal epileptiform discharges to hypsarrhythmia.	Hypsarrhythmia (11 m); asynchronous slow waves with irregular spike-wave or polyspikes with and without waves (6 y).	Chaotic, high voltage, polymorphic delta and theta rhythms with superimposed multifocal spikes and wave discharges.
Development delay	Severe	Severe	Severe	Moderate to severe
Seizures refractory to AEDs or required multiple AEDs use	Yes	Yes	Yes	Yes
Seizure prognosis	Difficult to control	Difficult to control	Controlled with ACTH	Favorable to KD
Brain MRI	Cortical atrophy, hypoplastic CC	Hydrocephalus, cortical atrophy	Cortical atrophy, agenesis of the CC	Unremarkable
References	[15–18]	[15]	[18]	The present study

CFC Cardiofaciocutaneous syndrome, *CFC3* Cardiofaciocutaneous syndrome 3, *GTCS* generalized tonic-clonic seizure, *sGTCS* secondarily generalized tonic-clonic seizure, *CPS* complex partial seizure, *Abs* absence seizure, *Myo* myoclonic seizure, status epilepticus, *SE*, *IS* infantile spasms, *AEDs* antiepileptic drugs, *ACTH* adrenocorticotropic hormone, *KD* ketogenic diet, *MRI* magnetic resonance image, *CC* corpus callosum, m: months, *y* years hypoglycemia; hyperuricemia; hypoproteinemia; hypomagnesemia; hyponatremia; hepatitis and metabolic acidosis; nephrolithiasis; osteopenia, osteoporosis and bone fractures; growth failure. Fortunately, our patient further proves the efficacy of the ketogenic diet for PPP1CB-related Noonan syndrome presenting as infantile spasms and no obvious side effects were observed [24]. However, whether the KD would also have been effective in our patient for treating earlier seizure occurrences could not be investigated. Moreover, limited data for epileptic seizures associated with PPP1CB mutations are available in the worldwide population. However, more in-depth studies with additional patient data to explore the efficacy of the KD for treating epileptic seizures caused by PPP1CB mutations are essential. In conclusion, our study expands the clinical spectrum of NSLH2 and strengthens the association between the PPP1CB gene and epileptic spasms. Furthermore, we suggest that the KD be considered when seizures are *medically refractory*. Additional investigations are warranted to clarify the genotype–phenotype correlations of several genes in the RAS/MAPK signaling pathway and their associations with epileptic seizures or encephalopathies.

Abbreviations

AEDs: antiepileptic drugs; EEG: electroencephalogram; HC: head circumference; KD: ketogenic diet; MAPK: mitogen-activated protein kinase; NSLH2: Noonan syndrome-like disorder with loose anagen hair-2; WES: whole-exome sequencing

Acknowledgments

We would like to thank the Genetic Medicine Laboratory of China Medical University Hospital for giving support and assistance to this work. We also want to thank Ni-Chung (Nina) Lee because she stimulated our enthusiasm for neurogenetics and provided assistance for this work.

Authors' contributions

SYH provided treatment to the patient, collected the data and wrote the draft. CHL and WDL participated in the design of the case report and wrote the manuscript. ICC provided her experience for the patient' s treatment, especially the use of ketogenic diet and modified the manuscript accordingly. ICL and HCF made the new Table 2 to meet the requirements of reviewers and participated in the editing and revising the manuscript and supervised this publication. All authors read and approved the final manuscript.

Competing interests

The authors declare that they have no competing interests.

Author details

[1]Division of Pediatrics Pulmonology, China Medical University, Children's Hospital, Taichung, Taiwan. [2]Department of Medical Research, China Medical University Hospital, Taichung, Taiwan. [3]Division of Pediatrics Neurology, China Medical University, Children's Hospital, Taichung, Taiwan. [4]Graduate Institute of Integrated Medicine, College of Chinese Medicine, China Medical University, Taichung, Taiwan. [5]Department of Pediatrics, Chung Shan Medical University Hospital and Institute of Medicine, School of Medicine, Chung Shan Medical University, Taichung, Taiwan. [6]Department of Pediatrics, Tungs' Taichung Metroharbor Hospital, Wuchi, 435 Taichung, Taiwan. [7]Department of Nursing, Jen-Teh Junior College of Medicine, Nursing and Management, 356 Miaoli, Taiwan. [8]Department of Pediatrics, China Medical University Hospital, 2 Yuh-Der Road, Taichung 404, Taiwan.

References

1. Barker HM, Brewis ND, Street AJ, Spurr NK, Cohen PT. Three genes for protein phosphatase 1 map to different human chromosomes: sequence, expression and gene localisation of protein serine/threonine phosphatase 1 beta (PPP1CB). Biochim Biophys Acta. 1994;1220:212–8.
2. Bordelon JR, Smith Y, Nairn AC, Colbran RJ, Greengard P, Muly EC. Differential localization of protein phosphatase-1alpha, beta and gamma1 isoforms in primate prefrontal cortex. Cereb Cortex. 2005;15(12):1928–37.
3. Ma L, Bayram Y, McLaughlin HM, Cho MT, Krokosky A, Turner CE, et al. De novo missense variants in PPP1CB are associated with intellectual disability and congenital heart disease. Hum Genet. 2016;135:1399–409.
4. Hamdan FF, Srour M, Capo-Chichi JM, Daoud H, Nassif C, Patry L, et al. De novo mutations in moderate or severe intellectual disability. PLoS Genet. 2014;10:e1004772.
5. Gripp KW, Aldinger KA, Bennett JT, Baker L, Tusi J, Powell-Hamilton N, et al. A novel rasopathy caused by recurrent de novo missense mutations in PPP1CB closely resembles Noonan syndrome with loose anagen hair. Am J Med Genet A. 2016;170:2237–47.
6. Chang X, Wang K. wANNOVAR: annotating genetic variants for personal genomes via the web. J Med Genet. 2012;49:433–6.
7. Yang H, Wang K. Genomic variant annotation and prioritization with ANNOVAR and wANNOVAR. Nat Protoc. 2015;10:1556–66.
8. Adzhubei IA, Schmidt S, Peshkin L, Ramensky VE, Gerasimova A, Bork P, et al. A method and server for predicting damaging missense mutations. Nat Methods. 2010;7:248–9.
9. Neal EG, Chaffe H, Schwartz RH, Lawson MS, Edwards N, Fitzsimmons G, et al. The ketogenic diet for the treatment of childhood epilepsy: a randomised controlled trial. Lancet Neurol. 2008;7:500–6.
10. Bertola D, Yamamoto G, Buscarilli M, Jorge A, Passos-Bueno MR, Kim C. The recurrent PPP1CB mutation p.Pro49Arg in an additional Noonan-like syndrome individual: broadening the clinical phenotype. Am J Med Genet A. 2017;173:824–8.
11. Zambrano RM, Marble M, Chalew SA, Lilje C, Vargas A, Lacassie Y. Further evidence that variants in PPP1CB cause a rasopathy similar to Noonan syndrome with loose anagen hair. Am J Med Genet A. 2017;173:565–7.
12. Garg S, Brooks A, Burns A, Burkitt-Wright E, Kerr B, Huson S, et al. Autism spectrum disorder and other neurobehavioural comorbidities in rare disorders of the Ras/MAPK pathway. Dev Med Child Neurol. 2017;59:544–9.
13. Kruszka P, Porras AR, Addissie YA, Moresco A, Medrano S, Mok GTK, et al. Noonan syndrome in diverse populations. Am J Med Genet A. 2017;173:2323–34.
14. Romano AA, Allanson JE, Dahlgren J, Gelb BD, Hall B, Pierpont ME, et al. Noonan syndrome: clinical features, diagnosis, and management guidelines. Pediatrics. 2010;126:746–59.
15. Yoon G, Rosenberg J, Blaser S, Rauen KA. Neurological complications of cardio-facio-cutaneous syndrome. Dev Med Child Neurol. 2007;49:894–9.
16. Wakusawa K, Kobayashi S, Abe Y, Tanaka S, Endo W, Inui T, et al. A girl with cardio-facio-cutaneous syndrome complicated with status epilepticus and acute encephalopathy. Brain Dev. 2014;36:61–3.
17. Adachi M, Abe Y, Aoki Y, Matsubara Y. Epilepsy in RAS/MAPK syndrome: two cases of cardio-facio-cutaneous syndrome with epileptic encephalopathy and a literature review. Seizure. 2012;21:55–60.
18. Aizaki K, Sugai K, Saito Y, Nakagawa E, Sasaki M, Aoki Y, et al. Cardio-facio-cutaneous syndrome with infantile spasms and delayed myelination. Brain Dev. 2011;33:166–9.
19. Arya R, Peariso K, Gaínza-Lein M, Harvey J, Bergin A, Brenton JN, et al. Efficacy and safety of ketogenic diet for treatment of pediatric convulsive refractory status epilepticus. Epilepsy Res. 2018;144:1–6.
20. Li T, Cheng M, Wang J, Hong S, Li M, Liao S, et al. De novo mutations of STXBP1 in Chinese children with early onset epileptic encephalopathy. Genes Brain Behav. 2018:e12492. https://doi.org/10.1111/gbb.12492.
21. Su DJ, Lu JF, Lin LJ, Liang JS, Hung KL. SCN2A mutation in an infant presenting with migrating focal seizures and infantile spasm responsive to a ketogenic diet. Brain Dev. 2018;40:724–7.
22. Wirrell E, Eckert S, Wong-Kisiel L, Payne E, Nickels K. Ketogenic diet therapy in infants: efficacy and tolerability. Pediatr Neurol. 2018;82:13–8.
23. Martin HC, Kim GE, Pagnamenta AT, Murakami Y, Carvill GL, Meyer E, et al. Clinical whole-genome sequencing in severe early-onset epilepsy reveals new genes and improves molecular diagnosis. Hum Mol Genet. 2014;23:3200–11.

23

Uremic encephalopathy with isolated brainstem involvement revealed by magnetic resonance image

Li-jing Jia[1,2,3*], Zhen-zhen Qu[1,2,3], Xue-qian Zhang[1], Yu-juan Tian[1] and Ying Wang[1]

Abstract

Background: Uremic Encephalopathy (UE) is a neurological complication associated with acute or chronic renal failure. Imaging findings of UE may present involvement of the basal ganglia, cortical or subcortical regions, and white matter. We report a rare case of UE caused by neurogenic bladder with isolated brainstem involvement revealed by magnetic resonance imaging (MRI). Immediate therapy resulted in full recovery of neurological signs and changes on MRI.

Case presentation: A 14-year-old Han Chinese woman with a history of chronic renal failure caused by neurogenic bladder. On admission, she was unconscious and her pupils presented different sizes, while her vital signs were normal. MRI showed high signal in the dorsal pontine base and in the mid brain on fluid-attenuated inversion-recovery (FLAIR) imaging and on T2-weighted imaging while the signal was normal on diffusion-weighted images (DWI). Blood analysis revealed renal failure and acidosis. After urinary retention treatment and acidosis correction, the patient soon recovered. Follow-up MRI 2 months after the discharge revealed complete resolution of UE in the brainstem.

Conclusion: We reported a rare case of a patient with UE that had unusual imaging manifestations for whom timely diagnosis and treatment assured recovery.

Keywords: Uremic encephalopathy, Magnetic resonance images, Brainstem, Renal failure, Posterior reversible encephalopathy syndrome

Background

Uremic encephalopathy (UE) may result from multiple disorders associated with acute or chronic renal failure and is characterized by acute or subacute onset of reversible neurological symptoms. There are 3 patterns of imaging findings in patients with UE: involving the basal ganglia, cortical or subcortical regions, and white matter [1]. Cortical involvement of UE is a category of posterior reversible encephalopathy syndrome (PRES) and basal ganglia involvement is rare [1, 2], the white matter involvement is limited to case reports [3, 4]. We came across a reported case of UE caused by neurogenic bladder that presented isolate involvement of the brainstem on magnetic resonance imaging (MRI). To our knowledge, only two other reported cases had MRI findings similar to this patient [5, 6]. We report a rare case of UE with unusual imaging manifestation to encourage timely diagnosis and treatment of this condition.

Case presentation

A 14-year-old Han Chinese woman with a history of neurogenic bladder for more than 10 years was admitted to our Department because of coma for 12 h. The patient complained for diplopia without fever or diarrhea 4 days before her coma with no incentive. She had no limb weakness and was treated with Vitamin B1and mecobalamine. Her previous medical history included neurogenic bladder caused by spina bifida occulta for 12 years and hydronephrosis diagnosed 1 year before. Sometimes she had urine retention, but she received no treatment for the neurogenic bladder except for urethral catheterization occasionally. She had no seizures and no fever. On admission, physical examination revealed that she was unconscious. The pupils did not react to light

* Correspondence: jlj997@126.com
[1]Department of Neurology, The Second Hospital of Hebei Medical University, Hebei, Shijiazhuang 050000, People's Republic of China
[2]Institution of Cardiocerebrovascular Disease, Hebei, West Heping Road 215, Shijiazhuang 050000, People's Republic of China
Full list of author information is available at the end of the article

and presented different sizes in each eye (left pupil diameter, 2.5 mm; right pupil diameter, 4 mm). On stimulation, she could move her 4 limbs spontaneously. There were exaggerated deep tendon reflexes over both legs and the right Barbinski sign was positive. However, her vital signs were stable: Blood Pressure (BP) was 120/81 mmHg; pulse rate, 76 beats/min; body temperature, 36.5 °C; breath, 12 times/min. Non-contrast brain computed tomography (CT) after the onset of her coma revealed diffuse brain stem hypodensity. Brain MRI acquired 4 h after the coma onset in the county hospital showed high signal at the dorsal part of the pontine base and the mid brain on fluid-attenuated inversion-recovery (FLAIR) imaging and T2-weighted imaging. However, diffusion-weighted images presented normal signal (Fig. 1). The non- contrast abdominal CT preformed on the next day of admission showed chronic obstructive uropathy with a distended bladder, severe hydronephrosis and dual renal atrophy.

Blood analysis immediately after admission revealed renal failure [Urea nitrogen: 23.87 mmol/L, Creatinine: 566.8 μmol/L], and anemia [RBC: 2.5 × 10^{12}/L, HGB: 79 g/L]. Arterial blood gas analysis revealed metabolic acidosis [pH 7.09 (7.35–7.45)]. Liver function was normal.

The patient was diagnosed with UE due to chronic renal failure and metabolic acidosis. She was immediately treated with 200 ml of bicarbonate at 5% conducted by quick intravenous injection, followed by 100 ml intravenous injection of bicarbonate at 5% once a day and 1.0 g of bicarbonate administered orally three times per day for 3 days. Simultaneously, she underwent urethral catheterization to relieve the urine retention. She was revived without diplopia 3 days after admission and the reviewed blood analysis after urethral catheterization showed that her renal function was returning to a normal level (Urea nitrogen: 13.10 mmol/L, Creatinine: 294 μmol/L); hence, dialysis was not necessary. She was treated with hypodermically administered erythropoietin 3000u twice a day, and ferrous sulfate 0.3 g orally thrice a day for the anemia. She was discharged 14 days after the admission without diplopia and any mental disturbance. She was still with the ureteral catheter because of the hydronephrosis. Two weeks after the discharge, the catheter was removed when abdomen ultrasonic showed decreased hydronephrosis. Follow-up MRI performed 2 months after the discharge revealed complete resolution of the brainstem UE (Fig. 2). Reviewed blood analysis after 2 months of discharge showed that her renal failure still persisted (Urea nitrogen: 13.10 mmol/L, Creatinine: 190.3 μmol/L). However, she had no neurological disturbance or urinary retention. She underwent the comprehensive bladder-retraining program to avoid urinary retention and her renal function was regularly assessed once a month.

Discussion and conclusions

Clinical manifestations of UE are variable and alterations in brain images play an important role in the diagnosis of the condition. Unusual for typical UE imaging manifestations, the imaging findings of our patient showed isolated brainstem hyperintensity on FLAIR and T2WI without basal ganglia and cortical or subcortical involvement. As opposed to the typical posterior reversible encephalopathy syndrome (PRES), central-variant posterior reversible encephalopathy syndrome had been described as brain stem or basal ganglia involvement that spares the cerebral cortex and subcortical white matter [7], which had similar imaging features with our patient. Approximately one-third of PRES cases are reported to have involved the brainstem and basal ganglia, accompanied by involvement of the parieto-occipital regions [8] and only 4% of these patients did not have cortical involvement [7]. As for UE, there were few reports on the isolated brain stem involvement detectable through MRI. Although the brainstem was involved and the patient presented severe symptoms, timely and accurate therapy resulted in clinical recovery.

Although the pathophysiological changes are not fully understood, UE and PRES share similar clinical and MRI features. The pathophysiology of PRES is thought to be

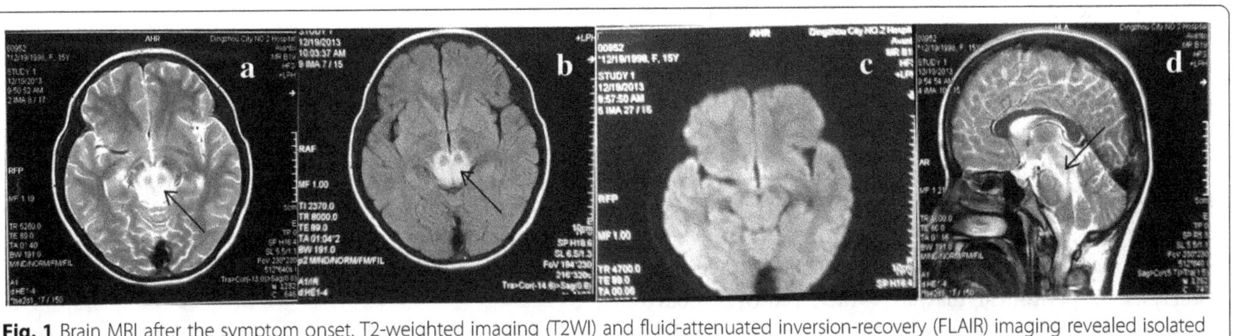

Fig. 1 Brain MRI after the symptom onset. T2-weighted imaging (T2WI) and fluid-attenuated inversion-recovery (FLAIR) imaging revealed isolated hyperintense signals in the dorsal part of the pons and the midbrain in axial view (**a**, **b**) and sagittal view (**d**). Diffusion-weighted imaging (DWI), however, showed normal intensity (**c**)

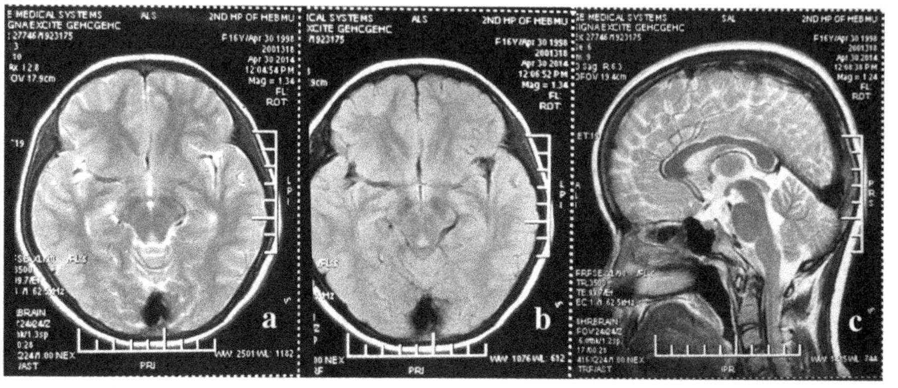

Fig. 2 Follow up magnetic resonance imaging (MRI) showed significant decrease in signal intensity in the brainstem on axial T2-weighted imaging (T2WI) (**a**), axial fluid-attenuated inversion-recovery (FLAIR) imaging (**b**), and sagittal T2WI (**c**)

the dysfunction of vascular autoregulation whereas UE is likely caused by the effects of neurotoxic compounds [1]. Regardless the reason, the breakdown of the blood-brain barrier is the key factor of the imaging manifestations [9]. MRI predominantly reveals vasogenic edema but cytotoxic edema has been reported in UE and PRES [1, 3, 4]. The imaging manifestations of our patient showed hyperintensity on T2WI and FLAIR but normal intensity on DWI, which represented vasogenic edema. We assumed that this image finding may be caused by the breakdown of the blood-brain barrier related to the uremic toxin or acidosis. When the acidosis was corrected (PH 7.42) and the renal failure decreased (Urea nitrogen: 14.6 mmol/L (1.7–7.1 mmol/L), Creatinine: 294 μmol/L (0.1–136 μmol/L), after the urinary obstruction was relieved 3 days after the admission, the clinical symptoms of the patient resolved. Follow-up images acquired 2 months after the discharge showed complete resolution of the brainstem even though the renal failure was not completely recovered (Urea nitrogen: 13.10 mmol/L, Creatinine: 190.3 μmol/L). However, we are not able to comment on why the lesion was located in the brain stem without cortical or basal ganglia involved.

The brainstem CT and MRI findings in our patient should be differentiated from Wernicke's encephalopathy, central pontine myelinolysis, and infectious brainstem encephalitis. The lack of no increased signal in periaqueductal regions and medial thalami make Wernicke's encephalopathy unlikely. Infectious encephalitis was ruled out, because there was no fever and other signs of infection. The reversibility of symptoms and imaging findings coupled with a negative history of rapid correction of hyponatremia makes central pontine myelinolysis less likely.

UE in renal failure is reversibly associated with hemodialysis or peritoneal dialysis, which removes neurotoxic compounds. Regarding our patient, her renal failure was caused by neurogenic bladder related to spina bifida occulta. It is reported that among nearly 60,000 patients with neurogenic bladder, the incidence of lower urinary tract infections was 29–36%, urinary retention was 9–14%, and urinary tract obstructions was 6–11% [10]. Our patient had urinary retention and urinary tract obstruction and she presented UE when the renal function got very severe. After the urinary retention was relieved by urethral catheterization and the acidosis was corrected, the renal function improved and the clinical manifestations were recovered without dialysis.

In summary, MRI manifestations are important for the diagnosis of UE. Neurotoxic compounds and metabolic acidosis may play roles in the pathophysiology of this disease. We reported a rare case of a patient with UE that had isolated brainstem vasogenic edema detectable through MRI, assuring timely diagnosis and treatment of the condition.

Abbreviations

MRI: Magnetic resonance imaging; PRES: posterior reversible encephalopathy syndrome; UE: uremic encephalopathy, renal failure

Acknowledgements

We thank the patient and her father for their collaboration.

Funding

The design of the study and collection, analysis, and interpretation of data and in writing the manuscript was supported by research grants from the second hospital of Hebei medical university foundation (2h1201612).

Authors' contributions

Study concept and design: LJJ, Acquisition of data: ZZQ, XQZ, YJT. YW. All authors read and approved the final manuscript.

Competing interests

The authors declare that they have no competing interests.

Author details
[1]Department of Neurology, The Second Hospital of Hebei Medical University, Hebei, Shijiazhuang 050000, People's Republic of China. [2]Institution of Cardiocerebrovascular Disease, Hebei, West Heping Road 215, Shijiazhuang 050000, People's Republic of China. [3]Neurological Laboratory of Hebei Province, Hebei, Shijiazhuang 050000, People's Republic of China.

References

1. Kim DM, Lee IH, Song CJ. Uremic encephalopathy: MR imaging findings and clinical correlation. Am J Neuroradiol. 2016;37:1604–9.
2. Graham BR, Pylypchuk GB. Posterior reversible encephalopathy syndrome in an adult patient undergoing peritoneal dialysis: a case report and literature review. BMC Nephrol. 2014;15:10.
3. Kang E, Jeon SJ, Choi SS. Uremic encephalopathy with atypical magnetic resonance features on diffusion-weighted images. Korean J Radiol. 2012; 13(6):808–11.
4. Pruss H, Siebert E, Masuhr F. Reversible cytotoxic brain edema and facial weakness in uremic encephalopathy. J Neurol. 2009;256:1372–3.
5. Osman Y, Imam Y Z, Salem K, Al-Hail H, Uthman B, Deleu D. Isolated brainstem involvement in a patient with hypertensive encephalopathy. Case Rep Neurol Med. 2013; Article ID 540947.
6. Shiga Y, Kanaya Y, Kono R, Takeshima S, Shimoe Y, Kuriyama M. Posterior reversible encephalopathy syndrome of the midbrain and hypothalamus - a case report of uremic encephalopathy presenting with hypersomnia. Rinsho Shinkeigaku. 2016;56:43–7.
7. Makinney AM, Jagadeesan BD, Truwit CL. Central-variant posterior reversible encephalopathy syndrome: brainstem or basal ganglia involvement lacking cortical or subcortical cerebral edema. AJR. 2013;201:631–8.
8. Liman TG, Bohner G, Heuschmann PU. The clinical and radiological spectrum of posterior reversible encephalopathy syndrome: the retrospective Berlin PRES study. J Neurol. 2012;259:155–64.
9. Fugate JE, Rabinstein AA. Posterior reversible encephalopathy syndrome: clinical and radiological manifestations, pathophysiology, and outstanding questions. Lancet Neurol. 2015;14:914–5.
10. Manack A, Motsko SP, Haag-Molkenteller C. Epidemiology and healthcare utilization of neurogenic bladder patients in a US claims database. Neurourol Urodyn. 2011;30:395–401.

24

A case report of rigidity and recurrent lower limb myoclonus: progressive encephalomyelitis rigidity and myoclonus syndrome, a chameleon

Aurélie Degeneffe[1*], Marie Dagonnier[1], Alain D'hondt[2] and Jose Antonio Elosegi[1]

Abstract

Background: Progressive encephalomyelitis with rigidity and myoclonus (PERM) syndrome is a rare neurological condition. Its clinical characteristics include axial and limb muscle rigidity, myoclonus, painful spasms and hyperekplexia. Diagnosis of this disease can be very challenging and optimal long-term treatment is unclear.

Case presentation: We report a case of a 62 year old patient admitted for repetitive myoclonus and rigidity in the lower limbs progressing since 10 years, associated with a fluctuating encephalopathy requiring stays in Intensive Care Unit. Multiple diagnostics and treatment were proposed, unsuccessfully, before the diagnosis of PERM syndrome was established. In association with the clinical presentation, a strong positive result for GAD (glutamic acid decarboxylase) antibodies lead to the diagnosis of PERM syndrome.

Conclusions: PERM syndrome is a rare disease and its diagnosis is not easy. Once the diagnosis is established, the correct treatment should follow and could be lifesaving, regardless of a delayed diagnosis. Maintenance of long-term oral corticotherapy is suggested to prevent relapses.

Keywords: PERM, Myoclonus, Rigidity, Stiff person, Stiff man

Background

Progressive encephalomyelitis with rigidity and myoclonus (PERM) syndrome is a rare neurological condition. PERM is suggested to be a more severe variant of the stiff person syndrome (SPS) [1–6]. Its clinical characteristics include muscle rigidity (both axial and limb), myoclonus often stimulus-sensitive and painful spasms [1, 2, 4–9]. This condition is often associated with hyperekplexia due to brainstem dysfunction [3, 10–12]. This brainstem dysfunction is manifesting in alteration of consciousness, cerebellar ataxia and respiratory insufficiency due to breathing and swallowing difficulties [6, 13, 14].

Seizures are often observed [1, 3, 6, 14–21]. This syndrome can present with an insidious onset, as well as an acute or subacute presentation, or exacerbations on a chronic course [3–5, 11, 14, 20]. This condition has previously been associated with the glutamic acid decarboxylase (GAD), dipeptidyl-peptidase-like protein-6 (DPPX) antibodies and glycine receptor (GlyR) serum antibodies [3, 14, 22]. The latter is associated with a disruption of the inhibitory glycinergic synaptic transmission, which is prominent in the spinal cord and brainstem [5, 13]. Abnormal cerebrospinal fluid (CSF) is seen and additional denervation on the electromyography (EMG) [2, 3, 6, 11, 18, 23, 24]. Immunomodulation using corticosteroids, intravenous (IV) immunoglobulin, plasma exchange or cyclophosphamide are described as an effective treatment [1, 24]. Intrathecal Bacflofen has also successfully been applied [1, 2]. Initial diagnosis of PERM is not easy and literature is limited regarding the long-term course of the syndrome. Herein, we report an unusual presentation of PERM in a patient with previous diagnosis of spinal myoclonus, neuroleptic malignant syndrome (NMS) and multiple episodes of relapse.

* Correspondence: aurelie.degeneffe@erasme.ulb.ac.be
[1]Department of Neurology, CHU Ambroise Paré Hospital, Boulevard John Fitzgerald Kennedy 2, 7000 Mons, Belgium
Full list of author information is available at the end of the article

Case presentation

The clinical story of this 62 year old woman started in 2007 with lower back pain, lumbar muscular contractures and back rigidity. After being examined by an orthopaedic surgeon, she was diagnosed with congenital scoliosis. A lumbar interbody fusion was subsequently performed with no significant impact on the symptoms.

Between 2007 and 2014, she presented multiple episodes of lower limb myoclonus. Episodes were often associated with hyperthermia. A diagnosis of spinal myoclonus was suggested and a treatment with clonazepam began.

In 2014, she presented with lower limb myoclonus, confusion, hyperthermia and acute respiratory failure. She was admitted to the intensive care unit (ICU). Differential diagnoses at the time included NMS versus meningoencephalitis. Nevertheless, no past history of neuroleptic use was identified and multiple attempts of lumbar puncture were unsuccessful. Large spectrum antibiotics were administered with favourable clinical evolution.

She finally presented in our hospital in our emergency department (ED) in January 2017 for recurrent myoclonus and a sudden onset of bilateral leg weakness in the context of an influenza infection. Upon arrival at the ED, moderate hypotension and fever (39.4 °C) were observed. Neurological examination showed bradyphrenia, however she followed one-step commands. There was a motor deficit of the lower extremities scored 4 on the Medical Research Council scale (MRC) [25], diminished and symmetrical knee and ankle jerks, myoclonus and rigidity in the lower limbs. Initial laboratory tests showed normal white cell count with moderately increased C reactive protein (CRP; 39 mg/l, normal: < 5 mg/l). Creatine kinase (CPK) was elevated at 52144 U/L (normal: 10–170 UI/l) with an acute renal insufficiency (clearance of 14 ml/min). Clonazepam doses were increased from 1 mg to 2 mg three times daily and antibioc therapy with amoxicillin/clavulanic acid was empirically started.

The day after admission in the neurology ward alteration of the level of consciousness, persistent hypotension and respiratory distress were observed and the patient was subsequently admitted to ICU. In the following days, there was a progressive deterioration of the motor function in the lower limbs until paraplegia was reached while lower limb rigidity and myoclonus persisted. Patient contact was lost with respiratory failure, necessitating invasive mechanical ventilation during one week.

Brain and spinal magnetic resonance imaging (MRI) revealed a pituitary adenoma, cervical osteoarthritis and thoraco-lumbar discopathy without stenosis. EMG showed continuous rhythmic motor unit activity within the axial muscles. CPK continued to rise in the following days to peak of 74,410 U/L. CSF analysis was normal, polymerase chain reaction (PCR) for herpes simplex virus 1 (HSV1), HSV 2 and enterovirus were negative (Table 1).

In doubt, anti-epileptic treatment with levetiracetam (2 g twice daily) was started. Nonetheless, a consecutive twenty-four-hour electroencephalogram (EEG) demonstrated numerous muscular artefacts but no epileptic activity (Table 1).

An extensive blood investigation (Table 1) was performed including: human immunodeficiency virus (HIV), anti-nuclear antibody (ANA), anti-neutrophil cytoplasmic antibody (ANCA), Anti-double-stranded DNA antibody, antibody to extractable nuclear antigens, anti-mitochondrial antibody (AMA), anti-smooth muscle antibody (ASMA), Anti-actin antibody (AAA), Anti-glomerular basement membrane antibody (anti-GBM Ab), paraneoplastic syndromes, complement C3 and C4, mycoplasma, influenza, enterovirus, adenovirus, borrelia burgdorferi, cytomegalovirus, cardiolipine antibody, lupus anticoagulant, thyroid function and paraneoplastic neurological antibodies (anti-Amphiphysin, anti-Hu, anti-Yo, anti-CV2, anti-Ri, anti-Ma2/Ta, anti-Sox1 and anti-Titin). All test results were either normal or negative. However, our patient was tested strongly positive for the antibodies to GAD (95; normal values 0–5). Together with the clinical presentation this ultimately led to the diagnosis of PERM syndrome.

Initial treatment was therefore started with gammaglobulins (0.4 g/kg/day) during 5 days with poor results. Concomitant corticotherapy was started with IV hydrocortisone (50 mg, three times daily) for 10 days, which was then continued orally. The treatment was continued with five sessions of plasma exchange (2 L). Recovery of her consciousness followed within days and myoclonus ceased. She was extubated one week after the end of plasma exchange sessions. Total duration of the ICU stay accounted 33 days. The patient was then transferred to the neurology ward where she recovered progressively with respect to motor function; she was able to walk with a walker when discharged to a rehabilitation centre.

While still in rehabilitation, our patient had a short relapse of the myoclonus in March 2017, only after she was already shortened on her corticosteroids and anti-epileptics. Decision was made to keep her on a regimen of levetiracetam 2 g twice a day and hydrocortisone 20 mg twice daily. She left the rehabilitation centre in May 2017 with a favourable evolution despite persistent mild lower proximal limb weakness (scored 4 on the MRC scale) and gait ataxia.

In August 2017, seven months after admission, she had no relapse of the myoclonus nor the rigidity and was able to walk without assistance. Hydrocortisone was reduced to 10 mg twice daily.

In October, she was again admitted for intermittent episodes of myoclonus (less than 60 min). Myoclonus

Table 1 Diagnostic work-up

Imaging	Brain MRI	Pituitary adenoma
	Spinal MRI	Cervical osteoarthritis and thoraco-lumbar discopathy without stenosis
EMG	Continuous rhythmic motor unit activity within the axial muscles	
EEG	No epileptic activity	
CSF	Normal	
Laboratory tests	CRP	39 mg/L
	CPK	74,410 U/L
	CrCl	14 ml/min
	HIV	Negative
	ANA	Negative
	ANCA	Negative
	Anti-double-stranded DNA AB	Negative
	Antibody to extractable nuclear antigens	Negative
	ASMA	Negative
	AAA	Negative
	Anti-GBM Antibody	Negative
	Paraneoplastic syndromes	Negative
	Complement C3 and C4	Negative
	Mycoplasma	Negative
	Influenza	Negative
	Enterovirus	Negative
	Adenovirus	Negative
	Borrelia Burgdorferi	Negative
	Cytomegalovirus	Negative
	Cardiolipine antibody	Negative
	Lupus anticoagulant	Negative
	Thyroid function	Normal
	Paraneoplastic neurological antibodies (anti-Amphiphysin, anti-Hu, anti-Yo, anti-CV2, anti-Ri, anti-Ma2/Ta, anti-Sox1, anti-Titin)	Negative
	GAD65	95

rapidly disappeared after treatment with IV methylprednisolone (1 g) for three consecutive days. Steroids dose were increased again to 20 mg twice daily. She is now followed monthly at the outpatient clinic and levetiracetam treatment has been progressively stopped while hydrocortisone is maintained at the same dose.

Discussion and conclusions

PERM is a challenging diagnosis due to several reasons. The condition, firstly described by Whitely et al. in 1976, is relatively rare [7]. Diagnosis is mainly clinical, as (in most cases) there is an absence of signs on imaging. Increased signal intensity of the cervical cord and lower brainstem in T2 MRI sequences was reported in only two cases [8, 26]. EMG and antibodies in serum and CSF could help to confirm the diagnosis. Initial clinical presentation can be very unspecific and uncommon, and this case is no exception. Common differential diagnoses of PERM syndrome are stiff person syndrome, paraneoplastic SPS and NMS [9, 17]. In this case, we can also add spinal myoclonus to the list and potentially scoliosis.

In retrospect, the initial lower back pain and rigidity could have been the premises of the PERM syndrome symptoms. Lumbar spinal fusion was performed in regards to the scoliosis indication. Unfortunately, it had no efficacy on the rigidity symptoms. Moreover, the patient later developed recurrent episodes of lower limb myoclonus. These were, in association with the past history of spinal fusion, wrongly diagnosed as spinal myoclonus.

The episode of myoclonus presented by our patient in 2014, associated with hyperthermia, was considered as an episode of NMS. It was previously reported by Xu et al. that PERM could be mimicking NMS due to its significant overlap in symptoms [17]. In this case, muscle rigidity, fever, autonomic nervous system dysfunction and altered mental status, common to both entities, could have been taken in favour of NMS. Nevertheless, generalised myoclonus, especially its history of recurrent pattern, and even more the lack of evidence of neuroleptic use should have alerted the clinician to intensify the diagnostics.

Elevation of CPK in NMS is reported up to at least four times the upper limit. In the context of PERM, elevation of CPK is less frequently described. Literature is not particularly rich on the topic, but we identified three reported cases with normal CPK values [5, 21, 27], while five described elevated CPK values between 408 IU/l and 4779 IU/l [4, 11, 17, 23, 28].

Besides the clinical presentation, antibodies can be determinative in diagnosing this syndrome. Initially both SPS and PERM syndromes were associated with the GAD antibodies. The most recent literature estimates that there is a 60–80% correlation between GAD positive antibodies and SPS [2, 10, 18, 19, 23, 29, 30]. According to Schmidt et al. GAD positive antibodies would only be present in 25% of the PERM cases [19, 30]. Discovered in association with PERM cases in 2008, GlyR antibodies are absent in most cases of SPS [31]. Unfortunately, GlyR antibodies testing was not available in our institution at the time.

Presumably, GAD antibodies cause a reduced brain GABA, which is consistent with the occurrence of seizures. A four channel EMG study showed defective inhibition and exaggerated excitation of the brainstem reflexes mediated by dysfunction of the inhibitory GABA and glycine neurons [32]. Interestingly, post-mortem analysis of PERM cases shows inflammation of the brainstem [23].

Brainstem involvement can be used to differentiate SPS from PERM. There is a controversy about PERM being part of the spectrum of SPS and considered as SPS-plus version of the main syndrome pain [33]. Initial clinical presentation does indeed show significant overlap in symptoms. Nevertheless, the fluctuating course of our patient with severe relapses definitely supports the diagnosis of PERM.

The presence of GAD antibodies is not specific to PERM syndrome. It is associated with a number of other conditions such as diabetes mellitus, schizophrenia or bipolar disease, Parkinson disease, cerebellar disorders and neuropathic conditions. Patients with type 1 diabetes mellitus usually show GAD65 antibody titers at only less than 20, while patients with neurological autoimmune disorders have serum antibody values greater than 20, usually even greater than 100 [22]. Level of GAD65 antibodies in our patient was increased to 95. However, its association with the clinical features of our case and its evolution leave little doubt to our final diagnosis.

Treatment recommended for PERM patients includes immunomodulation using corticosteroids, IV immunoglobulins, plasma exchange or cyclophosphamide [1, 24]. Intrathecal Bacflofen has also been used successfully [1, 2]. The prognosis after treatment can be fluctuating.

Literature is more limited regarding long-term clinical course of PERM. It has been suggested that the syndrome might stay latent during several years and suddenly decompensate by an infection. Up to 18% of PERM cases are reported with chronic course and acute exacerbations [14, 17]. Recurrence has been reported from a few weeks after disease onset up to nine years [1, 4, 8, 11, 12, 31, 34, 35]. In most cases, relapses are related to corticosteroid discontinuation, as in our case. Often, the dosage of corticosteroids is increased at the time of relapse [8, 11, 22]. However, when there is no satisfactory response, more aggressive immunosuppressive therapy may be required, such as cyclosporine, azathioprine and rituximab [5, 12, 14, 31, 35]. Also other immunotherapies have been described at the time of relapse: plasma exchange and cyclophosphamide [36]. Long-term treatment is described with oral corticosteroids variating from 8 mg/day to 20 mg/day combined with Azathioprine 50 mg/day to 150 mg/day [1, 6, 24, 35]. The combination of oral corticosteroids with Diazepam or Clonazepam and intrathecal Baclofen has also been reported [1, 24].

In the current case nearly 10 years went by, after onset of initial symptoms, before the right diagnosis was found. Cases reporting delayed diagnosis PERM are very rare in the literature. One case was identified with a six month delayed diagnosis of PERM, also with good response to immunoglobulin treatment [17]. After literature review we found three case reports with a delayed diagnosis of SPS, with delays ranging from four months up to three years. The first patient responded well to a treatment combination of diazepam, baclofen, dexamethasone, azathioprine and plasma exchange, the patient maintained moderate rigidity without spasms at a follow-up of five months [37]. The second case was treated by immunoglobulins with good response at a follow-up of two months [38]. The third case received an IV treatment of diazepam, no relapse at six months follow-up [39].

In conclusion, PERM syndrome is a rare disease and its diagnosis is not easy, which is underlined by this case report. Once the diagnosis is established, the correct treatment should follow, which could be lifesaving.

Maintenance of long term oral corticotherapy is suggested to prevent relapses. Moreover, it appears that regardless of a delayed diagnosis, a good response may be obtained with adequate treatment in autoimmune central nervous system (CNS) disorders such as PERM. However this report only describes a single case, more data need to be examined in order to generalize these conclusions.

Abbreviations

AAA: Anti-actin antibody; ANA: Anti-nuclear antibody; ANCA: Anti-neutrophil cytoplasmic antibody; anti-GBM Ab: anti-glomerular basement membrane antibody; CNS: Central nervous system; CPK: Creatine kinase; CSF: Cerebrospinal fluid; DPPX: Dipeptidyl-peptidase-like protein-6; ED: Emergency department; EMG: Electromyography; GAD: Glutamic acid decarboxylase; GlyR: Glycine receptor; HIV: Human immunodeficiency virus; HSV: Herpes simplex virus; ICU: Intensive care unit; IV: Intravenous; MRC: Medical Research Counsil; MRI: Magnetic resonance imaging; NMS: Neuroleptic malignant syndrome; PCR: Polymerase chain reaction; PERM: Progressive encephalomyelitis with rigidity and myoclonus; SPS: Stiff person syndrome

Acknowledgements

The authors would like to thank the patient for letting us publish her case and all the contributors for their input and work. Additionally we would like to express our gratitude to Dr. Laurence Verdickt who provided additional information regarding the interpretation of the anti-GAD65 antibodies by the immunoblot technique.

Authors' contributions

All authors were involved in the clinical care of the patient. ADE collected the clinical data, conducted the literature search, drafted the manuscript and participated in the conception and design of the case report. MD helped interpreting the findings, gave input into the discussion, drafted the manuscript and participated in the conception and design of the case report. ADH gave input into the discussion. JAE helped interpreting the findings and supervised the writing of the manuscript. All authors read and approved the final manuscript.

Competing interests

The authors declare that they have no competing interests.

Author details

[1]Department of Neurology, CHU Ambroise Paré Hospital, Boulevard John Fitzgerald Kennedy 2, 7000 Mons, Belgium. [2]Intensive Care Unit, CHU Ambroise Paré Hospital, Mons, Belgium.

References

1. Stern WM, Howard R, Chalmers RM, Woodhall MR, Waters P, Vincent A, et al. Glycine receptor antibody mediated progressive encephalomyelitis with rigidity and myoclonus (PERM): a rare but treatable neurological syndrome. Pract Neurol. 2014;14:123–7.
2. Barker RA, Revesz T, Thom M, Marsden CD, Brown P. Review of 23 patients affected by the stiff man syndrome: clinical subdivision into stiff trunk (man) syndrome, stiff limb syndrome, and progressive encephalomyelitis with rigidity. J Neurol Neurosurg Psychiatry. 1998;65:633–40. https://doi.org/10.1136/jnnp.65.5.633.
3. Martinez-Hernandez E, Ariño H, McKeon A, Iizuka T, Titulaer MJ, Simabukuro MM, et al. Clinical and immunologic investigations in patients with stiff-person Spectrum disorder. JAMA Neurol. 2016;73:E1–7. https://doi.org/10.1001/jamaneurol.2016.0133.
4. Damasio J, Leite MI, Coutinho E, Waters P, Woodhall M, Santos MA, et al. Progressive encephalomyelitis with rigidity and myoclonus. JAMA Neurol. 2013;70:498–501. https://doi.org/10.1001/jamaneurol.2013.1872.
5. Ueno S, Miyamoto N, Shimura H, Ueno Y, Watanabe M, Hayashi A, et al. Successful immune moderation treatment for progressive encephalomyelitis with rigidity and myoclonus. Intern Med. 2015;54:219–21. https://doi.org/10.2169/internalmedicine.54.3760.
6. Shugaiv E, Leite MI, Şehitoğlu E, Woodhall M, Çavuş F, Waters P, et al. Progressive encephalomyelitis with rigidity and myoclonus: a syndrome with diverse clinical features and antibody responses. Eur Neurol. 2013;69:257–62.
7. Whiteley AM, Swash M, Urich H. Progressive encephalomyelitis with rigidity. Brain. 1976;99:27–42.
8. Baraba R, Jušić A, Sruk A. Progressive encephalomyelitis with Rigidity : a case report. I Spinal Cord Med. 2010;33:73–6.
9. Kraemer M, Berlit P. Progressive encephalomyelitis with rigidity and myoclonus in an 81-year-old patient. Clin Neurol Neurosurg. 2008;110:279–81.
10. De Blauwe SN, Santens P, Vanopdenbosch LJ. Anti-glycine receptor antibody mediated progressive encephalomyelitis with rigidity and myoclonus associated with breast cancer. Case Rep Neurol Med. 2013;2013:589154. https://doi.org/10.1155/2013/589154.
11. Peeters E, Vanacker P, Woodhall M, Vincent A, Schrooten M, Vandenberghe W. Supranuclear gaze palsy in glycine receptor antibody-positive progressive encephalomyelitis with rigidity and myoclonus. Mov Disord. 2012;27:1830–2.
12. Iizuka T, Leite MI, Lang B, Waters P, Urano Y, Miyakawa S, et al. Glycine receptor antibodies are detected in progressive encephalomyelitis with rigidity and myoclonus (PERM) but not in saccadic oscillations. J Neurol. 2012;259:1566–73.
13. Papadopoulou A, Samuels TL, Dassanayake A, Spring C, Willers J, Uncles DR. Progressive encephalomyelitis with rigidity and myoclonus: anesthesia and glycine receptor antibodies. A A Case Reports. 2014;2:81–2.
14. Carvajal-Gonzalez A, Leite MI, Waters P, Woodhall M, Coutinho E, Balint B, et al. Glycine receptor antibodies in PERM and related syndromes : characteristics , clinical features and outcomes. Brain. 2014;137:2178–92.
15. Magira EE, Alexopoulos H, Charitatos E, Michas D, Dalakas MC. Progressive encephalomyelitis with rigidity and myoclonus (PERM): brucellosis as a possible triggering factor and long-term follow-up therapy with rituximab. Ther Adv Neurol Disord. 2016;9:69–73. https://doi.org/10.1177/1756285615614812.
16. Patel A, Boyd S, Amin B, Robinson R, Woodhall M, Vincent A, et al. Glycine receptor antibody mediated progressive encephalomyelitis with rigidity and myoclonus (PERM) presenting as an abnormal startle response in an adolescent girl. Eur J Paediatr Neurol. 2015;19:S62. https://doi.org/10.1016/S1090-3798(15)30205-1.
17. Xu Z, Prasad K, Yeo T. Progressive encephalomyelitis with rigidity and myoclonus in an intellectually disabled patient mimicking neuroleptic malignant syndrome. J Mov Disord. 2017;10:99–101.
18. Dalakas MC, Fujii M, Li M, Mcelroy B. syndrome The clinical spectrum of anti-GAD antibody-positive patients with stiff- person syndrome. Neurology. 2000;55(10):1531–5.
19. Schmidt C, Freilinger T, Lieb M, Rémi J, Klein M, Straube A, et al. Progressive encephalomyelitis with rigidity and myoclonus preceding otherwise asymptomatic Hodgkin ' s lymphoma. J Neurol Sci. 2010;291:118–20. https://doi.org/10.1016/j.jns.2009.12.025.
20. Leite MI, Waters P, Carvajal A, Woodhall M, Vincent A. Expanding the phenotypic spectrum of progressive encephalomyelitis with rigidity and myoclonus syndrome (PERMS) associated with glycine receptor antibody: clinical and laboratory study of 20 patients. J Neurol Neurosurg Psychiatry. 2012;83:8. https://doi.org/10.1136/jnnp-2011-301993.26.
21. Turner MR, Irani SR, Leite MI, Nithi K, Vincent A, Ansorge O. Progressive encephalomyelitis with rigidity and myoclonus. Glycine and NMDA receptor antibodies. Neurology. 2011;77:439–43. https://doi.org/10.1007/s00415-010-5575-7.
22. McKeon A, Tracy JA. GAD65 neurological autoimmunity. Muscle Nerve. 2017;56:15–27.
23. Cabre P, Smadja D, Humbel RL, Merle H, Vernant JC, West F. Progressive encephalomyelitis with rigidity, diabetes mellitus and retinopathy: an anti-GAD syndrome. Eur J Neurol. 1996;3:98–101.
24. Fogan L. Progressive encephalomyelitis with rigidity responsive to plasmapheresis and immunosuppression. Ann Neurol. 1996;40:451–3.

25. Medical Research Council: Nerve Injuries Committee. Aids to the investigation of peripheral nerve injuries. London: His Majesty's Stationery Office; 1942.
26. McCombe PA, Chalk JB, Searle JW, Tannenberg AEG, Smith JJ, Pender MP. Progressive encephalomyelitis with rigidity: a case report with magnetic resonance imaging findings. J Neurol Neurosurg Psychiatry. 1989;52:1429–31. https://www.ncbi.nlm.nih.gov/pmc/articles/PMC1031606/.
27. Burn DJ, Ball J, Lees AJ, Behan PO, Morgan-Hughes JA. A case of progressive encephalomyelitis with rigidity and positive antiglutamic acid decarboxylase antibodies [corrected]. J Neurol Neurosurg Psychiatry. 1991;54:449–51 https://www.ncbi.nlm.nih.gov/pmc/articles/PMC488547/.
28. Clerinx K, Breban T, Schrooten M, Leite MI, Vincent A, Verschakelen J, et al. Progressive encephalomyelitis with rigidity and myoclonus: resolution after thymectomy. Neurology. 2011;76:303–4.
29. Saidha S, Elamin M, Mullins G, Chaila E, Tormey VJ, Hennessy MJ. Treatment of progressive encephalomyelitis with rigidity and myoclonic jerks with rituximab: a case report. Eur J Neurol. 2008;15:e33.
30. Meinck HM, Thompson PD. Stiff man syndrome and related conditions. Mov Disord. 2002;17:853–66.
31. Hutchinson M, Waters P, McHugh J, Gorman G, O'Riordan S, Connolly S, et al. Progresive encephalomyelitis, rigidity, and myoclonus: a novel glycine receptor antibody. Neurology. 2008;71:1291–2.
32. Khasani S, Becker K, Meinck H-M. Hyperekplexia and stiff-man syndrome: abnormal brainstem reflexes suggest a physiological relationship. J Neurol Neurosurg Psychiatry. 2004;75:1265–9. https://doi.org/10.1136/jnnp.2003.018135.
33. Sarva H, Deik A, Ullah A, Severt WL, Disease P, Sinai M, et al. Clinical Spectrum of stiff person Syndrome : a review of recent reports. Tremor and Other Hyperkinetic Movements. 2016;4:340.
34. Mas N, Saiz A, Leite MI, Waters P, Baron M, Sabater L, et al. Antiglycine-receptor encephalomyelitis with rigidity. J Neurol Neurosurg Psychiatry. 2011;82:1399–402.
35. Kenda J, Švigelj V, Rodi Z, Koritnik B, Graus F, Kojović M. Glycine receptor antibodies and progressive encephalomyelitis with rigidity and myoclonus with predominant motor neuron degeneration - expanding the clinical spectrum. J Neurol Sci. 2015;353:177–8.
36. Balint B, Jarius S, Nagel S, Haberkorn U, Probst C, Blöcker IM, et al. Progressive encephalomyelitis with rigidity and myoclonus: a new variant with DPPX antibodies. Neurology. 2014;82:1521–8.
37. Ehler E, Latta J, Mandysova P, Havlasova J, Mrklovsky M. Stiff-person syndrome following tick-borne meningoencephalitiS. Acta Med (Hradec Kralove). 2011;54:170–4.
38. Razmeh S, Habibi AH, Sina F, Alizadeh E, Eslami M. Stiff person case misdiagnosed as conversion disorder: a case report. Casp J Intern Med. 2017;8:329–31.
39. Andreadou E, Kattoulas E, Sfagos C, Vassilopoulos D. Stiff person syndrome: avoiding misdiagnosis. Neurol Sci. 2007;28:35–7.

Mortality & recurrent seizure risk after new-onset seizure in HIV-positive Zambian adults

Melissa A. Elafros[1*], Brent A. Johnson[2], Omar K. Siddiqi[3,4], Jason F. Okulicz[5], Izukanji Sikazwe[6], Christopher M. Bositis[7], Michael J. Potchen[8], Igor J. Koralnik[9], William H. Theodore[10], Lisa Kalungwana[11] and Gretchen L. Birbeck[12,13]

Abstract

Background: Recurrent seizure risks in HIV-positive people with new-onset seizure are largely unknown, making it challenging to offer optimal recommendations regarding antiepileptic drug (AED) initiation. Existing outcomes data is limited, and risk factor identification requires a diagnostic assessment, which is often unavailable in regions heavily effected by HIV, like sub-Saharan Africa.

Methods: HIV-positive Zambian adults with new-onset seizure were enrolled in a prospective cohort study to determine seizure recurrence and risk factors for recurrence. Seizure etiology was evaluated, and recurrent seizures and medication usage were assessed during clinic visits. Due to unexpectedly high mortality rates, predictors of death were evaluated using proportional hazards with Gray's test to compare cumulative incidence functions for recurrent seizure across groups adjusting for the competing outcome of death.

Results: 95 patients were enrolled (mean age 37 years, 43% female, 83% with Karnofsky > 50) and followed for a mean of 293 days (median 241 (IQR: 29–532)). At presentation, 50 (53%) were in *status epilepticus*. The majority (91, 85%) had advanced HIV disease and 65 (68%) were not on combined antiretroviral therapy (cART). After extensive workup, seizure etiology remained unknown in 16 (17%). Average time to cART initiation after enrollment was 61 days. During follow up, 37 (39%) died and 23 (24%) had recurrent seizure. Most deaths (25/37, 68%) occurred in the first 60 days post-index seizure. Individuals with advanced HIV were more likely to die (HR: 19.1 [95% CI: 1.1–333.4]) as were those whose seizure etiology remained unknown (HR: 2.2 [95% CI: 1.1–4.4]). Among participants that survived from enrolment to the end of data collection on 10 May 2013 ($n = 58$), 20 (34%) experienced recurrent seizures.

Conclusions: New-onset seizure among HIV-positive Zambian adults is associated with high mortality despite good functional status prior to presentation. Advanced HIV infection and failure to identify an underlying seizure etiology are associated with greater mortality. Recurrent seizures occur in over a third of survivors within only 2 years of follow-up. This provides evidence to support AED initiation after first seizure in HIV-positive individuals with advanced HIV disease at the time of presentation though the risks of AED-cART interactions remain a concern and warrant further study.

* Correspondence: melafro1@jhmi.edu
[1]Department of Neurology, Johns Hopkins Hospital, Sheik Zayed Tower, Room 6005, 1800 Orleans Street, Baltimore, MD 21287, USA
Full list of author information is available at the end of the article

Background

HIV infection is a recognized seizure risk factor [1]. Hospital-based studies suggest convulsions are a presenting symptom in 2–13% of HIV-positive adults regardless of treatment status with combination antiretroviral the rapy (cART) [2–4]. Often, no underlying seizure etiology is identified despite a thorough workup including electroencephalogram (EEG), neuroimaging, and cerebrospinal fluid (CSF) analysis and HIV's effects on the central nervous system (CNS) is the presumed cause [5]. Unfortunately, very limited diagnostic capacity is available in resource-limited settings and existing data on seizure etiology in HIV-positive individuals is frequently limited to a small subset of individuals with a complete workup limiting generalizability [2–4, 6].

Retrospective [3, 4, 6] and prospective [2, 7–10] studies have examined new-onset seizure etiology in HIV-positive individuals, but few assess long-term health outcomes, including mortality and the risk of recurrent seizure [11]. Follow up is often incomplete [4, 12] or for unknown duration [3, 5, 9, 10]. Two U.S. studies conducted prior to cART and one Spanish study after cART tracked patients on average for 5 months [4, 6, 7]. Data from India showed that 65% of HIV-positive inpatients with new-onset seizure experienced recurrent seizure, however, it is un clear whether these observed seizures occurred during or after the initial hospitalization [2]. Since initiating antiepileptic drugs (AEDs) with cART may adversely affect HIV virologic suppression due to enzyme-induction, predispose to AED- and cART-associated toxicity, and decrease overall medication adherence due to increased pill burden, accurately characterizing the need for chronic AED treatment in this population is imperative, particularly in resource-limited settings where enzyme-inducing AEDs continue to be the mainstay of epilepsy care [13, 14].

We are conducting a prospective cohort study of HIV-positive individuals presenting with new-onset se izure in Zambia to determine seizure etiology and follow the cohort for relevant outcomes, including seizure recurrence and death [15]. Here, we examine seizure recurrence and death among a subset of patients enrolled in Phase I of our cohort study to summarize the timeline for repeated seizure events while properly accounting for the competing risk of death.

Methods

The Cohort for HIV-Associated Seizures and Epilepsy (CHASE) Study is an ongoing prospective observational study that enrolled urban adult participants from 8 August 2011 to 10 May 2013. HIV-infected Zambian adults presenting to the University of Zambia's University Tea ching Hospital (UTH) inpatient medical wards and outpatient HIV clinic and to Chreso Ministries ART clinic, a faith-based nongovernmental clinic in Lusaka, were assessed for eligibility. A study nurse went bed-to-bed in the UTH emergency room and inpatient wards to assess admitted patients while a study investigator screened all patients presenting to UTH's HIV clinic for eligible partici pants [15]. One of the investigators confirmed each pa tient's eligibility and informed consent was obtained from the patient or health care proxy in English or a local la nguage (Nyanja or Bemba) by a trained Zambian nurse.

Eligible participants included patients ≥18 years with documented HIV-infection, presenting within 2 weeks of new-onset seizure. Patients with a history of seizure other than childhood febrile seizures were excluded. To facilitate follow up, participants received their HIV care through the Adult Infectious Disease Centre (AIDC), which includes UTH's adult HIV clinic. All subjects recruited in Phase I of the CHASE Study are included in this outcomes assessment study.

Measures at enrolment

The following was collected via structured interview: age; gender; presenting clinical symptoms; and past medical history. Past medical history included seizure-related risk factors and HIV history, which captured duration of diagnosis and treatment. A neurologist characterized seizure type according to Fisher et al's 2017 operational classification of seizure types using patient and/or witness descriptions of the event or a focal neurologic exam at enroll ment [16]. Seizure severity was determined using duration of the index seizure based on clinical report. Status epilepticus included tonic-clonic seizures lasting more than 5 minutes or focal seizures lasting more than 10 minutes [17]. Consciousness at the time of enrolment was characterized with the Glasgow Coma Scale [18]. The WHO Clinical Staging Criteria were used to stage HIV infection [19]. Etiologic assessment included serum testing for: $CD4^+$ T-cell count; sodium; glucose; malaria infection using the *P. falciparum* rapid diagnostic antigen test; rapid plasma reagin test for syphilis and, if needed, a confirmatory Treponema pallidum hemagglutination assay. Among patients who consented to a lumbar puncture, CSF testing included: cell count and differential; glucose; total protein; gram stain; Venereal Disease Research Laboratory (VDRL) testing for neurosyphilis; and cryptococcal antigen testing. DNA PCR analysis included: *Mycobacterium tuberculosis*; Epstein-Barr virus (EBV); JC virus; varicella zoster virus; cytomegalovirus; herpes simplex virus type 1; herpes simplex virus type 2; and *Toxoplasma gondii* [15]. Patients who did not consent to a lumbar puncture had serum cryptococcal antigen testing.

Patients sufficiently stable for transportation to the outpatient EEG lab completed a 16-channel EEG using Biologic CEEGgraph equipment. EEGs were per formed in accordance with the American Clinical Neurophysiology Society Guidelines using silver-silver chloride electrodes applied with collodion using the international 10–20 electrode placement [20]. Filters were set at 1 and 70 Hz and impedances were below 10 k-ohms. EEGs were interpreted by two neurologists with EEG fellowship training [21, 22]. EEG findings, in addition to patient/witness descriptions and physical exam findings, were used to identify any seizure focality. Neuroimaging was obtained on patients who either had it as part of their routine clinical care or, whose seizure etiology remained unknown after CSF evaluations [23]. All results were shared with the patient's inpatient and outpatient providers.

Underlying seizure etiology was independently classified into the following categories by two investigators blinded to outcome with external consensus mediation, as needed. Categories delineated post hoc included: CNS OI; other infection such as bacterial meningitis, malaria, or syphilis; structural lesion on neuroimaging; hyponatremia; and unknown. A serum sodium < 135 mmol/L was considered hyponatremia, which was further classified as either primary or secondary [15]. More than one possible underlying seizure assignment was permitted.

Measures during follow-up

Patients were followed through their hospitalization and, after discharge, via the AIDC. AIDC providers directed all treatment-related decisions. Patients were followed until death, withdrawal, or closure on 18 December 2013. Reminder phone calls and a transport reimbursement of 20 kwacha (~US $4.00) were provided to participants to assist with transportation costs to attend the AIDC appointments. The study facilitated transportation for patients not well enough to use public transportation. Patients were also offered rescheduling assistance for missed appointments. If a patient could not be located, a research assitant and/or study investigator attempted to trace participants using phone numbers patients provided during enrolment or in their clinic file. These phone calls continued once a week until the patient was located, staff were informed the patient had died, the patient withdrew, or the study closed.

At each encounter with patients or close contacts, seizure recurrence data and major medical events, including death, were collected. Among participants experiencing recurrent seizure, the number, date, and a description of each seizure were recorded. In the event of death, circumstances surrounding the event were obtained from a close contact, specifically to determine whether any seizures occurred around the time of death. Data regarding medication use and changes was abstracted from patient files at the time of interview and confirmed by patients.

Statistical analysis

Baseline demographic and clinical data, seizure etiologies, and follow up data, including duration of follow up and medication changes, were summarized using frequencies and means. The primary outcomes of interest were seizure recurrence and death. Proportional hazards models were used to evaluate clinical and demographic predictors of death. Gray's method, which accounts for a competing event when comparing the cumulative incidence of an event across risk factors, was used to compare the incidence for recurrent seizure during follow up based on clinical and demographic risk factors, while controlling for the competing risk of death. Characteristics associated with death and seizure recurrence were then examined using the entire study cohort. A subsequent sensitivity analysis was performed using only patients who had CSF available for DNA PCR and, thus, had a complete laboratory workup. All analyses were performed using SAS 9.4 (SAS Institute, Cary, North Carolina). A p-value of < 0.05 was considered statistically significant.

Ethical approval

Ethical approval was obtained from the University of Zambia's Biomedical Research Ethics Committee (UNZA BREC) as well as Michigan State University's Biomedical Institutional Review Board (MSU BIRB). All participants or their proxies provided written, informed consent. If a proxy provided initial consent, patient consent was obtained once the patient was well enough to provide it.

Results

Baseline

Ninety-five patients (43% female, mean age 36.9 years, SD 10.2 years) participated in the CHASE Study. All were black Zambians. Seventy-nine (83%) patients had a Karnofsky Scale Score > 50 at enrolment. There was no difference in gender ($p = 0.61$), age ($p = 0.40$), presenting seizure severity ($p = 0.15$), or $CD4^+$ T-cell count at enrolment ($p = 0.55$) between patients with a Karnofsky Scale Score > 50 and those with a Karnofsky Scale Score < 50.

As shown in Table 1, most patients (78%) presented with tonic-clonic seizures, 33 (35%) with focal onset. Seizure type could not be classified for six (6%) participants. 43 (45%) participants with tonic clonic seizures and 6 (6%) participants with focal clonic seizures met criteria for *status epilepticus*. 54 (57%) had multiple seizures prior to presenting for care, of which 31 (31/54, 57%) had multiple seizures within 24 h. Eleven (12%) patients had an immediate family member with epilepsy; two (2%) had a prior head injury. The majority (85%) of study participants had advanced HIV infection (WHO

Table 1 Demographics and clinical characteristics of HIV-positive adults with new-onset seizure ($n = 95$)

Demographic	
Gender, female n (%)	41 (43)
Age, mean (SD)	36.9 (10.2)
Family history of epilepsy n (%)	11 (12)
History of head injury n (%)	2 (2)
History of severe malaria n (%)	6 (6)
History of meningitis/encephalitis n (%)	7 (7)
History of coma n (%)	1 (1)
History of opportunistic infection ($n = 94$)[a] n (%)	5 (5)
History of stroke (n = 94) [a] n (%)	4 (4)
Clinical	
Seizure type n (%)	
Focal clonic	13 (14)
Focal onset to bilateral tonic-clonic	33 (35)
Tonic clonic	1 (1)
Unknown onset bilateral tonic-clonic	42 (44)
Unclassified	6 (6)
Presenting seizure severity n (%)[b]	
Status epilepticus	50 (53)
Glasgow Coma Score, mean (SD)	14.3 (1.9)
Karnofsky score < 50 at enrollment n (%)	16 (17)
WHO clinical stage n (%)[a]	
I or II	12 (13)
III or IV	81 (85)
Current cART use n (%)	
Yes, less than a year	13 (14)
Yes, more than a year	17 (18)
No, defaulted	7 (7)
No, never	58 (61)
$CD4^+$ T-cell count at enrolment, mean cells/mm^3($n = 89$) [a] (SD)	179 (185)
Underlying seizure etiology[c]	
CNS opportunistic infection n (%)	21 (22)
Other infection n (%)	8 (8)
Structural lesion n (%)	25 (26)
Hyponatremia ($n = 91$) n (%)	47 (49)
Likely secondary to another etiology	17/47 (36)
Unknown, n (%)	20 (21)

Data is presented as number (%), mean (SD), or median (IQR), as appropriate. *WHO* World Health Organization, *cART* combination antiretroviral therapy, *CNS* central nervous system. [a]Patient unable to provide information. [b]Missing data for 6 participants [c]More than one seizure etiology possible

Stage III or IV) at enrolment. Among those able to provide information regarding their HIV history ($n = 85$), the index seizure led to HIV diagnosis among 46 (54%) patients and, thus, most participants were cART-naïve. Among those on cART at enrolment, 27/32 (84%) were on their initial cART regimen, which in this setting includes a non-nucleoside reverse transcriptase inhibitor, often efavirenz (19/27; 70%). The remaining five patients had failed their initial regimen and had been switched to a regimen containing a protease inhibitor.

Eighty-one (85%) participants had CSF collected as part of their workup. There were no significant demographic or clinical differences between patients who underwent a lumbar puncture and those who did not, including time to death ($p = 0.95$). Sixty-one patients (61/81; 75%) had sufficient CSF collected for DNA PCR testing. Eighty-one (85%) participants had an EEG. Of the remaining 14 patients, 12 (86%) died before EEG could be completed. Fifty-five (55/81; 68%) EEGs were abnormal. 23 (33%) had background slowing, 27 (34%) had generalized slowing, and 16 (20%) had focal slowing. Nine (11%) had interictal focal discharges and four (5%) had interictal general discharges. Six (8%) patients had seizures captured during EEG. Sleep architecture was captured on two EEGs. Forty (42%) participants had neuroimaging (38 CT, 2 MRI), of which 70% had an abnormality. White matter abnormalities, primarily vasogenic edema, were the most common abnormality detected (24/40; 56%). Some of these findings have been reported elsewhere in papers dedicated to these specific risk factors [22, 23].

Twenty-one (22%) patients had a CNS OI, eight (10%) had another identified infection (bacterial meningitis (4), malaria (1), and neurosyphilis (3)), and 47 (49%) were hyponatremic (Table 1). Of those with neuroimaging ($n = 40$), 25 (63%) had a structural lesion. Twenty (21%) patients had multiple potential etiologies (14 with two etiologies and 6 with three etiologies), including seventeen (17/47; 36%) with secondary hyponatremia. Etiology remained unknown in 20 (21%) participants.

Participants were followed, on average, 236 days (7.7 months; median 4.4 months [IQR: 0.8–12.5 months]). Follow up was abbreviated for those who died (2.3 versus 11.3 months, $p < 0.001$). Patients had an average of seven follow-up encounters with a mean of 42 days between encounters. Two (2/95 2%) participants withdrew due to relocation; the remainder were followed until death or study closure.

Seizure recurrence and associated factors

Twenty-three (23/95; 24%) patients experienced at least one, and 9/23 (10%) more than one recurrent seizure during follow up. Of those who presented with new-onset seizures limited to a 24-h period prior to enrolment ($n = 72$), 21 (30%) experienced recurrent seizure during follow up. Although time to first recurrent seizure varied substantially, 14/23 recurrent seizures occurred within four months after enrolment. Death was a significant competing risk for seizure recurrence. Among participants that survived until study closure ($n = 58$), 20 (34%) experienced recurrent seizures whereas 3/37 (8%) of patients who died during follow up experienced recurrent seizure. One participant died in status epilepticus. After controlling for death, presenting in status epilepticus was associated with recurrent seizure during follow up ($p < 0.003$). Individuals who presented initially in status epilepticus experienced seizures on average later during follow up (Table 2). However, this association is likely complicated by increased frequency of recurrent seizure among individuals presenting in status epilepticus compared to individuals who did not present in status and early AED initiation after presentation. Neither an abnormal EEG nor a structural brain lesion on neuroimaging was associated with recurrent seizure ($p = 0.205$ and $p = 0.627$, respectively).

Twenty-two (22/95; 23%) participants initiated an AED. Carbamazepine was the most commonly used AED ($n = 21$), followed by phenobarbital (1) and valproic acid (1). Twelve (13%) initiated an AED during hospitalization and continued it during follow up. Of those that began an AED during hospitalization, 6/12 (50%) experienced recurrent seizure during follow up. A post hoc analysis indicated that AED initiation during hospitalization was not associated with presenting with status epilepticus ($p = 0.251$), multiple seizures prior to presentation ($p = 0.548$), advanced HIV infection ($p = 0.651$), $CD4^+$ T-cell count at enrolment ($p = 0.929$), or seizure focality ($p = 0.129$). However, it is likely that this analysis was underpowered. Of those not on an AED at discharge ($n = 83$), 17 (20%) experienced recurrent seizure. Eleven (11/17, 65%) initiated an AED as a result. Six participants did not initiate an AED despite recurrent

Table 2 Demographics and clinical characteristics of patients associated with seizure recurrence, controlling for the competing risk of death ($n = 95$)

	Median time to seizure recurrence [IQR]	*P-value*[a]
Gender		0.960
Male ($n = 13$)	3.1 [1.2–9.3]	
Female ($n = 10$)	3.3 [0.5–14.6]	
Presenting seizure severity ($n = 89$)		**< 0.01**
Status epilepticus ($n = 17$)	3.1 [1.2–9.3]	
Not status epilepticus ($n = 4$)	1.5 [0.4–8.8]	
Evidence of seizure focality		0.339
Yes ($n = 14$)	3.1 [1.2–9.3]	
No ($n = 9$)	1.1 [0.5–8.8]	
WHO clinical stage		0.334
I or II ($n = 4$)	6.4 [1.4–13.5]	
III or IV ($n = 19$)	3.1 [0.9–9.3]	
cART use		0.105
Yes ($n = 8$)	1.4 [0.3–6.3]	
No, defaulted ($n = 4$)	2.8 [1.5–10.0]	
No, never ($n = 11$)	8.6 [1.2–15.9]	
CSF collected for analysis		0.845
Yes ($n = 20$)	3.5 [0.7–12.6]	
No ($n = 3$)	2.6 [2.2–3.7]	
CNS opportunistic infection		0.788
Yes ($n = 5$)	9.3 [8.7–15.9]	
No ($n = 18$)	5.0 [0.9–8.6]	
Unknown seizure etiology		0.230
Yes (n = 3)	1.2 [0.03–1.8]	
No (n = 20)	3.8 [1.1–12.6]	

Data is presented as median (IQR). [a]Gray's test of cumulative incidence functions. *WHO*, World Health Organization. *cART* combination antiretroviral therapy. *CSF* cerebrospinal fluid. *CNS* central nervous system seizure as providers considered their seizures to be provoked by alcohol withdrawal (3), the participant refused (2), or the participant died (1). Few of the patients were seen by health care providers outside of the AIDC, therefore, AEDs were typically managed in this setting. Of those prescribed AEDs, five (23%) stopped their AED either because they ran out of drug or chose to stop independently without consulting a provider. One stopped after consulting a provider.

Risk of death and associated factors

During follow up, 37 (39%) patients died (Fig. 1). Eighteen (18/95, 19%) participants did not survive their initial hospitalization. Twenty-two (59%) were not on cART at the time of death. Of those on cART at the time of death, 9/15 had been on it less than a year. Among those who survived hospitalization yet died during follow up, median time to death after enrolment was 2 months (IQR: 1.3–6.3 months). Death during initial hospitalization or during follow up was associated with WHO Stage III or IV HIV infection at enrolment (HR: 19.1 [95% CI: 1.1–333.4], $p = 0.01$) (Table 3). Death was also associated with an unknown seizure etiology (HR: 2.2 [95%CI: 1.1–4.4], $p = 0.025$, Fig. 2). Death was not associated with an abnormality on EEG or neuroimaging ($p = 0.173$ and $p = 0.56$, respectively). Among participants with a full etiologic workup, including CSF DNA PCR ($n = 61$), the trend for this association remained but it was no longer significant (HR: 2.1 [95% CI: 0.8–5.3], $p = 0.129$). In a post hoc analysis, no demographic or clinical variables, including CSF collection, were associated with an unknown seizure etiology.

Table 3 Individual characteristics at enrollment and their association with death ($n = 95$)

Characteristic	Hazard Ratio [95% CI]	*P-value*[a]
Gender, female	0.9 [0.5–1.7]	0.745
Age, mean	1.01 [0.98–1.05]	0.383
WHO HIV clinical stage III or IV[b]	19.1 [1.1–333.4]	0.01
cART use at enrollment	1.5 [0.8–2.9]	0.240
Karnofsky score < 50 at enrollment	1.8 [0.9–3.8]	0.125
Seizure severity at enrollment		
Brief, Single	Referent	0.173
Multiple, prolonged	1.7 [0.7–3.9]	
Status epilepticus	2.6 [0.96–7.3]	
CNS opportunistic infection	0.9 [0.4–2.2]	0.889
Unknown etiology	2.2 [1.1–4.4]	0.025
Among those with CSF ($n = 61$)	2.1 [0.8–5.3]	0.129

Data is presented as the hazards ratio for the listed characteristic versus the null with a hazards ratio of 1.0 indicating no difference. *CI* confidence interval, *WHO* World Health Organization, *cART* combination antiretroviral therapy, *CNS* central nervous system, *CSF* cerebrospinal fluid
[a]Log-Rank Tests [b]As compared to WHO clinical stage I or II

During follow up, six (6%) patients were readmitted to UTH for non-seizure related illness. Thirty-nine participants not on cART at enrolment initiated treatment (39/65; 55%); average time to initiation was 61 days. Twenty-two (23%) participants never started cART. One participant declined cART despite having a $CD4^+$ T-cell count < 250 cells/mm^3, while the remaining 22 died before cART could be initiated. Time to cART initiation was not associated with a diagnosis of AIDS at study enrolment ($p = 0.30$). During follow up, four patients on

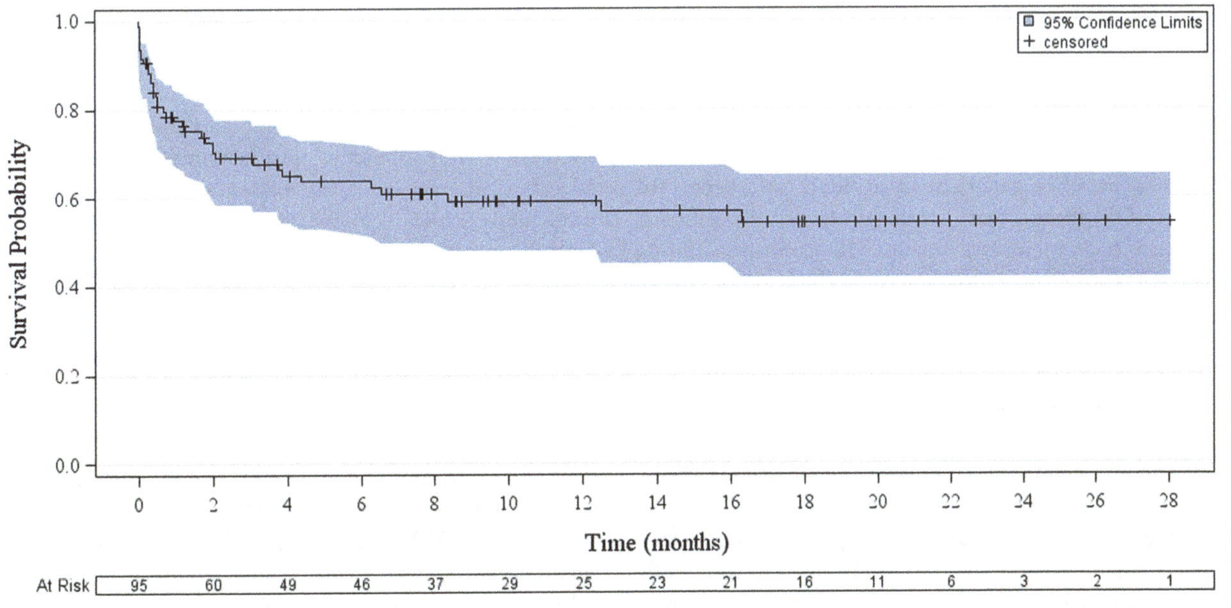

Fig. 1 Mortality after new-onset seizure in HIV^+ Zambian adults

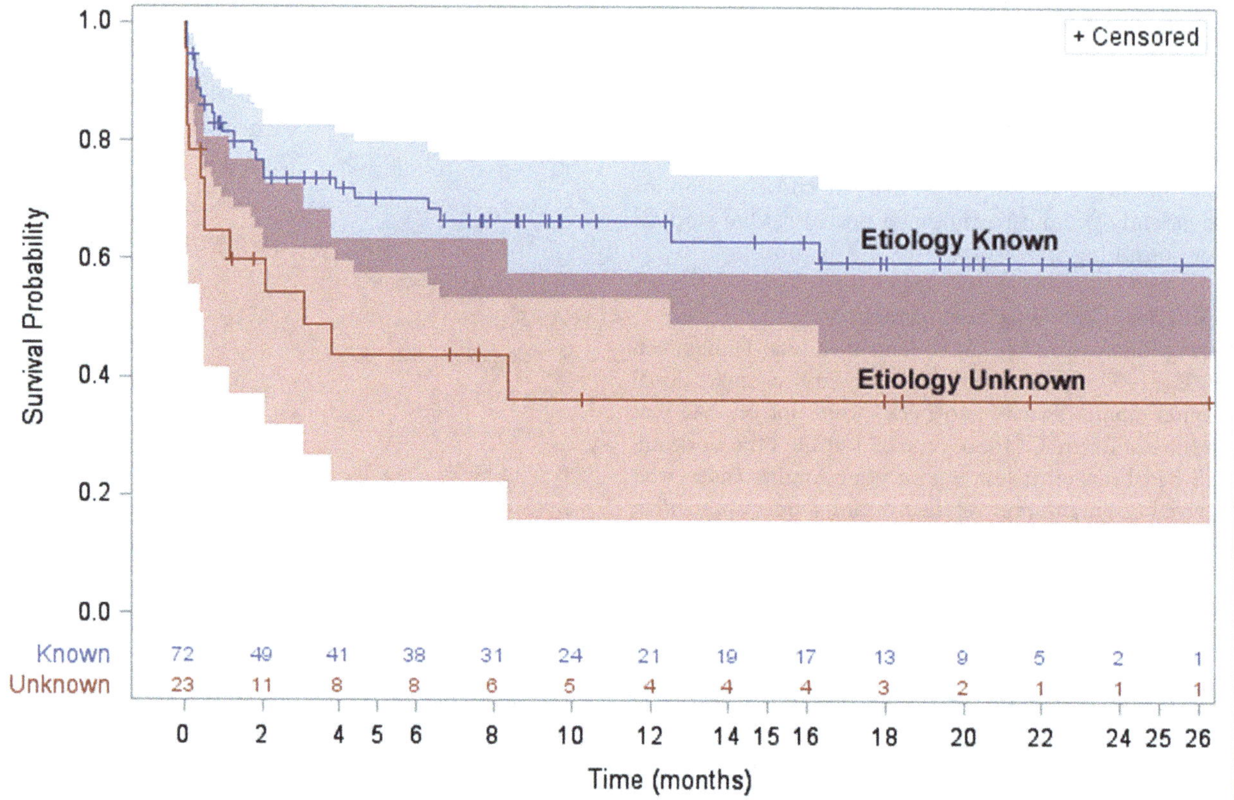

Fig. 2 Mortality after new-onset seizure by etiology among HIV+ Zambian adults

cART at enrolment (4/30; 13%) defaulted treatment. AIDC clinical providers switched eight (8/69; 12%) participants to different cART regimens due to clinical or virologic treatment failure.

Discussion

Assessment of seizure recurrence among HIV-positive Zambian adults after new-onset seizure is complicated by mortality, despite good functional status at baseline. We followed all patients for an average of 7.7 months and tracked survivors for 11.3 months. During that time, 23 (24%) patients experienced at least one recurrent seizure. Of those that survived to study closure, one-third had recurrent seizure. In contrast, among Nigerians seen at an outpatient HIV clinic, 13/20 (65%) developed recurrent seizures within a year of their index seizure [10]. These patients were likely healthier than the CHASE cohort as they were recruited from the outpatient setting and had a higher seizure recurrence primarily due to survival.

Death was a significant competing risk for seizure recurrence and, as a result, few predictors of seizure recurrence were identified. Initial seizure focality and severity were based on patient and witness report, which inherently limits classification using the 2017 International League Against Epilepsy seizure classification. Further, application of the International League Against Epilepsy's practical clinical definition of epilepsy was limited by participant mortality and cART initiation, both of which likely reduced seizure recurrence during follow up [24]. A larger sample size, including adults with WHO stage I and II HIV infection, is warranted to examine recurrent seizure predictors among this extremely ill patient population. Initiating an AED in a patient with new-onset seizures has significant implications. In addition to lifestyle modifications required to ensure medication adherence, AEDs may decrease overall adherence to other medications and may adversely interact with the patient's other medications, particularly cART [14]. While newer AEDs available in high-income settings are not associated with enzyme-induction, in resource-limited settings like Zambia, en zyme-inducing AEDs such as carbamazepine and phenobarbital continue to be the most available therapies. Additional research is needed to determine the pharmacologic and virologic effects of AED and cART co-usage [13]. Further, recognizing adverse effects associated with co-usage of AEDs and cART is imperative [25], particularly in resource-limited settings where there is a shortage of neurologists and AED use is frequently left to primary care providers with limited neurologic training.

In Phase I of the CHASE study, 39% of urban adult participants died during follow up, nearly half of which occurred during their initial hospitalization. Our mortality rate is similar to a 10-year primarily retrospective inpatient review of HIV-positive patients with new-onset seizure in Cameroon [26], yet lower than inpatient data reported from developed countries prior to the availability of cART [4]. CHASE mortality was associated with advanced infection, consistent with a prospective study of 17 patients in Spain [7]. Death was also associated with failure to identify an underlying seizure etiology at presentation. Diagnostic limitations, such as an inability to obtain regular $CD4^+$ counts and viral loads, limited our ability to confidently identify immune reconstitution syndrome (IRIS) in participants. While 15/37 participants who died were not on cART at the time of death, 11/22 participants on cART had been on it less than a year.

The generalizability of the outcomes and risk factor data relying on CSF analysis, EEG, and neuroimaging may be inadequate, particularly where diagnostic measures are scarce and, when available, limited by cost or capacity. While we employed all the available laboratory and imaging to assess seizure etiology in our setting, a negative CSF PCR assay does not guarantee the absence of infection, particularly for conditions like tuberculosis, where testing sensitivity is less than ideal [15]. Unfortunately, not all patients consented to a lumbar puncture, therefore, to improve the external validity of our findings, we performed a sensitivity analysis with only patients who had CSF available to assess the impact of lumbar puncture refusal on findings as prior data from this setting required CSF analysis for inclusion [27]. Because of this, we were unable to apply select clinical terms, such as new-onset refractory status epilepticus (NORSE), to our study population. Similarly, unlike prior studies in this setting, patients with a family history of epilepsy or a personal history of head trauma were eligible for inclusion [8, 10]. Given the documented challenges associated with obtaining consent for lumbar puncture in many resource-limited settings, efforts to improve procedure understanding and uptake may be warranted [28–30].

Whether more expedited HIV diagnosis and cART initiation could have decreased the high mortality rate in this population is unclear. Among CHASE participants, the average time to cART initiation was 61 days and this was likely abbreviated by staff advocating for follow up visits at AIDC. While earlier initiation of cART among patients with OIs decreases mortality [31, 32], a diagnosis of AIDS was not associated with earlier cART initiation in our patient population. Twenty-two participants survived their initial hospitalization yet died before cART was initiated, despite meeting national eligibility criteria to initiate treatment. As resource-limited countries implement universal treatment access irrespective of WHO stage or $CD4^+$ T-cell count, the number of HIV-positive individuals eligible for cART will grow and delays in cART initiation may increase substantially due to an overwhelmed primary health system. Efforts dedicated to shortening these treatment delays are imperative, particularly for extremely ill patients.

Conclusions

New-onset seizure among HIV-positive Zambian adults is associated with a nearly 40% mortality rate despite good functional status prior to presentation. Patients with advanced HIV infection or an unknown underlying seizure are most likely to die during follow up. Death is a significant competing risk factor for the development of epilepsy and, as a result, we were unable to identify significant risk factors for future seizures. Among survivors, 24% experience recurrent seizures often less than a year after the index seizure.

Abbreviations

AED: Antiepileptic drug; AIDC: Adult Infectious Disease Centre; AIDS: Acquired immunodeficiency syndrome; cART: Combination antiretroviral therapy; CHASE: Cohort for HIV-Associated Seizures and Epilepsy; CI: Confidence interval; CNS: Central nervous system; CSF: Cerebrospinal fluid; DNA PCR: Deoxyribonucleic acid polymerase chain reaction; EBV: Epstein-Barr virus; EEG: Electroencephalogram; HIV: Human immunodeficiency virus; IQR: Interquartile range; IRIS: Immune reconstitution inflammatory syndrome; MSU BIRB: Michigan State University's Biomedical Institutional Review Board; OI: Opportunistic infection; UNZA BREC: University of Zambia Biomedical Research Ethics Committee; UTH: University Teaching Hospital; VDRL: Venereal disease research laboratory; WHO: World Health Organization

Acknowledgements

We thank the UTH staff of the Adult Infectious Diseases Clinic and the Neurology Research Office for their support and assistance. We are also grateful to the patients and families who participated in this study.

Funding

Fogarty International Center and the National Institute of Neurological Disorders and Stroke (NINDS), Award Number 1R21NS073509 and R01NS094037. Content is the responsibility of the authors and does not represent the views of the Department of Defense, or the Departments of the Army, Navy or Air Force or National Institutes of Health. MAE: MD/PhD Fellowship from Spectrum Health, the AMA Foundation, and the Lois C. Walker Endowed Fund for Student Research in the Michigan State University College of Human Medicine. OKS: American Academy of Neurology Clinical Research Fellowship. IJK: NINDS R01 047029 and 074995. WHT: International League against Epilepsy.

Authors' contributions

MAE assisted with data collection, analysis, and manuscript writing. BAJ assisted with data analysis and manuscript writing. OKS assisted with participant recruitment, data collection, and analysis. JFO assisted with study design. IS assisted with participant recruitment and data collection. CMB, MJP, IJK, WHT assisted with study design, data collection, and analysis. LK assisted with data collection. GLB conceived the study design, data collection, analysis and manuscript writing. All authors read and approved the final manuscript.

Competing interests
OKS, IJ, MJP, IJK, and GLB have received funding from the NIH. OKS also received grant funding from the American Academy of Neurology. MJP also received funding from the Dana Foundation. GLB has also played a role in writing guidelines relevant to this patient population. MAE, BAJ, JFO, CMB, WHJ, and LK report no competing interests.

Author details
[1]Department of Neurology, Johns Hopkins Hospital, Sheik Zayed Tower, Room 6005, 1800 Orleans Street, Baltimore, MD 21287, USA. [2]Department of Biostatistics and Computational Biology, University of Rochester, 265 Crittenden Boulevard, CU 420-630, Rochester, NY 14642-0630, USA. [3]Global Neurology Program, Division of Neuroimmunology, Department of Neurology, E/CLS 1017B Beth Israel Deaconess Medical Center, 330 Brookline Avenue, Boston, MA 02215, USA. [4]Department of Internal Medicine, University of Zambia School of Medicine, Lusaka, Zambia. [5]Infectious Disease Service, Brooke Army Medical Center, 3851 Roger Brooke Dr., Fort Sam Houston, San Antonio, TX 78234, USA. [6]Center for Infectious Disease Research in Zambia, 5032 Great North Road, P.O. Box 34681, Lusaka, Zambia. [7]Greater Lawrence Family Health Center, 34 Haverhill St, Lawrence, MA 01841, USA. [8]Neuroradiology Division, Department of Imaging Sciences, University of Rochester Medical Center, 601 Elmwood Ave, Box 648, Rochester, NY 14642, USA. [9]Department of Neurological Sciences, Rush University Medical Center, 1725 W. Harrison Street, Suite 1106, Chicago, IL 60612, USA. [10]Clinical Epilepsy Section, National Institute of Neurological Disorders and Stroke, NINDS NIH Building 10 Room 7D-43, Bethesda, MD 20892, USA. [11]Department of Psychology, University of Zambia, P.O. BOX 32379, 10101 Lusaka, Zambia. [12]Epilepsy Division, Department of Neurology, University of Rochester School of Medicine & Dentistry, 265 Crittenden Blvd, CU420694, Rochester, NY 14642–0694, USA. [13]Epilepsy Care Team, Chikankata Hospital, Private Bag S2, Mazabuka, Zambia.

References

1. Mateen FJ, Shinohara RT, Carone M, Miller EN, McArthur JC, Jacobson LP, Sacktor N, Multicenter ACSI. Neurologic disorders incidence in HIV+ vs HIV- men: Multicenter AIDS cohort study, 1996-2011. Neurology. 2012;79(18):1873–80.
2. Chadha DS, Handa A, Sharma SK, Varadarajulu P, Singh AP. Seizures in patients with human immunodeficiency virus infection. J Assoc Physicians India. 2000; 48(6):573–6.
3. Kellinghaus C, Engbring C, Kovac S, Moddel G, Boesebeck F, Fischera M, Anneken K, Klonne K, Reichelt D, Evers S, et al. Frequency of seizures and epilepsy in neurological HIV-infected patients. Seizure. 2008;17(1):27–33.
4. Wong MC, Suite ND, Labar DR. Seizures in human immunodeficiency virus infection. Arch Neurol. 1990;47(6):640–2.
5. Dore GJ, Law MG, Brew BJ. Prospective analysis of seizures occurring in human immunodeficiency virus type-1 infection. J NeuroAIDS. 1996;1(4):59–69.
6. Holtzman DM, Kaku DA, So YT. New-onset seizures associated with human immunodeficiency virus infection: causation and clinical features in 100 cases. Am J Med. 1989;87(2):173–7.
7. Pascual-Sedano B, Iranzo A, Marti-Fabregas J, Domingo P, Escartin A, Fuster M, Barrio JL, Sambeat MA. Prospective study of new-onset seizures in patients with human immunodeficiency virus infection: etiologic and clinical aspects. Arch Neurol. 1999;56(5):609–12.
8. Modi G, Modi M, Martinus I, Saffer D. New-onset seizures associated with HIV infection. Neurology. 2000;55(10):1558–61.
9. Millogo A, Lankoande D, Yameogo I, Yameogo AA, Sawadogo A, Sawadogo AB. new-onset seizures in patients with immunodeficiency virus infection in Bobo-Dioulasso hospital (Burkina Faso). Bull Soc Pathol Exot. 2004;97(4):268–70.
10. Olajumoke O, Akinsegun A, Njideka O, Oluwadamilola O, Olaitan O, Adedoyin D, Adewumi A, Akinola D, Sarah A. New-onset seizures in HIV patients on antiretroviral therapy at a tertiary Centre in South-West, Nigeria. World J AIDS. 2013;03(02):67–70.
11. Romanelli F, Pomeroy C. Concurrent use of antiretrovirals and anticonvulsants in human immunodeficiency virus (HIV) seropositive patients. Curr Pharm Des. 2003;9(18):1433–9.
12. Van Paesschen W, Bodian C, Maker H. Metabolic abnormalities and new-onset seizures in human immunodeficiency virus-seropositive patients. Epilepsia. 1995;36(2):146–50.
13. Birbeck G, Chomba E, Ddumba E, Kauye F, Mielke J. Lack of appropriate treatment for people with comorbid HIV/AIDS and epilepsy in sub-Saharan Africa. Epilepsia. 2007;48(7):1424–5.
14. Birbeck GL, French JA, Perucca E, Simpson DM, Fraimow H, George JM, Okulicz JF, Clifford DB, Hachad H, Levy RH, et al. Antiepileptic drug selection for people with HIV/AIDS: evidence-based guidelines from the ILAE and AAN. Epilepsia. 2012;53(1):207–14.
15. Siddiqi OK, Elafros MA, Bositis CM, Koralnik IJ, Theodore WH, Okulicz JF, Kalungwana L, Potchen MJ, Sikazwe I, Birbeck GL. New-onset seizure in HIV-infected adult Zambians: a search for causes and consequences. Neurology. 2017;88(5):477–82.
16. Fisher RS, Cross JH, French JA, Higurashi N, Hirsch E, Jansen FE, Lagae L, Moshe SL, Peltola J, Roulet Perez E, et al. Operational classification of seizure types by the international league against epilepsy: position paper of the ILAE Commission for Classification and Terminology. Epilepsia. 2017;58(4):522–30.
17. Trinka E, Cock H, Hesdorffer D, Rossetti AO, Scheffer IE, Shinnar S, Shorvon S, Lowenstein DH. A definition and classification of status epilepticus--report of the ILAE task force on classification of status epilepticus. Epilepsia. 2015;56(10): 1515–23.
18. Teasdale G, Jennett B. Assessment of coma and impaired consciousness. A practical scale. Lancet. 1974;2(7872):81–4.
19. WHO: Consolidated guidelines on the use of antiretroviral drugs for treating and preventing HIV infection. In: A Public Health Approach. Geneva 2013. http://apps.who.int/iris/bitstream/handle/10665/208825/9789241549684_eng.pdf;jsessionid=C62C9F39CB8AAC6B5534321F6B139FB5?sequence=1/
20. Sinha SR, Sullivan L, Sabau D, San-Juan D, Dombrowski KE, Halford JJ, Hani AJ, Drislane FW, Stecker MM. American clinical neurophysiology society guideline 1: minimum technical requirements for performing clinical electroencephalography. J Clin Neurophysiol. 2016;33(4):303–7.
21. NINDS Common Data Elements [online].
22. Siddiqi OK, Elafros MA, Sikazwe I, Birbeck GL, Kalungwana L, Potchen MJ, Bositis CM, Koralnik IJ, Theodore WH. Acute EEG findings in HIV-infected Zambian adults with new-onset seizure. Neurology. 2015;84(13):1317–22.
23. Potchen MJ, Siddiqi OK, Elafros MA, Koralnik IJ, Theodore WH, Sikazwe I, Kalungwana L, Bositis CM, Birbeck GL. Neuroimaging abnormalities and seizure recurrence in a prospective cohort study of zambians with human immunodeficiency virus and first seizure. Neurol Int. 2014;6(4):5547.
24. Fisher RS, Acevedo C, Arzimanoglou A, Bogacz A, Cross JH, Elger CE, Engel J Jr, Forsgren L, French JA, Glynn M, et al. ILAE official report: a practical clinical definition of epilepsy. Epilepsia. 2014;55(4):475–82.
25. Elafros MA, Birbeck GL, Gardiner JC, Siddiqi OK, Sikazwe I, Paneth N, Bositis CM, Okulicz JF. Patient-reported adverse effects associated with combination antiretroviral therapy and Coadministered enzyme-inducing antiepileptic drugs. Am J Trop Med Hyg. 2017;96(6):1505–11.
26. Mbonda PC, Kuate C, Njamnshi AK, Fogang Y, Fonsah J, Muna W. Etiologic aspects of epileptic seizures of recent onset in HIV-AIDS infected subjects at the Yaounde central hospital (Cameroon). World J AIDS. 2013;03(02):160–7.
27. Modi M, Mochan A, Modi G. New onset seizures in HIV--seizure semiology, CD4 counts, and viral loads. Epilepsia. 2009;50(5):1266–9.
28. Thakur KT, Mateyo K, Hachaambwa L, Kayamba V, Mallewa M, Mallewa J, Nwazor EO, Lawal T, Mallum CB, Atadzhanov M, et al. Lumbar puncture refusal in sub-Saharan Africa: a call for further understanding and intervention. Neurology. 2015;84(19):1988–90.
29. Sikazwe I, Elafros MA, Bositis CM, Siddiqi OK, Koralnik IJ, Kalungwana L, Theodore WH, Okulicz JF, Potchen MJ, Birbeck GL. HIV and new onset seizures: slipping through the cracks in HIV care and treatment. HIV Med. 2016;17(2):118–23.
30. Kambugu A, Meya DB, Rhein J, O'Brien M, Janoff EN, Ronald AR, Kamya MR, Mayanja-Kizza H, Sande MA, Bohjanen PR, et al. Outcomes of cryptococcal meningitis in Uganda before and after the availability of highly active antiretroviral therapy. Clin Infect Dis. 2008;46(11):1694–701.
31. Blanc FX, Sok T, Laureillard D, Borand L, Rekacewicz C, Nerrienet E, Madec Y, Marcy O, Chan S, Prak N, et al. Earlier versus later start of antiretroviral therapy in HIV-infected adults with tuberculosis. N Engl J Med. 2011;365(16):1471–81.
32. Zolopa A, Andersen J, Powderly W, Sanchez A, Sanne I, Suckow C, Hogg E, Komarow L. Early antiretroviral therapy reduces AIDS progression/death in individuals with acute opportunistic infections: a multicenter randomized strategy trial. PLoS One. 2009;4(5):e5575.

26

LARGE expression in different types of muscular dystrophies other than dystroglycanopathy

Burcu Balci-Hayta[1*], Beril Talim[2], Gulsev Kale[2] and Pervin Dincer[1]

Abstract

Background: Alpha-dystroglycan (αDG) is an extracellular peripheral glycoprotein that acts as a receptor for both extracellular matrix proteins containing laminin globular domains and certain arenaviruses. An important enzyme, known as Like-acetylglucosaminyltransferase (LARGE), has been shown to transfer repeating units of -glucuronic acid-β1,3-xylose-α1,3- (matriglycan) to αDG that is required for functional receptor as an extracellular matrix protein scaffold. The reduction in the amount of LARGE-dependent matriglycan result in heterogeneous forms of dystroglycanopathy that is associated with hypoglycosylation of αDG and a consequent lack of ligand-binding activity. Our aim was to investigate whether LARGE expression showed correlation with glycosylation of αDG and histopathological parameters in different types of muscular dystrophies, except for dystroglycanopathies.

Methods: The expression level of *LARGE* and glycosylation status of αDG were examined in skeletal muscle biopsies from 26 patients with various forms of muscular dystrophy [Duchenne muscular dystrophy (DMD), Becker muscular dystrophy (BMD), sarcoglycanopathy, dysferlinopathy, calpainopathy, and merosin and collagen VI deficient congenital muscular dystrophies (CMDs)] and correlation of results with different histopathological features was investigated.

Results: Despite the fact that these diseases are not caused by defects of glycosyltransferases, decreased expression of *LARGE* was detected in many patient samples, partly correlating with the type of muscular dystrophy. Although immunolabelling of fully glycosylated αDG with VIA4–1 was reduced in dystrophinopathy patients, no significant relationship between reduction of *LARGE* expression and αDG hypoglycosylation was detected. Also, Merosin deficient CMD patients showed normal immunostaining with αDG despite severe reduction of *LARGE* expression.

Conclusions: Our data shows that it is not always possible to correlate *LARGE* expression and αDG glycosylation in different types of muscular dystrophies and suggests that there might be differences in αDG processing by LARGE which could be regulated under different pathological conditions.

Keywords: *LARGE*, Alpha-dystroglycan, Hypoglycosylation, Muscular dystrophy, Skeletal muscle

Background

Dystroglycan (DG), a heterodimeric transmembrane glycoprotein, is a central component of the dystrophin-glycoprotein complex (DGC) and responsible for a variety of physiological and developmental processes, including muscle stabilization, basement membrane assembly, cell migration and signalling [1]. The protein is synthesized as a precursor molecule that is post-translationally cleaved into a cell surface α- and a transmembrane β-subunits [2]. The extracellular subunit, alpha-dystroglycan (αDG), is a highly glycosylated basement membrane protein that acts as a receptor for non-collagenous proteins in the extracellular matrix (ECM) containing laminin globular domains, and for Old World arenaviruses [1, 3–5]. Mutations in the DG-encoding gene *(DAG1)* [6, 7] and several other genes whose products are involved, directly or indirectly, in glycosylation pathway of αDG [8] have been identified in

* Correspondence: burcub@hacettepe.edu.tr
[1]Department of Medical Biology, Hacettepe University Faculty of Medicine, 06100 Sihhiye, Ankara, Turkey
Full list of author information is available at the end of the article

various forms of congenital and limb-girdle muscular dystrophies (CMD/ LGMDs). These disorders are all associated with hypoglycosylation of αDG and a consequent lack of ligand-binding activity and thus are collectively termed as dystroglycanopathies [9].

Although the precise glycosylation pathway of αDG is not fully understood, the function of Like-acetylglucosaminyltransferase (LARGE) enzyme has been of particular interest. It is encoded by one of the largest genes (*LARGE*) in the human genome [10–12], which is mutated in the myodystrophy mouse (LARGE-myd) [10, 13] and in patients affected by MDC1D, a subclass of CMD associated with skeletal muscle and structural brain involvement [11]. The mentioned enzyme is a bifunctional glycosyltransferase, with both xylosyltransferase and glucuronyltransferase activities and plays an important role in the glycosylation pathway of αDG. It transfers a novel heteropolysaccharide structure, repeating units of -glucuronic acid-β1,3-xylose-α1,3- to the basement membrane receptor DG [14]. This structure has been recently termed as matriglycan, which is bound to the αDG through a phosphorylated *O*-mannosyl glycan anchored at Thr317 and Thr319 in the mucin-like domain [8, 15, 16]. It is required for the αDG to bind laminin-G domain-containing ECM ligands including laminin, agrin, perlecan and neurexin [4, 17–19]. It has been reported that LARGE-dependent matriglycan structure plays an important role for normal skeletal muscle function and the consequent reduction in the amount of glycans on αDG causes structural alterations of the basement membrane, immature neuromuscular junctions and dysfunctional muscle predisposed to dystrophy [20]. Uniquely, transient overexpression of *LARGE* has been shown to increase glycosylation of αDG as evaluated by increased immunoreactivity to antibodies IIH6 and VIA4–1 both of which are known to recognize carbohydrate moieties and leads to a recovery of receptor function in cells derived from patients diagnosed as Fukuyama CMD (FCMD), muscle-eye-brain disease (MEB) and Walker–Warburg syndrome (WWS) [17]. Also, the identical results has been reported in vivo, after adenovirus or adeno-associated virus mediated gene transfer of *LARGE* in *Fukutin (FKTN), Fukutin-related protein (FKRP)* and *Protein-O-mannose β2-N-acetylglucosaminyltransferase 1 (POMGNT1)* deficient mice models [21–23]. Although a recent study demonstrates that fukutin is required for the ability of LARGE to hyperglycosylate αDG [24], this strategy is already regarded as a promising therapeutic approach for preventing/slowing progression of a broad range of dystroglycanopathies regardless of the causative gene defects. However, it remains crucial to analyze such a strategy in different types of muscular dystrophies other than dystroglycanopathy.

In this study, we analyzed the influence of *LARGE* gene expression profile on VIA4–1 immunoreactivity in different types of muscular dystrophies, except for dystroglycanopathies [i.e. Duchenne muscular dystrophy (DMD), Becker muscular dystrophy (BMD), sarcoglycanopathy, dysferlinopathy, calpainopathy, and merosin and collagen VI deficient CMDs]. Correlation between different histopathological features, *LARGE* expression profile and glycosylation status of αDG was investigated. We detected reduced expression level of *LARGE* in different types of muscular dystrophies, partly correlating with the severity of dystrophic changes, but we did not find any significant relationship between reduction of *LARGE* expression and VIA4–1 immunoreactivity.

Methods

Patients and muscle biopsies

The study protocol was approved by the Hacettepe University Faculty of Medicine Ethical Review Board (FON 10/35–11). As the legal age of consent is 18 years of age in Turkey, written informed consent was obtained from patients' parents or legal guardians at the time of diagnostic muscle biopsy. Skeletal muscle biopsies from 3 controls and 26 patients with clinicopathological and/or molecular diagnosis of various forms of muscular dystrophy other than dystroglycanopathy were included in this study. The number of patients in each disease type is indicated in parentheses; DMD (3), BMD (4), sarcoglycanopathy (5), dysferlinopathy (1), calpainopathy (1), Merosin deficient CMD (4), Collagen VI deficient CMD (3), unclassified CMD (2), and unclassified MD (3). All patients have been investigated in the Department of Pediatrics at Hacettepe University Faculty of Medicine and open biopsies were taken from vastus lateralis muscle at the time of diagnosis. The muscle biopsy specimens were rapidly frozen in isopentane cooled in liquid nitrogen and kept at − 80 °C until use. Serial transverse muscle sections were cut by cryostat for histochemical staining. Standard histological and histochemical techniques were applied to cryostat sections, including Haematoxylin and eosin (H&E), modified Gomori trichrome, periodic acid Schiff, oil-red-O, nicotinamide adenine dinucleotide dehydrogenase-tetrazolium reductase, succinic dehydrogenase, cytochrome-c oxidase and ATPase. Immunohistochemical and/or immunofluorescent studies were done at the time of diagnosis, using antibodies against dystrophins, sarcoglycans, dysferlin, laminin α2 (merosin), collagen VI, and αDG, as appropriate.

Histopathological evaluation

H&E stained archive sections were examined to identify the severity of various dystrophic changes, including necrosis, regeneration, adiposis, endomysial and perimysial fibrosis and inflammation. These pathological changes were scored from 0 (absent) to 4 (severe).

Immunofluorescent staining

For immunofluorescent staining, skeletal muscle cryosections of 7 μm were immunostained with primary antibodies [1/10 for mouse anti-α-Dystroglycan antibody (clone VIA4–1 against fully glycosylated form of αDG, Millipore), 1/50 for sheep anti-α-Dystroglycan core antibody (R&D Systems: AF6868), 1/100 for mouse anti-Spectrin (NCL-SPEC1 Clone: RBC2/3D5, Novocastra), 1:20 for anti-Beta-Dystroglycan (βDG) (NCL-b-DG Clone 43DAG1/8D5, Novocastra) and 1:1000 for mouse anti-laminin α2 (MAB1922 Chemicon (Millipore)] for 1 h at room temperature, followed by incubation with Alexa Fluor 488 goat anti-mouse or donkey anti-sheep IgG antibodies (Molecular Probes) at 1:1000 dilution for 45 min at room temperature. All dilutions and washing steps were made in phosphate buffered saline. Immunostained sections were then mounted and observed with epifluorescence using a Nicon Eclipse E400 microscope. The fluorescent labeling was scored from 0 (absent) to 3 (intense) using a scale based on the proportion of positive fibers and intensity relative to the control muscle sections.

Quantitative real-time PCR (qRT-PCR)

In order to assess the expression of *LARGE*, total RNA was extracted from liquid nitrogen fresh-frozen skeletal muscle tissues (3 mm^3) from 26 patiens and 3 control samples using RNeasy® fibrous tissue mini kit (Qiagen) and cDNA was synthesized from 500 ng RNA using QuantiTect Reverse Transcription kit (Qiagen) according to manufacturer's guidelines. Real-time PCR was then performed using SYBR Green JumpStart TaqReadyMix kit (Sigma) on Rotor-Gene 6000™ (Corbett Research) with the following conditions: 2 min at 94 °C, followed by 40 cycles of 5 s at 94 °C, 10 s at 58 °C, and 15 s at 72 °C. Reactions were performed in a total volume of 10 μL, including 5 μL SYBR Green JumpStart TaqReadyMix kit (Sigma), 1.2 μl of 25 mM $MgCl_2$ (Sigma), 0.4 μl each of 10 mM forward and reverse primers and 1 μl of template cDNA. Mastermix with no cDNA was used as the no template control whereas water was used as the negative control. The relative amount of mRNA, normalized to an internal control human beta-actin *(ACTB)* and relative to a calibrator (control), was calculated by $2^{-\Delta\Delta CT}$. Primers used were as follows: *LARGE*-F: 5'-TGAGCCGTATGTTGTTGTG AGAC-3'; *LARGE*-R: 5'-GATGCGGTATTGCTTGTTG GAAC-3' and *ACTB*-F: 5'- CGCAAAGACCTGTACGC CAAC -3'; *ACTB*-R: 5'- GAGCCGCCGATCCACACG -3'. All reactions were performed in triplicate and optimal threshold in 95–100% efficiency. All data was analyzed using Rotor-Gene 6000 Series Software 1.7 (Corbett Research).

Statistical analysis

All experiments performed at least three times and data were evaluated as means ± SD. The significance of differences between experimental groups was determined using Mann-Whitney U test. p values less than 0.05 were considered statistically significant.

Results

We assessed human muscle biopsies from DMD, BMD, sarcoglycanopathy, calpainopathy, dysferlinopathy, and merosin and collagen VI deficient CMDs, in addition to unclassified CMDs and MDs. Scoring for the severity of histopathological features and age at biopsy for each patient are shown in Table 1. In each muscular dystrophy group, samples had variable severity of histopathological findings such as necrosis, regeneration, fibrosis, adiposis and inflammation. Even some patients with the same diagnosis and similar age of biopsy showed different severity of pathological changes.

We first assessed the expression level of *LARGE* by qRT-PCR and detected reduced expression level of *LARGE* gene in analyzed samples, partly correlating with the form of muscular dystrophy (Fig. 1). The reduction of *LARGE* expression was more significant in all cases of DMD (P1, P2 and P3) and merosin deficient CMD (P14, P15, P16 and P17) as compared to control skeletal muscle. Also, *LARGE* mRNA levels were markedly reduced in all BMD cases, except one (P6). The expression of *LARGE* was similarly reduced in two cases of unclassified CMD (P22 and P23) and MD (P24 and P25), who had similar histopathological patterns. However, decreased expression in one case of Collagen VI deficient CMD (P18) with mild dystrophic features remains unexplained. The results of our study revealed different expression profiles for *LARGE* also among patients with different types of sarcoglycanopathies. Reduced *LARGE* expression levels were found also in the single dysferlinopathy (P13) and calpainopathy (P21) patients compared with age-matched healthy controls, with more severe reduction in *LARGE* and more severe dystrophic features in the case with dysferlin deficiency.

In order to reveal a correlation between *LARGE* expression and functional glycosylation of αDG, skeletal muscle sections were immunostained using VIA4–1 antibody against fully glycosylated form of αDG, and evaluated together with αDG core protein (Fig. 2), beta-dystroglycan and laminin α2 immunostaining. The spectrum of VIA4–1 labeling was very variable and ranged from an absent to intense, compared with control skeletal muscle, whereas the immunoreactivity of core protein was indistinguishable between control and patients (Fig. 3). Therefore, the loss of VIA4–1 reactivity in some specimens reflects a reduction of α-DG glycosylation, rather than loss of α-DG core protein expression.

Table 1 The clinicopathological diagnosis and histopathological characteristics of the patients (Assessment scores: 0: absent; 1: rare; 2: mild; 3: moderate; 4: severe)

#	Necrosis	Regeneration	Endomysial fibrosis	Perimysial fibrosis	Adiposis	Inflammation	Age	Ambulatory status	Diagnosis
P1	1	2	4	4	4	2	8 yr	Ambulant	DMD
P2	2	2	2	3	2	2	8 yr	Ambulant	
P3	4	3	2	2	2	4	6 yr	Ambulant	
P4	3	3	3	4	2	3	8 yr	Ambulant	BMD
P5	3	3	2	2	2	2	7 yr	Ambulant	
P6	3	4	2	2	3	3	2 yr	Ambulant	
P7	1	3	3	4	4	2	10 yr	Ambulant	
P8	3	3	2	3	0	3	1 yr	Ambulant	Sarcoglycanopathy
P9	0	2	0	0	0	0	2,5 yr	Ambulant	
P10	3	3	0	0	2	3	6 yr	Ambulant	g-Sarcoglycanopathy
P11	0	2	0	0	2	0	4 yr	Ambulant	
P12	0	3	1	0	0	1	8 yr	Ambulant	
P13	4	4	3	2	1	4	15 yr	Ambulant	Dysferlinopathy
P14	1	3	3	3	3	3	7 mo	Non-ambulant (infant)	Merosin deficient CMD
P15	1	3	2	2	2	4	8 mo	Non-ambulant (infant)	
P16	1	1	2	3	4	2	3 yr	Non-ambulant	
P17	1	2	2	2	2	2	3 yr	Non-ambulant	
P18	1	2	2	2	3	1	5 yr	Ambulant	Collagen VI deficient CMD
P19	0	1	2	0	0	0	3,5 yr	Non-ambulant	
P20	0	0	0	0	0	0	6 mo	Non-ambulant (infant)	
P21	2	3	3	2	0	3	13 yr	Ambulant	Calpainopathy
P22	2	3	3	2	3	3	10 yr	Ambulant	CMD, unclassified
P23	2	3	3	3	3	3	4 yr	Ambulant	
P24	0	2	2	0	2	1	12 yr	Ambulant	MD, unclassified
P25	0	1	2	0	2	2	14 yr	Ambulant	
P26	2	3	2	0	0	3	9 yr	Ambulant	
Control-1	0	0	0	0	0	0	6 yr	Ambulant	---
Control-2	0	0	0	0	0	0	3 yr	Ambulant	
Control-3	0	0	0	0	0	0	17 yr	Ambulant	

The skeletal muscle of patients with DMD showed a marked depletion of αDG glycosylation. The reduction of VIA4–1 labeling in BMD group ranged from an absence on most fibres to a very mild reduction. Also, in some patients with sarcoglycanopathy, Collagen VI deficient CMD and unclassified MD, a mild reduction of sarcolemmal labelling with VIA4–1 antibody was detected. Interestingly, patient 8 and 18 displayed an almost total absence of αDG glycosylation relative to other patients within their group. Spectrin appeared normal in all cases indicating that the reduction in αDG hypoglycosylation was not due to non-specific damage of the plasma membrane. Except for merosin deficient CMDs, laminin α2 staining was also normal in all analyzed cases. Labeling of the transmembrane protein βDG was preserved in most cases, although a mild reduction has been reported in 9 of the 26 cases, mostly in dystrophinopathies. There was no significant relationship between reduction of *LARGE* expression and αDG hypoglycosylation, most obvious example being the merosin deficient CMD patients (P14, P15, P16 and P17) (Figs. 1 and 3) who showed normal immunostaining with αDG despite severe reduction of *LARGE* expression.

Discussion

In order to determine correlations between *LARGE* expression, glycosylation of αDG and histopathological parameters, we analyzed *LARGE* gene expression profile and glycosylation status of αDG in various forms of muscular dystrophies, except for dystroglycanopathies. The expression level of *LARGE* was analyzed by qRT-PCR in skeletal muscle biopsies from 26 patients diagnosed as different forms of muscular dystrophy with various histopathological phenotypes (Table 1). Our findings indicated that most of the patients with severe histopathological phenotype (DMD and merosin deficient CMD) have decreased *LARGE* expression levels compared to control skeletal muscle (Fig. 1). We then evaluated whether there was a relationship between *LARGE* expression and αDG glycosylation. The functional glycosylation of αDG is associated with the

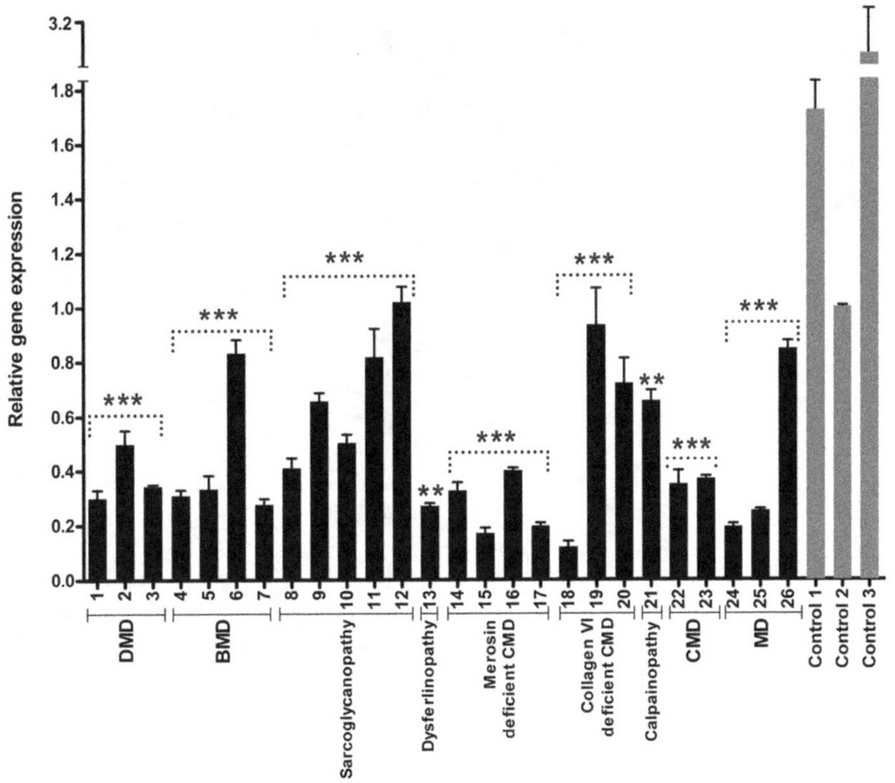

Fig. 1 Relative expression levels of *LARGE*, measured by quantitative real time PCR in different types of muscular dystrophies. Bar graph representations are shown of the mean ± SEM values of the expression levels of patients (dark grey) and controls (light grey), respectively. Each bar represents the combined relative expression of three independent experiments measured by triplicate. Control 2 is used as calibrator. Error bars indicate standard deviations. Asterisks denote statistical significance as compared to the average of control group (Mann-Whitney U test, $^{**}p < 0.01$, $^{***}p < 0.001$)

binding of either IIH6 and/or VIA4–1 antibodies to αDG. Thus, immunofluorescence staining was done using the widely used VIA4–1 antibody. Our findings indicate that irrespective of the muscular dystrophy type, the degree of hypoglycosylation varied (Figs. 2 and 3) and there was generally no correlation with clinical/histopathological severity. Similar results have previously been reported in dystroglycanopathy patients with *Protein-O-mannosyl transferase 1 (POMT1), Protein-O-mannosyl transferase 2 (POMT2), POMGnT1, FKTN* and *FKRP* mutations [25]. Also, our results were not consistent with the findings which suggests a correlation between a reduction in αDG labeling and the clinical severity in mild, late-onset LGMD type 2I and severe CMD [20, 26]. On the other hand, we observed a severe reduction of αDG glycosylation in skeletal muscle biopsies of dystrophinopathy patients as a secondary finding, which has already been shown in DMD patients and mdx mouse [27, 28]. In contrast to those findings, the labelling obtained using the αDG core antibody was preserved in all patients, which suggested that the glycosylation of αDG is affected independently of DG protein expression.

In dystroglycanopathies, the effects of decreased glycosylation on laminin binding are variable [4, 11]. Therefore, further studies are necessary to evaluate if hypoglycosylation of αDG affects laminin binding or other functions of αDG in different types of muscular dystrophies other than dystroglycanopathy. Campbell and colleagues have previously demonstrated that short LARGE-glycan repeats reduces normal physiological function of muscle and predisposes it to dystrophy and showed that upregulation of *LARGE* and DG facilitates extension of LARGE-glycan repeat chains in differentiating mouse muscle [20]. However, consistent with our preliminary findings [29], we did not find any significant relationship between reduction of *LARGE* expression and αDG hypoglycosylation (Figs. 1 and 3), except for DMD. Our results suggest that LARGE enzyme may have an additional function in skeletal muscle fibers that is probably distinct from adding a critical sugar chain onto αDG. Equally likely is that the RNA changes in LARGE, while present, are not related at all to the MD phenotype. Transcriptional changes are difficult to interpret in prediction effects downstream.

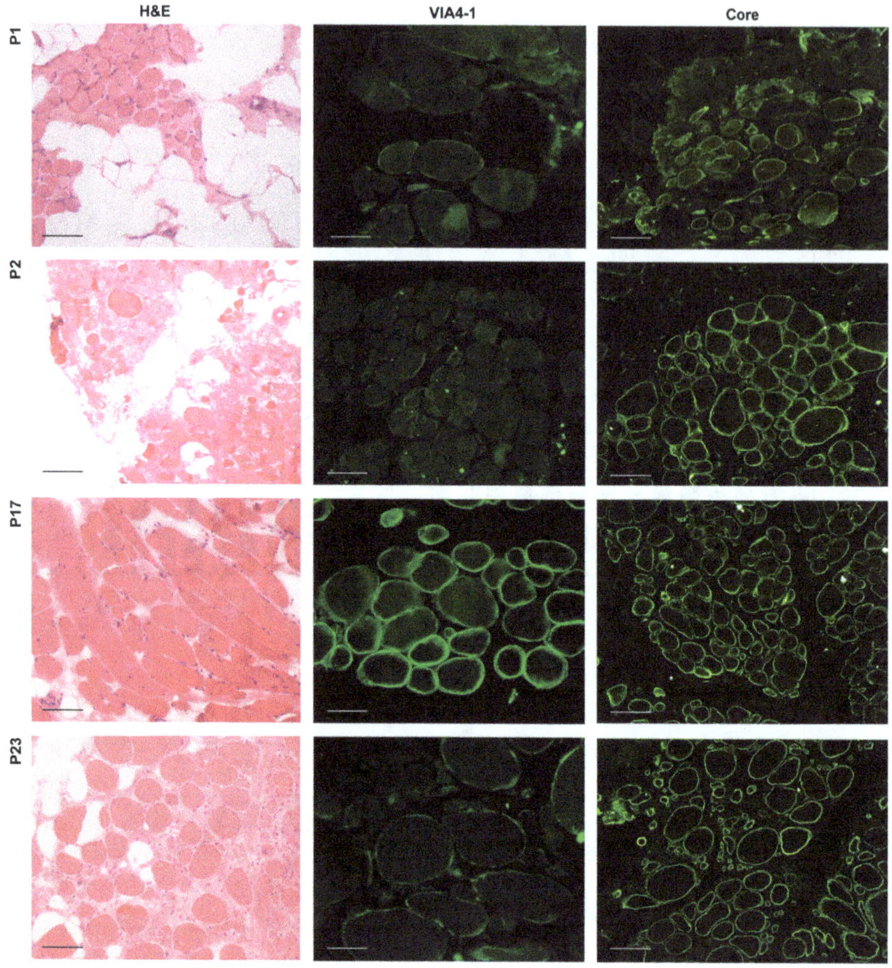

Fig. 2 Illustrative images of muscle sections with hematoxylin and eosin staining (left-hand panel; scale bars: 40 μm.), glycosylated αDG labeling with VIA4–1 antibody (middle panel; scale bars: P1, P17 and P23: 20 μm.; P2: 40 μm.) and α-DG core antibody (right-hand panel; scale bars: 40 μm.). αDG labeling was normal in merosin deficiency (P17), mildly reduced in CMD (P23), but severely reduced/absent in cases with dystrophin deficiency (P1 and P2). Expression of the core αDG protein was well preserved in all samples

	DMD			BMD				Sarcoglycanopathy					Dysferlinopathy	Merosin deficient CMD				Collagen VI deficient CMD			Calpainopathy	CMD		MD					
PATIENTS	1	2	3	4	5	6	7	8	9	10	11	12	13	14	15	16	17	18	19	20	21	22	23	24	25	26	C-1	C-2	C-3
VIA4-1	1	0	0	0	1	2	2	0	3	2	3	2	3	3	3	3	3	0	2	3	3	2	2	3	2	3	3	3	3
βDG	3	2	2	2	2	2	3	2	3	3	3	3	3	3	3	3	3	2	3	2	3	3	3	3	3	2	3	3	3
Laminin α2	3	3	3	3	3	3	3	3	3	3	3	3	3	0	0	0	0	3	3	3	3	3	3	3	3	3	3	3	3
Spectrin	3	3	3	3	3	3	3	3	3	3	3	3	3	3	3	3	3	3	3	3	3	3	3	3	3	3	3	3	3
Core	3	3	3	3	3	3	3	3	3	3	3	3	3	3	3	3	3	3	3	3	3	3	3	3	3	3	3	3	3

Fig. 3 Representative results of immunofluorescence staining with VIA4–1, βDG, Laminin, Spectrin and αDG core antibodies. Immunolabeling scores were assigned to a scale of 0 to 3: (0 = absent; 1 = faint staining; 2 = moderate staining; 3 = intense staining)

Conclusions

Glycosylation of αDG undergoes tissue and developmental stage specific changes, which indicates that it may have different roles in developing and fully differentiated skeletal muscle [4, 30]. αDG glycosylation is likely to be regulated by developmental and differential expression of numerous enzymes, including LARGE. Therefore the detected *LARGE* expression profiles in various form of muscular dystrophies may still reflect responses to pathological processes of skeletal muscle related to αDG glycosylation. Our cohort encompassed a wide range of muscular dystrophies, suggesting that a different pathomechanism may explain the relationship between *LARGE* expression and αDG glycosylation in the pathogenesis of different types of muscular dystrophies and highlighting the need for further studies.

Abbreviations

ACTB: Beta-actin; BMD: Becker muscular dystrophy; CMD: Congenital muscular dystrophy; *DAG1*: DG-encoding gene; DG: Dystroglycan; DGC: Dystrophin-glycoprotein complex; DMD: Duchenne muscular dystrophy; ECM: Extracellular matrix; FCMD: Fukuyama congenital muscular dystrophy; *FKRP*: Fukutin-related protein; *FKTN*: Fukutin; H&E: Haematoxylin and eosin; *LARGE*: Like-acetylglucosaminyltransferase; LARGE-myd: myodystrophy mouse; LGMD: Limb-girdle muscular dystrophy; MEB: Muscle-eye-brain disease; *POMGNT1*: Protein-O-mannose ß2-N-acetylglucosaminyltransferase 1; *POMT1*: Protein-O-mannosyl transferase 1; *POMT2*: Protein-O-mannosyl transferase 2; qRT-PCR: Quantitative real-time PCR; WWS: Walker–Warburg syndrome; αDG: Alpha-dystroglycan

Acknowledgements

Not applicable.

Funding

This study was supported by a grant from Hacettepe University Scientific Research Projects Coordination Unit (grant number 011 D01 101 003).

Authors' contributions

BBH drafted the manuscript, obtained funding for this study, designed and performed the experiments. BT provided biopsy specimens, evaluated the histopathological data and revised the manuscript. PD contributed to the design and implementation of the study. GK contributed to the evaluation of the histopathological data and made a significant intellectual contribution to this study. All authors discussed the results and contributed to the final manuscript.

Competing interests

The authors declare that they have no competing interests.

Author details

[1]Department of Medical Biology, Hacettepe University Faculty of Medicine, 06100 Sihhiye, Ankara, Turkey. [2]Department of Pediatrics, Pathology Unit, Hacettepe University Faculty of Medicine, 06100 Sihhiye, Ankara, Turkey.

References

1. Barresi R, Campbell KP. Dystroglycan: from biosynthesis to pathogenesis of human disease. J Cell Sci. 2006;119:199–207.
2. Ibraghimov-Beskrovnaya O, Ervasti JM, Leveille CJ, Slaughter CA, Sernett SW, Campbell KP. Primary structure of dystrophin-associated glycoproteins linking dystrophin to the extracellular matrix. Nature. 1992;355:696–702.
3. Cao W, Henry MD, Borrow P, Yamada H, Elder JH, Ravkov EV, Nichol ST, Compans RW, Campbell KP, Oldstone MB. Identification of α-dystroglycan as a receptor for lymphocytic choriomeningitis virus and Lassa fever virus. Science. 1998;282:2079–81.
4. Michele DE, Barresi R, Kanagawa M, Saito F, Cohn RD, Satz JS, Dollar J, Nishino I, Kelley RI, Somer H, Straub V, Mathews KD, Moore SA, Campbell KP. Post-translational disruption of dystroglycan-ligand interactions in congenital muscular dystrophies. Nature. 2002;418:417–22.
5. Spiropoulou CF, Kunz S, Rollin PE, Campbell KP, Oldstone MB. New World arenavirus clade C, but not clade A and B viruses, utilizes alpha-dystroglycan as its major receptor. J Virol. 2002;76:5140–6.
6. Dinçer P, Balci B, Yuva Y, Talim B, Brockington M, Dinçel D, Torelli S, Brown S, Kale G, Haliloglu G, Gerçeker FO, Atalay RC, Yakicier C, Longman C, Muntoni F, Topaloglu H. A novel form of recessive limb girdle muscular dystrophy with mental retardation and abnormal expression of alpha-dystroglycan. Neuromuscul Disord. 2003;13:771–8.
7. Hara Y, Balci-Hayta B, Yoshida-Moriguchi T, Kanagawa M, Beltrán-Valero de Bernabé D, Gündeşli H, Willer T, Satz JS, Crawford RW, Burden SJ, Kunz S, Oldstone MB, Accardi A, Talim B, Muntoni F, Topaloğlu H, Dinçer P, Campbell KP. A dystroglycan mutation associated with limb-girdle muscular dystrophy. N Engl J Med. 2011;364:939–46.
8. Yoshida-Moriguchi T, Campbell KP. Matriglycan: a novel polysaccharide that links dystroglycan to the basement membrane. Glycobiology. 2015; 25:702–13.
9. Godfrey C, Foley AR, Clement E, Muntoni F. Dystroglycanopathies: coming into focus. Curr Opin Genet Dev. 2011;21:278–85.
10. Grewal PK, Hewitt JE. Mutation of Large, which encodes a putative glycosyltransferase, in an animal model of muscular dystrophy. Biochim Biophys Acta. 2002;1573:216–24.
11. Longman C, Brockington M, Torelli S, Jimenez-Mallebrera C, Kennedy C, Khalil N, Feng L, Saran RK, Voit T, Merlini L, Sewry CA, Brown SC, Muntoni F. Mutations in the human LARGE gene cause MDC1D, a novel form of congenital muscular dystrophy with severe mental retardation and abnormal glycosylation of alpha-dystroglycan. Hum Mol Genet. 2003;12:2853–61.
12. van Reeuwijk J, Grewal PK, Salih MA, Beltrán-Valero de Bernabé D, JM ML, Michielse CB, Herrmann R, Hewitt JE, Steinbrecher A, Seidahmed MZ, Shaheed MM, Abomelha A, Brunner HG, van Bokhoven H, Voit T. Intragenic deletion in the LARGE gene causes Walker-Warburg syndrome. Hum Genet. 2007;121:685–90.
13. Grewal PK, Holzfeind PJ, Bittner RE, Hewitt JE. Mutant glycosyltransferase and altered glycosylation of alpha-dystroglycan in the myodystrophy mouse. Nat Genet. 2001;28:151–4.
14. Inamori K, Yoshida-Moriguchi T, Hara Y, Anderson ME, Yu L, Campbell KP. Dystroglycan function requires xylosyl- and glucuronyltransferase activities of LARGE. Science. 2012;335:93–6.
15. Hara Y, Kanagawa M, Kunz S, Yoshida-Moriguchi T, Satz JS, Kobayashi YM, Zhu Z, Burden SJ, Oldstone MB, Campbell KP. Like-acetylglucosaminyltransferase (LARGE)-dependent modification of dystroglycan at Thr-317/319 is required for laminin binding and arenavirus infection. Proc Natl Acad Sci U S A. 2011;108:17426–31.
16. Yoshida-Moriguchi T, Yu L, Stalnaker SH, Davis S, Kunz S, Madson M, Oldstone MB, Schachter H, Wells L, Campbell KP. O-mannosyl phosphorylation of alpha-dystroglycan is required for laminin binding. Science. 2010;327:88–92.
17. Barresi R, Michele DE, Kanagawa M, Harper HA, Dovico SA, Satz JS, Moore SA, Zhang W, Schachter H, Dumanski JP, Cohn RD, Nishino I, Campbell KP. LARGE can functionally bypass α-dystroglycan glycosylation defects in distinct congenital muscular dystrophies. Nature Med. 2004;10:696–703.
18. Sato S, Omori Y, Katoh K, Kondo M, Kanagawa M, Miyata K, Funabiki K, Koyasu T, Kajimura N, Miyoshi T, Sawai H, Kobayashi K, Tani A, Toda T, Usukura J, Tano Y, Fujikado T, Furukawa T. Pikachurin, a dystroglycan ligand, is essential for photoreceptor ribbon synapse formation. Nature Neurosci. 2008;11:923–31.
19. Willer T, Valero MC, Tanner W, Cruces J, Strahl S. O-mannosyl glycans: from yeast to novel associations with human disease. Cur Opin Struct Biol. 2003;13:621–30.

20. Goddeeris MM, Wu B, Venzke D, Yoshida-Moriguchi T, Saito F, Matsumura K, Moore SA, Campbell KP. LARGE glycans on dystroglycan function as a tunable matrix scaffold to prevent dystrophy. Nature. 2013;503:136–40.
21. Kanagawa M, Nishimoto A, Chiyonobu T, Takeda S, Miyagoe-Suzuki Y, Wang F, Fujikake N, Taniguchi M, Lu Z, Tachikawa M, Nagai Y, Tashiro F, Miyazaki J, Tajima Y, Takeda S, Endo T, Kobayashi K, Campbell KP, Toda T. Residual laminin-binding activity and enhanced dystroglycan glycosylation by LARGE in novel model mice to dystroglycanopathy. Hum Mol Genet. 2009;18:621–31.
22. Vannoy CH, Xu L, Keramaris E, Lu P, Xiao X, Lu QL. Adeno-associated virus-mediated overexpression of LARGE rescues α-dystroglycan function in dystrophic mice with mutations in the fukutin-related protein. Hum Gene Ther Method. 2014;25:187–96.
23. Yu M, He Y, Wang K, Zhang P, Zhang S, Hu H. Adeno-associated viral-mediated LARGE gene therapy rescues the muscular dystrophic phenotype in mouse models of dystroglycanopathy. Hum Gene Ther. 2013;24:317–30.
24. Ohtsuka Y, Kanagawa M, Yu CC, Ito C, Chiyo T, Kobayashi K, Okada T, Takeda S, Toda T. Fukutin is prerequisite to ameliorate muscular dystrophic phenotype by myofiber-selective LARGE expression. Sci Rep. 2015;5:8316.
25. Jimenez-Mallebrera C, Torelli S, Feng L, Kim J, Godfrey C, Clement E, Mein R, Abbs S, Brown SC, Campbell KP, Kröger S, Talim B, Topaloglu H, Quinlivan R, Roper H, Childs AM, Kinali M, Sewry CA, Muntoni F. A comparative study of alpha-dystroglycan glycosylation in dystroglycanopathies suggests that the hypoglycosylation of alpha-dystroglycan does not consistently correlate with clinical severity. Brain Pathol. 2009;19:596–611.
26. Brown SC, Torelli S, Brockington M, Yuva Y, Jimenez C, Feng L, Anderson L, Ugo I, Kroger S, Bushby K, Voit T, Sewry C, Muntoni F. Abnormalities in alpha-dystroglycan expression in MDC1C and LGMD2I muscular dystrophies. Am J Pathol. 2004;164:727–37.
27. Ohlendieck K, Campbell KP. Dystrophin-associated proteins are greatly reduced in skeletal muscle from mdx mice. J Cell Biol. 1991;115:1685–94.
28. Pereira CC, Kiyomoto BH, Cardoso R, Oliveira AS. Duchenne muscular dystrophy: alpha-dystroglycan immunoexpression in skeletal muscle and cognitive performance. Arq Neuropsiquiatr. 2005;63:984–9.
29. Balci-Hayta B, Talim B, Topaloglu H, Kale G, Dincer P. Reduction of *LARGE* expression in different types of muscular dystrophies other than dystroglycanopathy. Neuromuscul Disord. 2013;23(9–10):p780.
30. Ervasti JM, Burwell AL, Geissler AL. Tissue-specific heterogeneity in alphadystroglycan sialoglycosylation. Skeletal muscle alpha-dystroglycan is a latent receptor for Vicia villosa agglutinin b4 masked by sialic acid modification. J Biol Chem. 1997;272:22315–21.

27

Myasthenia gravis following human papillomavirus vaccination

Ji Yeon Chung[1†], Seung Jae Lee[2†], Byoung-Soo Shin[3,4] and Hyun Goo Kang[3,4*]

Abstract

Background: Myasthenia gravis (MG), an autoimmune neuromuscular disorder, occurs owing to autoantibodies against acetylcholine receptors. MG symptoms can be triggered by various vaccines. Many studies have evaluated the safety and adverse events of the human papillomavirus (HPV) vaccine. Here, we present a life-threatening case of ocular and bulbar MG symptoms after HPV vaccination and a brief literature review.

Case presentation: A 23-year-old woman presented with binocular diplopia, ptosis, dysarthria, and dysphagia, which occurred on the 3rd day after the second HPV vaccine administration. She was diagnosed with MG based on history, clinical features, and test results. Her symptoms deteriorated on the 3rd day after admission, and she was transferred to the intensive care unit with mechanical ventilation. On the 7th day after admission, due to discomfort in the right chest, pulmonary embolism was suspected. A tracheostomy was performed on the 14th day of mechanical ventilation. In the 4th week, the tracheostomy tube was removed; all symptoms had completely resolved at discharge. She was followed up for 5 months without recurrence or further treatment.

Conclusion: HPV vaccination may cause MG owing to unexpected abnormal autoimmune responses. Additional studies are needed to clarify the possible causal relationship between the HPV vaccine and neurological complications and to evaluate the safety of the vaccine.

Keywords: Adverse event, Human papillomavirus vaccine, Myasthenia gravis, Myasthenia gravis crisis, Vaccination

Background

Myasthenia gravis (MG) is an autoimmune disease that causes a neuromuscular junction disorder owing to blockage of the nicotinic acetylcholine receptor (AChR). MG may be associated with autoimmune reactions, such as autoantibodies and autoimmune responses against AChR [1]. Furthermore, MG is related to thymus disorders and other autoimmune diseases [2]. The human papillomavirus (HPV) vaccination was developed to prevent cervical cancer and is recommended for female individuals aged 9–26 years. In South Korea, bi- and quad-rivalent vaccines have been used; however, since 2016, the nine-valent vaccine has been used, with no serious adverse effects reported to date. Here, we present a case of MG after HPV nine-valent vaccination in a patient whose condition rapidly progressed to MG.

* Correspondence: hgkang@jbnu.ac.kr
†Ji Yeon Chung and Seung Jae Lee contributed equally to this work.
3Department of Neurology, Chonbuk National University School of Medicine, Jeonju 54896, Republic of Korea
4Department of Neurology & Research Institute of Clinical Medicine of Chonbuk National University - Biomedical Research Institute of Chonbuk National University Hospital, 20 Geonji-ro, Deokjin-gu, Jeonju-si, Jeonbuk-do 54907, South Korea
Full list of author information is available at the end of the article

Case presentation

A 23-year-old woman with binocular vertical diplopia, bilateral ptosis (which worsened with left and down gazing), dysarthria, and dysphagia visited the outpatient department. She had received a primary HPV nine-valent vaccination 2 months prior and a second vaccination 5 days before the visit. The symptoms occurred on the 3rd day after the second vaccination. The muscular strength of her upper and lower extremities was normal, and the deep tendon reflex of both sides was normal. Her ptosis and diplopia temporarily improved with an ice pack and pyridostigmine test. The repetitive nerve stimulation (RNS) did not reveal a significant decrement in deltoid, abductor digiti minimi, flexor carpi, and orbicularis oculi muscles. The serum AChR antibody titer was 1.66 nmol/L. Other autoimmune disease tests, including rheumatoid factor and antinuclear antibody, were negative. A thyroid function test was normal, and no thymus abnormality was observed on chest computed tomography (CT).

She was diagnosed with MG, and pyridostigmine oral administration and high-dose intravenous steroid therapy were initiated. Her dyspnea became more severe on the 2nd day after admission, and oxygen saturation decreased; therefore, she received intravenous immunoglobulin therapy. Afterward, spontaneous breathing became more difficult, and the dysphagia and bilateral ptosis worsened. These symptoms were determined to demonstrate an MG crisis, and mechanical ventilation was initiated after endotracheal intubation (Fig. 1). Although muscle strength was normal at admission, the extension power of the distal fingers decreased.

On the 7th day after admission, sudden tachycardia was observed, the patient experienced persistent pressure in the right chest, and oxygen saturation decreased during mechanical ventilation. Chest CT revealed a low-density-filling defect of the pulmonary artery in the right lower lobe. Ischemic changes in the lung parenchyma and an increased D-dimer level (2199 ng/mL) were also observed. Therefore, heparin treatment was initiated owing to the possibility of pulmonary embolism. The D-dimer level decreased to within the normal range (99 ng/mL) in the 2nd week after the increase.

In the 4th week of hospitalization, the symptoms further improved such that she could walk and the AChR antibody titer decreased (0.99 nmol/L). However, right eye ptosis and binocular vertical diplopia persisted. She was discharged after the dysphagia had completely resolved. The AchR antibody titer was normal (0.05 nmol/L) at discharge. The patient has returned to daily life without symptom recurrence or further treatment.

Discussion

The HPV vaccination was first approved in 2006 for preventing cervical cancer. However, in Japan, serious adverse events, such as Guillain-Barré syndrome, acute disseminated encephalomyelitis, postural orthostatic tachycardia syndrome, and complex regional pain syndrome have been reported in patients receiving the HPV vaccination, which were suspected to be associated with the HPV vaccination [3]. The causal relationship between these adverse events and HPV vaccination has not yet been elucidated, and the underlying pathogenesis remains unclear. Studies in Japan have hypothesized that an antibody that cross-reacts with autonomic ganglia, neurons, and cardiac proteins or ß1/2-adrenergic and M2/3 muscarinic receptors could be synthesized owing to the epitope of the HPV vaccination [4], and that cytotoxic T cells could be

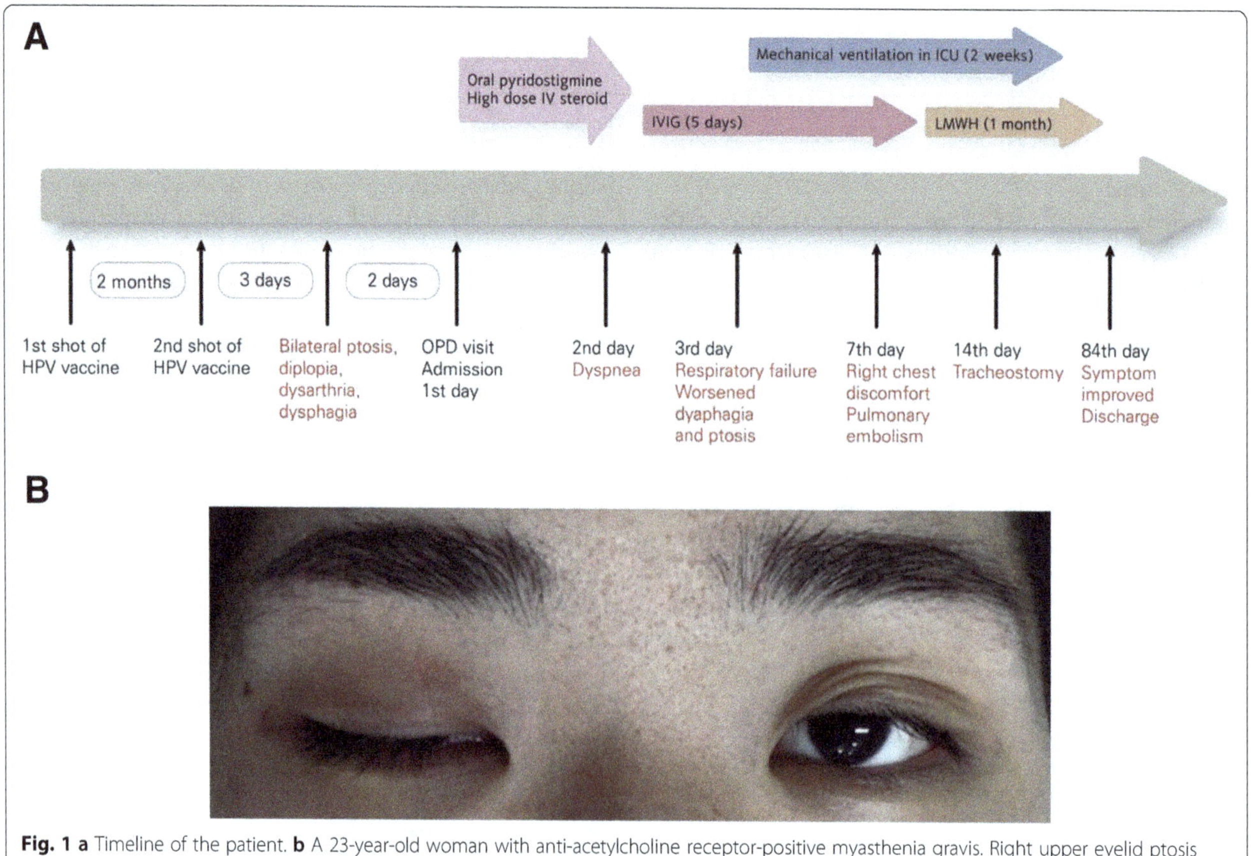

Fig. 1 a Timeline of the patient. **b** A 23-year-old woman with anti-acetylcholine receptor-positive myasthenia gravis. Right upper eyelid ptosis worsened to almost complete closure, and respiratory muscle weakness resulted in intubation and mechanical ventilation on hospital day 3

Table 1 Case reports of new-onset myasthenia gravis after vaccination

Author	Age/Sex	Vaccine Type	Time to onset	Initial symptoms	Treatment	Prognosis (Time to recovery)	Thymoma	MGFA Class
Biron [9]	48/M	HBV	1 mo after 2nd shot	Ocular	Edrophonium,, plasma exchange, cyclophosphamide, steroid	Improved. (After 30 PE)	+	I
Bahri [10]	46/F	HBV	1mo after 2nd shot	Ocular, bulbar	Pyridostigmine, steroid	Improved (Not mentioned)	+	IIb
Takizawa [8]	69/M	BCG	6 wks	Ocular	Pyridostigmine	Improved (70 days)	-	IIa
Our case	23/F	HPV	3 d after 2nd shot	Ocular, bulbar	Pyridostigmine, steroid, IVIG	Improved (84 days)	-	V

Mo months, *d* days, *HBV* hepatitis B vaccine, *BCG* Bacillus Calmette-Guerin, *HPV* human papillomavirus, *IVIG* intravenous immunoglobulin, *MGFA* myasthenia gravis foundation of America clinical classification

activated by stimulating the antibody production by binding to acetylcholine receptors [5]. A recent study reported a complex involving HPV and p53 pro-apoptotic tumor suppressor, and the inhibitory enzyme is degraded upon complex formation [6]. Viral oncoprotein E6 can recognize a short leucine-rich consensus sequence within ligase E6AP, and this complex finally degrades p53. The E6 domain has two zinc ions, which maintain structural features for the interactions. Non-specific interactions of HPV with AChR may result in the complex formation and unexpected side effects of HPV, which need to be investigated.

Our patient had no problems with the primary HPV vaccination but exhibited acute bilateral ptosis, dysarthria, and dysphagia on the 3rd day after the second vaccination. She also experienced acute respiratory failure and pulmonary embolism. In our case, blood stasis owing to immobilization while in the intensive care unit could be a risk factor for pulmonary embolism. However, because venous thromboembolism was reported as an adverse event of the HPV vaccination [7], pulmonary embolism could occur owing to the HPV vaccination.

In our patient, MG may have been induced by the HPV vaccination as an adverse event or incidentally without an association between the two factors. Therefore, it may be difficult to suggest a strong relationship between HPV vaccination and MG outbreak. However, previous studies have reported MG occurrence after inoculation with other vaccines [8–10], suggesting an association between symptoms and changes in immune responses in the body following vaccination. This study summarized the studies that reported the first occurrence of MG after vaccinations based on the available literature (Table 1). Additionally, there is no absolute contraindication to the use of the HPV vaccination. Our patient developed MG after receiving the nine-valent vaccine, and the relative risk of the nine-valent vaccine is unclear.

This case report implies that the HPV vaccination may cause MG. Other neurological manifestations may occur owing to unexpected abnormal autoimmune responses such as autonomic dysfunction and pain. It is important to inform patients prior to inoculation and observe the occurrence of abnormal symptoms. Moreover, it is critical to intervene promptly and treat the patient when fatal deterioration is observed. We believe that additional studies are needed to assess the possible causal relationship between the HPV vaccine and neurological complications and to evaluate the safety of the vaccine.

Abbreviations

AChR: Acetylcholine receptor; CT: Computed tomography; HPV: Human papillomavirus; MG: Myasthenia gravis

Acknowledgements

Not applicable.

Funding

This research was supported by the Basic Science Research Program through the National Research Foundation of Korea funded by the Ministry of Education (2017R1A1A03015876) and Ministry of Science and ICT (2017R1C1B5017293). The funders had no role in study design, data collection and analysis, decision to publish, or preparation of the manuscript.

Authors' contributions

JYC and HGK participated the design of this research. JYC, SJL, BSS and HGK collected and analyzed the raw clinical data. BSS, SJL, and HGK carried out computational studies and wrote the manuscript. JYC and SJL contributed equally to this work as co-first authors. All authors have read and approved the final manuscript.

Competing interests

The authors declare no conflicts of interest with respect to the research, authorship, funding, and/or publication of this article.

Author details

[1]Department of Neurology, Chosun University School of Medicine, Gwangju 61453, Republic of Korea. [2]Institute for Molecular Biology and Genetics and Department of Chemistry, Chonbuk National University, Jeonju 54896, Republic of Korea. [3]Department of Neurology, Chonbuk National University School of Medicine, Jeonju 54896, Republic of Korea. [4]Department of Neurology & Research Institute of Clinical Medicine of Chonbuk National University - Biomedical Research Institute of Chonbuk National University Hospital, 20 Geonji-ro, Deokjin-gu, Jeonju-si, Jeonbuk-do 54907, South Korea.

References

1. Carr AS, Cardwell CR, McCarron PO, McConville J. A systematic review of population based epidemiological studies in myasthenia gravis. BMC Neurol. 2010;18(10):46.
2. Oosterhuis HJ. The natural course of myasthenia gravis. J Neurol Neurosurg Psychiatry. 1989;52(10):1121–7.
3. Kinoshita T, Abe RT, Hineno A, Tsunekawa K, Nakane S, Ikeda S. Peripheral sympathetic nerve dysfunction in adolescent Japanese girls following immunization with the human papillomavirus vaccine. Intern Med. 2014;53: 2185–200.
4. Pinto LA, Castle PE, Roden RB, Harro CD, Lowy DR, Schiller JT, et al. HPV-16 L1 VLP vaccine elicits a broad-spectrum of cytokine responses in whole blood. Vaccine. 2005;23:3555–64.
5. Weber JS, Kahler KC, Hauschild A. Management of immune-related adverse events and kinetics of response with iplimumab. J Clin Oncol. 2012;30:2691–7.
6. Martinez-Zapien D, Ruiz FX, Poirson J, Mitschler A, Ramirez J, Forster A, et al. Structure of the E6/E6AP/p53 complex required for HPV-mediated degradation of p53. Nature. 2016;28;529(7587):541–5.
7. Slade BA. Postlicensure safety surveillance for quadrivalent human papillomavirus recombinant vaccine. JAMA. 2009;302(7):750–7.
8. Takizawa T, Kojima M, Suzuki S, Osada T, Kitagawa S, Nakahara J, et al. New onset of myasthenia gravis after intravesical Bacillus Calmette-Guerin: a case report and literature review. Medicine (Baltimore). 2017;96(46):e8757.
9. Stübgen JP. Neuromuscular disorders associated with hepatitis B vaccination. J Neurol Sci. 2010;292(1–2):1–4.
10. Louzir B, Othmani S, Battikh R, Ben Abdelhafidh N, Bahri M, Taalouche L, et al. Myasthenia after hepatitis B vaccination. Therapie. 2003;58(4):378–9.

28

Mutation m.15923A>G in the *MT-TT* gene causes mild myopathy – case report of an adult-onset phenotype

Mikko Kärppä[1,2,3], Laura Kytövuori[1,2,3*], Markku Saari[4] and Kari Majamaa[1,2,3]

Abstract

Background: Only five patients have previously been reported to harbor mutations in the *MT-TT* gene encoding mitochondrial tRNA threonine. The m.15923A > G mutation has been found in three severely affected children. One of these patients died within days after birth and two had a phenotype of myoclonic epilepsy with ragged red fibers (MERRF) in early childhood. We have now found the mutation in an adult patient with mild myopathy.

Case presentation: The patient is a 64-year-old Finnish man, who developed bilateral ptosis, diplopia and exercise intolerance in his fifties. Family history was unremarkable. Muscle histology showed cytochrome c-oxidase (COX) negative and ragged red fibres. The m.15923A > G mutation heteroplasmy was 33% in the skeletal muscle and 2% in buccal epithelial cells. The mutation was undetectable in the blood. Single-fibre analysis was performed and COX-negative fibres had a substantially higher heteroplasmy of 92%, than the normal fibres in which it was 43%.

Conclusions: We report the fourth patient with m. 15923A > G and with a remarkably milder phenotype than the previous three patients. Our findings and recent biochemical studies suggest that the mutation m.15923A > G is a definite disease-causing mutation. Our results also suggest that heteroplasmy of the m.15923A > G mutation correlates with the severity of the phenotype. This study expands the catalog of the phenotypes caused by mutations in mtDNA.

Keywords: Case report, Mitochondrial diseases, Mitochondrial $tRNA^{Thr}$, Neuromuscular disorders, Single-fibre analysis

Background

Mutations in mitochondrial DNA (mtDNA) were found to cause diseases for the first time in 1988 [1, 2], and since then, the number of new mutations and associated phenotypes has continuously increased. MtDNA contains 22 tRNAs, 2 rRNAs and 13 protein-coding genes and disease-causing mutations have been reported in all of them. Mitochondrial tRNA mutations are a well-established cause of mitochondrial disorder, and most of the patients carry the m.3243A > G mutation in *MT-TL1*. The prevalence of mt-tRNA mutations has been estimated to be 4.3 per 100,000 in U.K. [3]. Among these mutations, the prevalence of m.3243A > G solely has been reported to be 3.5 per 100,000. Interestingly, the prevalence is several fold, 16.3 per 100,000, in Finland [4].

While many tRNA genes seem to be mutational hotspots in patients with mitochondrial disorder, the mitochondrially encoded tRNA threonine (*MT-TT*) has been reported to be mutated in five patients only [5–10]. The m.15923A > G has previously been found in three patients; an infant dying from multisystem failure at the age of 2.5 days [5, 6], and two children with myoclonic epilepsy and ragged-red fibers (MERRF) syndrome [8, 10]. We report here the fourth patient with m.15923A > G and the first with an adult-onset phenotype.

Case presentation

Patient

The patient was a 64-year-old man, who had bilateral ptosis, diplopia and exercise intolerance. His early development had been normal and currently he had no regular medication. Ocular symptoms had started to develop at the age of 54 years, the right eye had been operated

* Correspondence: laura.kytovuori@oulu.fi
[1]Research Unit of Clinical Neuroscience, University of Oulu, P.O. Box 5000, FI-90014 Oulu, Finland
[2]Medical Research Center Oulu, Oulu University Hospital and University of Oulu, Oulu, Finland
Full list of author information is available at the end of the article

due to squint at the age of 58 years and ptosis surgery had been performed on the right at the age of 63 years. He had right clubfoot, which had been regarded as a complication of vaccination at the age of two years. There was muscle atrophy in the right leg and the leg movements were restricted. His parents, his seven siblings and his son were healthy. Patient's maternal uncle had ocular symptoms and, interestingly, uncle's granddaughter had ptosis and a 7.5 kb deletion in mtDNA.

On neurological examination, the patient limped slightly because of the right clubfoot. Ptosis was moderate on the right and mild on the left. Vertical gaze paresis and a slight restriction in horizontal movements was noted in both eyes. Otherwise, muscle examination was normal. Ankle reflexes were absent, while other tendon reflexes were normal.

Routine laboratory values including creatine kinase were normal. Blood lactate was 1.16 mmol/l (reference values 0.33–1.33 mmol/l) and pyruvate was 84 µmol/l (reference values 30–80 µmol/l). Brain MRI showed minimal nonspecific white matter lesions in the frontal lobe. Polyphasic units in frontal and nasal muscles were found in electromyography. Myasthenia gravis was first diagnosed at the age of 60 years and pyridostigmine was initiated. Because the treatment did not alleviate symptoms and all myasthenia studies were negative, treatment was discontinued. Lambert-Eaton myasthenic syndrome was excluded and *PABP2* gene test for repeat expansion causing dominantly inherited oculopharyngeal muscle dystrophy was negative.

Muscle biopsy from *vastus lateralis* was compatible with mitochondrial myopathy (Fig. 1). Ten percent of the muscle fibers were COX-negative and few RRFs were found as well. Ultrastructural examination revealed an increased number of mitochondria and changes in the internal structure of mitochondria.

Molecular methods and muscle histology

DNA of blood leucocytes and buccal epithelial cells was extracted by using QIAamp DNA Blood Mini Kit (QIAGEN, Hilden, Germany) and that of muscle by using Wizard® Genomic DNA purification kit (Promega Corporation, Madison, WI). Mitochondrial DNA was amplified and sequenced in twelve overlapping fragments. The amplification reactions were done by using *Phire Hot Start II* DNA polymerase (Thermo Fisher Scientific, Waltham, MA, U.S.A.) according to the provided protocol. Sequencing was carried out at Biocenter Oulu sequencing core facility.

The muscle sample for histological staining was fresh-frozen and cryostat sections (5 µm) were stained with routine histochemical techniques [11]. The stainings included hematoxylin and eosin and combined cytochrome c-oxidase and succinate dehydrogenase (COX-SDH). Laser-capture microdissection of COX-SDH stained frozen sections was done using Carl Zeiss P.A.L.M. microscope (Microlaser Technologies GmbH, Bernried, Germany) in Turku Centre for Biotechnology, University of Turku and Åbo Akademi University. Ten COX-negative and ten COX-positive fibers were collected into Carl Zeiss AdhesiveCap tubes (Carl Zeiss Gmbh, Göttingen, Germany) and DNA was released incubating fibers 30 min in 65 °C in lysis buffer containing 200 mM potassium hydroxide and 50 mM dithiothreitol followed by neutralization step with

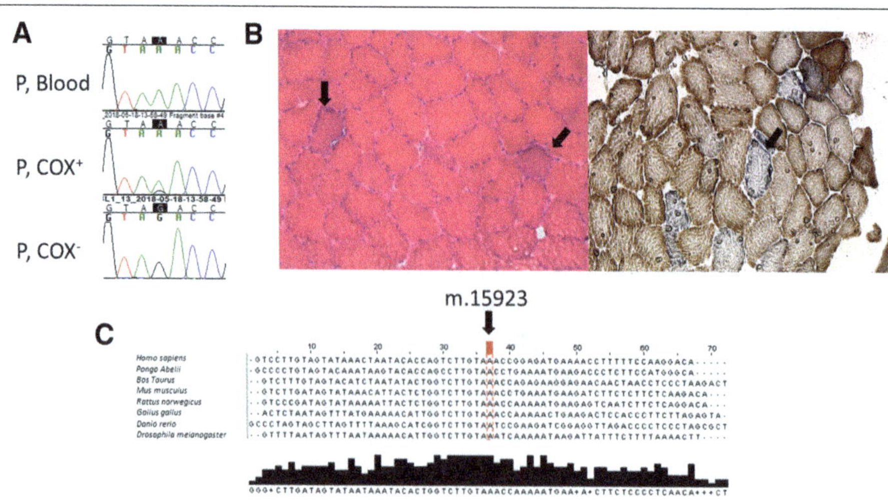

Fig. 1 Mutation m.15923A > G is situated in a conservative position and causes typical mitochondria myopathy. **a** Sequence chromatograms showing variable heteroplasmy. P, patient; COX$^+$, biochemically normal fibers; COX$^-$, cytochrome c-oxidase negative fibers. **b** Histology stainings. Left panel: Hematoxylin & eosin staining showing ragged red fibers. Right panel: Cytochrome c-oxidase staining showing COX-negative (blue) fibers. Arrows denote biochemically abnormal fibers. **c** Clustal Omega [15] alingnment for multiple sequences showing complete conservation between species

900 mM Tris-HCl, pH 8.3. Amplification was carried out using Phusion High-Fidelity DNA polymerase (Thermo Fisher Scientific). Heteroplasmy was determined by cloning using CloneJET PCR Cloning Kit with blunt-end cloning protocol and DH5α competent cells (Thermo Fisher Scientific). Colony screening was done by using FastDigest *XmiI* (Thermo Fisher Scientific). XL-PCR for whole mtDNA amplification was carried out using Phusion High-Fidelity DNA polymerase with GC Buffer according to the original protocol (Thermo Fisher Scientific).

We found the m.15923A > G mutation in *MT-TT* in the skeletal muscle of the patient. The heteroplasmy was determined and, interestingly, the mutation was undetectable in the blood of the patient, while it was present with a 33% heteroplasmy in the skeletal muscle and with 2% heteroplasmy in the buccal mucosa. In

Table 1 Patients harboring the m.15923A > G mutation in the *MT-TT* gene

	Patient 1	Patient 2	Patient 3	Patient 4
Reference	[5, 6]	[8]	[10]	present study
Age at onset	Day 2	Childhood	6 years	54 years
Age at the latest examination	Died at the age of 56 h	19 years	15 years	64 years
Hypoglycemia	yes	–	–	–
Lactic acidosis	yes	yes	yes	–
Multisystem failure	yes	–	–	–
Short stature	–	–	yes	–
Hearing impairment	–	yes	yes	Age-related
Exercise intolerance	–	yes	–	yes
Muscle weakness	–	yes	–	yes
Generalized seizures	–	yes	yes	–
Myoclonic seizures	–	yes	yes	–
Cognitive delay	–	yes	–	–
Migraine	–	yes	yes	–
Ataxia	–	yes	–	–
Dysmetry	–	yes	–	–
Dysarthria	–	yes	–	–
Vomiting	–	yes	–	–
Retinitis pigmentosa	–	yes	yes	–
Ptosis	–	–	–	yes
Diplopia	–	–	–	yes
MRI	–	Cortical and cerebellar atrophy	Basal ganglia calcifications	Nonspecific white matter lesions in frontal lobe
Family history	Several miscarriages of the mother	Deafness, maternal aunt	Negative	Nonspesific
RRF	n.a.	yes	yes	yes
COX-negative	n.a.	yes	yes	yes
Other	n.a.	Mitochondrial aggregates with abnormal structure	n.a.	Mitochondrial aggregates with abnormal structure
Functional studies	Decreased activity of complexes III and IV	Complex IV normal	Defect in tRNA modification	COX-negative fibres had higher mutation heteroplasmy than normal fibres
Heteroplasmy				
Blood	n.a.	10%	n.a.	< 1%[a]
Skeletal muscle	n.a.	78%	> 95%[b]	33%
Buccal epithelium	n.a.	n.a.	n.a.	2%

RRF Ragged red fibres, *COX* Cytochrome c-oxidase, *n.a.*, Not analyzed
[a]Undetectable by cloning, 100 colonies
[b]The mutation was reported to be homoplasmic in Sanger sequencing

pooled COX-negative fibers, the heteroplasmy was 92% while it was 43% in biochemically normal fibers. The investigation of mtDNA deletions remained negative.

Discussion and conclusions

We found the m.15923A > G mutation in an adult patient with ptosis and exercise intolerance. The pathogenicity of the mutation has been unclear, because the mutation has been found only in three patients before our study. Recent studies have shown, however, that m.15923A > G affects post-translational modification of tRNA threonine [10, 12]. The nucleotide in position 38 (m.15923A) has been shown to be crucial in N^6-threonylcarbamoyladenosine (t^6A) modification that occurs in position 37, and decreased level of t^6A-modified tRNA has been detected in patient cell lines [10]. In addition, according to the Yarham scoring [13], the m.15923A > G is classified as definitely pathogenic. The score includes evaluation of nucleotide site conservation, heteroplasmy and mutation segregation with disease, and evidence of biochemical defect from single-fiber studies and mitochondrial complex activity measurements [13].

Three children harboring m.15923A > G have been reported to suffer from severe mitochondrial disorder (Table 1) [5, 6, 10]. Patient 1 was a girl who died 2.5 after birth of a fatal cardiopulmonary arrest [5, 6]. The mother had a history of five miscarriages and a delivery of a boy who died within two days. The two pregnancies and deliveries and the first 24 h of the infants had been normal. The mutation was heteroplasmic in the girl, but samples were not available from her deceased brother. Patient 2 was a girl with symptoms from early childhood [8]. The patient had exercise intolerance, vomiting and generalized seizures during her early childhood. She developed deafness, migraine, retinitis pigmentosa, and cognitive delay. Her symptoms were progressive. Mutation heteroplasmy was 78% in the muscle, 10% in the blood and 18% in buccal mucosa. Patient 3 was a 15-year-old girl with bilateral hearing impairment as the first manifestation at the age of 6 years [10]. At the time of the latest clinical examination, she had retinitis pigmentosa, lactic acidosis, myoclonic epilepsy, proteinuria and migraine suggesting a MERRF syndrome.

Decreased activity of OXPHOS complexes is a common finding in patients with mitochondrial disorder. The activity of complexes III and IV have been reported to be decreased in the muscle, liver and kidney of patient 1 [5, 6], whereas the activity of complex IV was normal in the muscle of patient 2 with mutation heteroplasmy of 78% [8]. Unfortunately, lack of remaining muscle prevented us from carrying out these analyses. However, previous studies and our single-fibre analysis suggest that the heteroplasmy required to cause an OXPHOS defect is very high and, therefore, the heteroplasmy of 33% in our patient may not be sufficient to cause the defect.

Pathogenic mutations in *MT-TT* are rare. In addition to m.15923A > G in the three patients, two other mutations have been found previously in single patients [5–10]. The m.15915A > G mutation has been found in a 16-year-old boy, whose symptoms started at the age of 8 years [7]. He had muscle weakness, hearing impairment, seizures, ptosis, intellectual disability, growth failure, and mitochondrial myopathy in muscle histology. The m.15933G > A mutation has been found in an adult patient, who had exercise-induced muscle weakness, myalgia, dysphagia and ptosis with mitochondrial myopathy in the skeletal muscle [9].

We conclude that the pathogenicity of the m.15923A > G mutation is now confirmed on the basis of the following facts: The mutation has been found in three severely affected children [5, 6, 8] and we describe the first adult patient harboring the mutation and with a mild mitochondrial disorder. The mutation has not been reported in population controls or listed among polymorphisms in MITOMAP database [14]. Mutation heteroplasmy has been shown to be high in the children with fatal mitochondrial disorder, while it was lower in our patient with a milder phenotype. COX-negative and ragged red fibers have been found in the skeletal muscle in all the four patients and decreased OXPHOS enzyme activities have been reported in the most severely affected infant. Differences in mutation load between biochemically deficient and normal fibers in our study further confirm the functional consequences of the mutation.

Abbreviations

COX: Cytochrome c-oxidase; mtDNA: Mitochondrial DNA; *MT-TT*: Mitochondrialally encoded transferRNA threonine; OXPHOS: Oxidative phosphorylation

Acknowledgements

The authors gratefully acknowledge the expert technical assistance of Ms. Anja Heikkinen. Laser capture microdissection was performed at the Cell Imaging Core, Turku Centre for Biotechnology, University of Turku and Åbo Akademi University. The Cell Imaging Core is supported by Biocenter Finland infrastructure.

Funding

The study was supported by grants from the Sigrid Juselius Foundation, Medical Research Center, University of Oulu and Oulu University Hospital, and State research funding from Oulu University Hospital.

Authors' contributions

MK performed clinical examinations. LK carried out molecular analyses and wrote the first draft of the manuscript. MS designed and conducted the LCM protocol. KM participated in designing the project, and all investigations occurred under his supervision. All authors have revised the manuscript and approved the manuscript for submission.

Competing interests

The authors declare that they have no competing interests.

Author details

[1]Research Unit of Clinical Neuroscience, University of Oulu, P.O. Box 5000, FI-90014 Oulu, Finland. [2]Medical Research Center Oulu, Oulu University Hospital and University of Oulu, Oulu, Finland. [3]Department of Neurology, Oulu University Hospital, P.O. Box 20, FI-90029 OYS Oulu, Finland. [4]Turku Centre for Biotechnology, Cell Imaging Core, University of Turku, FI-20520 Turku, Finland.

References

1. Zeviani MI, Moraes CT, DiMauro S, Nakase H, Bonilla E, Schon EA, et al. Deletions of mitochondrial DNA in Kearns-Sayre syndrome. Neurology. 1988; 38:1339–46.
2. Wallace DC, Singh G, Lott MT, Hodge JA, Schurr TG, Lezza AM, et al. Mitochondrial DNA mutation associated with Leber's hereditary optic neuropathy. Science. 1988;242:1427–30.
3. Gorman GS, Schaefer AM, Ng Y, Gomez N, Blakely EL, Alston CL, et al. Prevalence of nuclear and mitochondrial DNA mutations related to adult mitochondrial disease. Ann Neurol. 2015;77:753–9.
4. Majamaa K, Moilanen JS, Uimonen S, Remes AM, Salmela PI, Kärppä M, et al. Epidemiology of A3243G, the mutation for mitochondrial encephalomyopathy, lactic acidosis, and strokelike episodes: prevalence of the mutation in an adult population. Am J Hum Genet. 1998;63:447–54.
5. Yoon KL, Aprille JR, Ernst SG. Mitochondrial tRNAThr mutation in fatal infantile respiratory enzyme deficiency. Biochem Biophys Res Commun. 1991;176:1112–5.
6. Yoon KL, Ernst SG, Rasmussen C, Dooling EC, Aprille JR. Mitochondrial disorder associated with newborn cardiopulmonary arrest. Pediatr Res. 1993; 33:433–40.
7. Nishino I, Seki A, Maegaki Y, Takeshita K, Horai S, Nonaka I, et al. A novel mutation in the mitochondrial tRNAThr gene associated with a mitochondrial encephalomyopathy. Biochem Biophys Res Commun. 1996;225:180–5.
8. Del Mar O'Callaghan M, Emperador S, Lopez-Gallardo E, Jou C, Bujan N, Montero R, et al. New mitochondrial DNA mutations in tRNA associated with three severe encephalopamyopathic phenotypes: neonatal, infantile, and childhood onset. Neurogenetics. 2012;13:245–50.
9. Soini HK, Vaisanen A, Karppa M, Hinttala R, Kytovuori L, Moilanen JS, et al. A novel MTTT mutation m.15933G>a revealed in analysis of mitochondrial DNA in patients with suspected mitochondrial disease. BMC Med Genet. 2017;18:14.
10. Lin H, Miyauchi K, Harada T, Okita R, Takeshita E, Komaki H, et al. CO_2-sensitive tRNA modification associated with human mitochondrial disease. Nat Commun. 1875;2018:9.
11. Dubowitz V, Sewry C, Oldfors A. Muscle biopsy: a practical approach. 4th edition. London: Saunders, Elsevier; 2006.
12. Wang Y, Zeng QY, Zheng WQ, Ji QQ, Zhou XL, Wang ED. A natural non-Watson-crick base pair in human mitochondrial $tRNA^{Thr}$ causes structural and functional susceptibility to local mutations. Nucleic Acids Res. 2018;46: 4662–76.
13. Yarham JW, Al-Dosary M, Blakely EL, Alston CL, Taylor RW, Elson JL, et al. A comparative analysis approach to determining the pathogenicity of mitochondrial tRNA mutations. Hum Mutat. 2011;32:1319–25.
14. MITOMAP: A human mitochondrial genome database. http://www.mitomap.org, 2018.
15. Sievers F, Wilm A, Dineen D, Gibson TJ, Karplus K, Li W, et al. Fast, scalable generation of high-quality protein multiple sequence alignments using Clustal omega. Mol Syst Biol. 2011;7:539.

29

Validation of a leg movements count and periodic leg movements analysis in a custom polysomnography system

Ambra Stefani, Anna Heidbreder, Heinz Hackner and Birgit Högl*

Abstract

Background: Periodic leg movements (PLM) during sleep (PLMS) are considered strongly related to restless legs syndrome (RLS), and are associated with polymorphisms in RLS risk genes. Various software for automatic analysis of PLMS are available, but only few of them have been validated. Aim of this study was to validate a leg movements count and analysis integrated in a commercially available polysomnography (PSG) system against manual scoring.

Methods: Twenty RLS patients with a PLMS index > 20/h and 20 controls with a PLMS index < 5/h were included. Manual and computerized scoring of leg movements (LM) and PLM was performed according to the standard American Academy of Sleep Medicine (AASM) criteria. LM and PLM indices during sleep and wakefulness, the rate of PLMS associated with respiratory events, intermovement interval and periodicity indices were manually and automatically scored.

Results: The correlation between manual and computerized scoring was high for all investigated parameters (Spearman correlation coefficients 0.751–0.996, $p < 0.001$; intraclass correlation coefficients 0.775–0.999, $p < 0.001$). Bland-Altman plots showed high agreement between manual and automatic analysis.

Conclusions: This study validated an automatic LM count and PLM analysis against the gold standard manual scoring according to AASM criteria. The data demonstrate that the software used in this study has an outstanding performance for computerized LM and PLM scoring, and LM and PLM indices generated with this software can be reliably integrated in the routine PSG report. This automatic analysis is also an excellent tool for research purposes.

Keywords: PLM, Restless legs syndrome, Sleep, PSG, Computerized scoring

Background

Periodic leg movements (PLM) during sleep (PLMS) are present in more than 80% of patients with restless legs syndrome (RLS) [1], represent a supportive diagnostic criterium, and are associated with polymorphism in various RLS risk genes (BTBD9, TOX3/BC034767, MEIS1, MAP2K5/SKOR1, and PTPRD) [2]. They have also been observed in other sleep-related or neurological disorders, such as narcolepsy [3], sleep-related breathing disorders [4], Parkinson's disease [5], multiple system atrophy [6] and REM sleep behaviour disorder [7], as well as in healthy subjects [8, 9].

Although several software programs for automatic detection and analysis of leg movements (LM) during sleep (LMS) have been developed and are commonly used in the clinical polysomnography (PSG) routine and research applications, only few of them have been validated and time-consuming visual detection and manual scoring of PLMS is still considered the gold standard for research purposes.

The aim of this study was to validate a LM detection and PLM analysis program integrated in a commercially available custom PSG system against manual scoring, which could be useful not only for clinical but also for research purposes.

* Correspondence: birgit.ho@i-med.ac.at
Department of Neurology, Medical University of Innsbruck, Anichstrasse 35, Innsbruck A-6020, Austria

Methods

Selection of participants

Routine PSG reports of the Sleep Disorders Unit, Department of Neurology, Innsbruck Medical University were screened to find 20 patients with RLS with an automatic-scored PLMS index higher than 20/h. RLS was diagnosed according to the International RLS Study Group (IRLSSG) criteria [10], based on an urge to move the legs, usually accompanied by unpleasant sensations, which begin or worsen during rest and is relieved by movement, worsen in the evening or night, and is not explained by other conditions. RLS mimics were excluded.

Control subjects were selected among patients without RLS who underwent PSG for other reasons, and had an automatic-scored PLMS index ≤ 5/h.

For both groups, exclusion criteria were an apnea-hypopnea index (AHI) higher than 5/h or the use of a continuous positive airway pressure (CPAP) therapy. RLS treatment did not represent an exclusion criterion.

This study was approved by the local ethic committee of Innsbruck Medical University. All participants granted written informed consent prior to study participation.

Video-PSG

All subjects underwent at least one night of 8-h video-PSG according to the American Academy of Sleep Medicine (AASM) 2012 standards [11]. In case of more nights of PSG, the second night was used for this study, unless technical reasons prevented this.

Video-PSG was recorded on a OSG BrainRT PSG device (OSG 2840 Rumst, Belgium; http://www.osg.be) and consisted of electrooculography, electroencephalography (F3, F4, C3, C4, O1, O2, M1 and M2 electrodes), cardiorespiratory recording [single channel electrocardiography, recording of nasal air flow (thermocouple), nasal pressure cannula, tracheal microphone, thoracic and abdominal respiratory movements (piezo), transcutaneous oxygen saturation], electromyography (EMG) included at least the mental, submental and both anterior tibialis muscles, and time-synchronized digital videography. The video was recorded with an infrared camera (Sony IP Camera ER521P).

Leg movements were recorded using surface electrodes placed longitudinally and symmetrically around the middle of the tibialis anterior muscle, 2–3 cm apart. For scoring of EMG activity, bipolar surface EMG was recorded with the low frequency filter at 50 Hz, the high frequency filter at 300 Hz, and a sampling rate of 1000 Hz. Amplification was set at 10 μV per mm. Impedance of surface EMG electrodes had to be lower than 10 kΩ.

Sleep and LM scoring criteria

Sleep was scored according to American Academy of Sleep Medicine (AASM) criteria [1].

According to the AASM criteria [11], the onset of a leg movement event is defined as the point at which there is an 8 μV increase in EMG voltage above resting EMG; the ending of a leg movement event is defined as the start of a period lasting at least 0.5 s during which the EMG does not exceed 2 μV above resting EMG. Bilateral leg movements separated by less than 5 s between movement onsets are counted as a single leg movement. Leg movements occurring during a period from 0.5 s preceding a respiratory event to 0.5 s following are not scored according to AASM criteria. We performed two separate analyses, one according to AASM and one including also respiratory-related leg movements.

Periodic limb movements (PLM) are defined as repetitive leg movements lasting from 0.5 to 10 s, separated by an intermovement interval (defined as the time between onsets of consecutive leg movements) ranging from 5 to 90 s, organized in series of at least 4 leg movements [11].

The periodicity index, which is an independent measure able to pick up the time structure of LM activity in patients with RLS and PLMS, was calculated as defined by Ferri et al. as the ratio of the number of periodic LM intervals (at least 3, 10–90 s) divided by the total number of intervals found [12].

Description of manual and computerized PLM quantification and analysis

PLMS indices in NREM, REM and total sleep, PLM during wakefulness (PLMW) index, the intermovement interval in NREM, REM and total sleep, and in wakefulness, index of PLMS associated with respiratory events and periodicity index were all scored manually and automatically as explained below, and inserted in a SPSS database for the statistical analysis. The manual scoring was performed first, without running the automatic analysis, blind for the automatic scoring.

Manual quantification of LM and PLM

LM and PLM during sleep and during wakefulness were manually analysed by a trained scorer (AS) according to AASM criteria [1]. All identified leg movements (LM) were tabulated in an excel spread-sheet, and associated to sleep stages manually. The duration of each LM and the interval between two consecutive LM were measured. Indices were calculated for PLMS during NREM, REM and total sleep, and for PLMW. Intermovement intervals for LMS and PLMS during NREM, REM and total sleep, as well as LM during wakefulness (LMW) and PLMW, were scored. The periodicity index according to Ferri et al. was also calculated [12].

PLMS associated with respiratory events were excluded from the analysis according to the AASM standard criteria [11]. All PLMS were however recorded in the excel spread-sheet, including informations about association or not with respiratory events, so that separate analysis including or excluding PLMS associated with respiratory events were possible. Indices of PLMS associated with respiratory events per hour of total sleep time were separately calculated.

Computerized scoring algorithm for PLM detection and analysis

The computerized software algorithm for detection and analysis of PLM is a feature of the Brain RT PSG system by OSG (2840 Rumst, Belgium; http://www.osg.be). The algorithm was developed by OSG and adjusted in several site visits and steps upon author's request, to automatically detect PLM according to AASM criteria.

For this study, LMS and PLMS indices in NREM, REM and total sleep, LMW and PLMW index, the intermovement interval in NREM, REM and total sleep, and in wakefulness were automatically calculated. In addition, the analysis was run again changing the settings in order to include also PLMS associated with respiratory events, and indices of PLMS associated with respiratory events per hour of total sleep time were automatically scored. No artefact correction was performed.

The analysis was then run changing in the settings the criterion for the interval between two consecutive PLMS from 5–90 s to 10–90 s, in order to be able to automatically calculate the periodicity index [12].

The settings of the software for detection and analysis of LM are shown in Additional file 1: Figure S1, and an example of the computerized detection of PLM is shown in Additional file 2: Figure S2.

Event per event analysis

An event per event analysis was performed for each LM. All LM detected by both manual and computerized analysis were counted as matched in case of overlap between a manually detected LM and at least half of the automatically detected LM. The LMs detected only manually, as well as those detected only by computerized analysis, were also counted. The sensitivity of the computerized detection was calculated as the percentage of manually scored leg movements also detected automatically. The false positive rate was calculated as the percentage of automatically detected LM that did not match manually detected LM.

Statistics

IBM SPSS 21 (SPSS, Inc., Chicago, IL) was used for all statistical analysis. Data were tested for normal distribution using the Shapiro-Wilk test. Descriptive statistics are given as numbers (percentages) as well as medians (range), as data were not normally distributed. Nonparametric statistics were applied. Correlations and agreement between manual and computerised quantification of LM and PLM were calculated by means of the Spearman correlation coefficients, the intraclass correlation coefficients and the Bland-Altman plots. P-values <0.05 were considered significant. In case of multiple comparisons, correction for Bonferroni was performed, and p-values were set accordingly ($p < 0.01$).

Results

Demographic, clinical and sleep characteristics of the RLS patients and the control group

Twenty patients with RLS (14 men, 6 women) with a median age of 51.5 (37–73) years were included in this study.

The control group included 13 men and seven women with a median age of 32 (20–60) years. The main reason for PSG examination was suspected sleep-related breathing disorder (11/20, 55%), followed by insomnia (6/20, 30%), NREM parasomnia (2/20, 10%) and suspected narcolepsy (1/20, 5%). In none of those patients sleep-related breathing disorder was confirmed by PSG, nor was narcolepsy confirmed by MSLT. The final diagnosis were primary snoring ($n = 7$), insomnia ($n = 5$), no sleep disorder ($n = 5$), NREM parasomnia ($n = 2$) and delayed sleep phase syndrome ($n = 1$). None of the patients included in the control group had relevant comorbidities, and none had central nervous system active medication.

The sleep parameters of the two groups are provided in Additional file 3: Table S1.

Comparison of manual versus computerized detection and analysis of PLM

For this analysis, a total of 10,269 PLM (median 172.5 per subject, range 8–979) were manually scored, 6731 PLMS (median 76.5 per subject, range 1–910) and 3538 PLMW (median 44 per subject, range 0–547).

Tables 1 and 2 provide the LM and PLM measures obtained by manual and computerized detection and analysis according to AASM criteria [11], as well as the manual and computerized calculation of the periodicity index according to Ferri et al. [12] Of note, all values calculated by manual and computerized analysis were very similar. In line with this, all Spearman correlation coefficients were between 0.751 and 0.996, and all intraclass correlation coefficients between 0.775 and 0.999. Correlations between manual and computerized detection and analysis of LM and PLM are also shown in Figs. 1 and 2. The limits of agreement between manual and computerized analysis for LMS indices in total sleep (left −6.22 to 5.58, right −4.82 to 4,93), and PLMS indices in total sleep, NREM and REM sleep, and for PLMW indices, which are −3.02 to 4.27, −3.13 to 4.53, −7.79 to 8.69 and −5.20 to 10.86, respectively, are shown in Fig. 3. The mean bias was −0.32 and 0.05 for the LMS indices left and right, respectively, 0.62 for the PLMS index in

Table 1 Agreement between manual and computerized detection and analysis of LM, evaluated with intraclass correlation coefficients

	Manual quantification	Computerized quantification	Intraclass correlation coefficient	*P* values
LM index right				
LMS/h, TST	12.3 (6–37.4)	13.9 (6.3–37.3)	0.997 (0.995–0.999)	**<0.001***
LMS/h, NREM sleep	13.8 (4.8–44)	13.9 (5.2–43.7)	0.998 (0.996–0.999)	**<0.001***
LMS/h, REM sleep	12.8 (6.1–33.7)	11.9 (5.4–33.5)	0.989 (0.979–0.994)	**<0.001***
LMW	59.7 (39.5–80)	63.7 (48.4–86.3)	0.911 (0.839–0.952)	**<0.001***
LM index left				
LMS/h, TST	12.9 (5.4–32)	13.1 (5.4–32.1)	0.995 (0.991–0.998)	**<0.001***
LMS/h, NREM sleep	13.3 (3.8–35.7)	13.5 (4.1–36.1)	0.996 (0.992–0.998)	**<0.001***
LMS/h, REM sleep	10.5 (7–24.1)	10.3 (7–25.1)	0.991 (0.982–0.995)	**<0.001***
LMW	57.8 (42.2–76.6)	55.2 (43.9–79.6)	0.939 (0.888–0.967)	**<0.001***

LM leg movements, *LMS* leg movements during sleep, *LMW* leg movements during wakefulness, *TST* total sleep time
*Significant *p*-values after correction for multiple comparisons according to Bonferroni are given in bold letters

TST, 0.76 for the PLMS index during NREM sleep, 0.45 for the PLMS index during REM sleep, and 2.83 for the PLMW index.

The event per event analysis showed a high agreement between the two methods, as shown by sensitivity percentages of the computerized LM and PLM analysis ranging from 95 to 100%, and false positive percentages between 0 and 11% (Additional file 4: Table S2).

Discussion

This study validated a software for the detection and analysis of LM integrated into a commercialy available PSG system, which quantifies different LM and PLM indices according to AASM criteria. The correlation between the computerized scoring of different LM and PLM indices and the standard visual detection and manual scoring was remarkable high. The validated integrated software allows the correlation of LM and PLM data with all other PSG data without needing to export data to another program or to run another analysis on the same platform, as the analysis can be done within the same single routine PSG report, and gives in addition visual informations. All LM and PLM parameters used not only in the routine but also for research purposes, including intermovement intervals and periodicity index, can be automatically scored with this software, and the scoring settings can be modified by the user.

Several software programs for the automatic detection and analysis of PLM are available. The first study evaluating an algorithm for automatic detection of PLM dates back to 1990 [13], and after that several algorithms for the automatic scoring of PLM were tested [14–20], but not adequately validated. To our knowledge only one [20] is included in a commercially available software for

Table 2 Agreement between manual and computerized detection and analysis of PLM, evaluated with intraclass correlation coefficients

	Manual quantification	Computerized quantification	Intraclass correlation coefficient	*P* values
PLM index				
PLMS/h, TST	16.5 (0.2–194.6)	16.6 (0.2–204.7)	0.999 (0.998–0.999)	**<0.001***
PLMS/h, NREM sleep	16.9 (0–195)	17.5 (0–205.2)	0.999 (0.998–0.999)	**<0.001***
PLMS/h, REM sleep	4.4 (0–172.5)	4.4 (0–195)	0.994 (0.989–0.994)	**<0.001***
PLMW	50.2 (0–128.5)	49 (0–134.8)	0.991 (0.965–0.996)	**<0.001***
PLMS associated with respiratory events/h	0 (0–4.5)	0.1 (0–3.8)	0.977 (0.955–0.988)	**<0.001***
Intermovement interval				
TST, sec	32.8 (17.2–59.8)	34.9 (17.2–61.3)	0.945 (0.886–0.973)	**<0.001***
NREM sleep, sec	35 (17.4–59.8)	34.5 (17–61.3)	0.878 (0.778–0.875)	**<0.001***
REM sleep, sec	28.9 (15.5–62.6)	29.1 (16.2–55.2)	0.831 (0.659–0.921)	**<0.001***
Wakefulness, sec	25.4 (14.7–35.3)	22.9 (16.3–34.7)	0.779 (0.617–0.877)	**<0.001***
Periodicity index	0.8 (0–1)	0.8 (0–1)	0.958 (0.918–0.978)	**<0.001***

PLM periodic leg movements, *PLMS* periodic leg movements during sleep, *PLMW* periodic leg movements during wakefulness, *TST* total sleep time
*Significant *p*-values after correction for multiple comparisons according to Bonferroni are given in bold letters

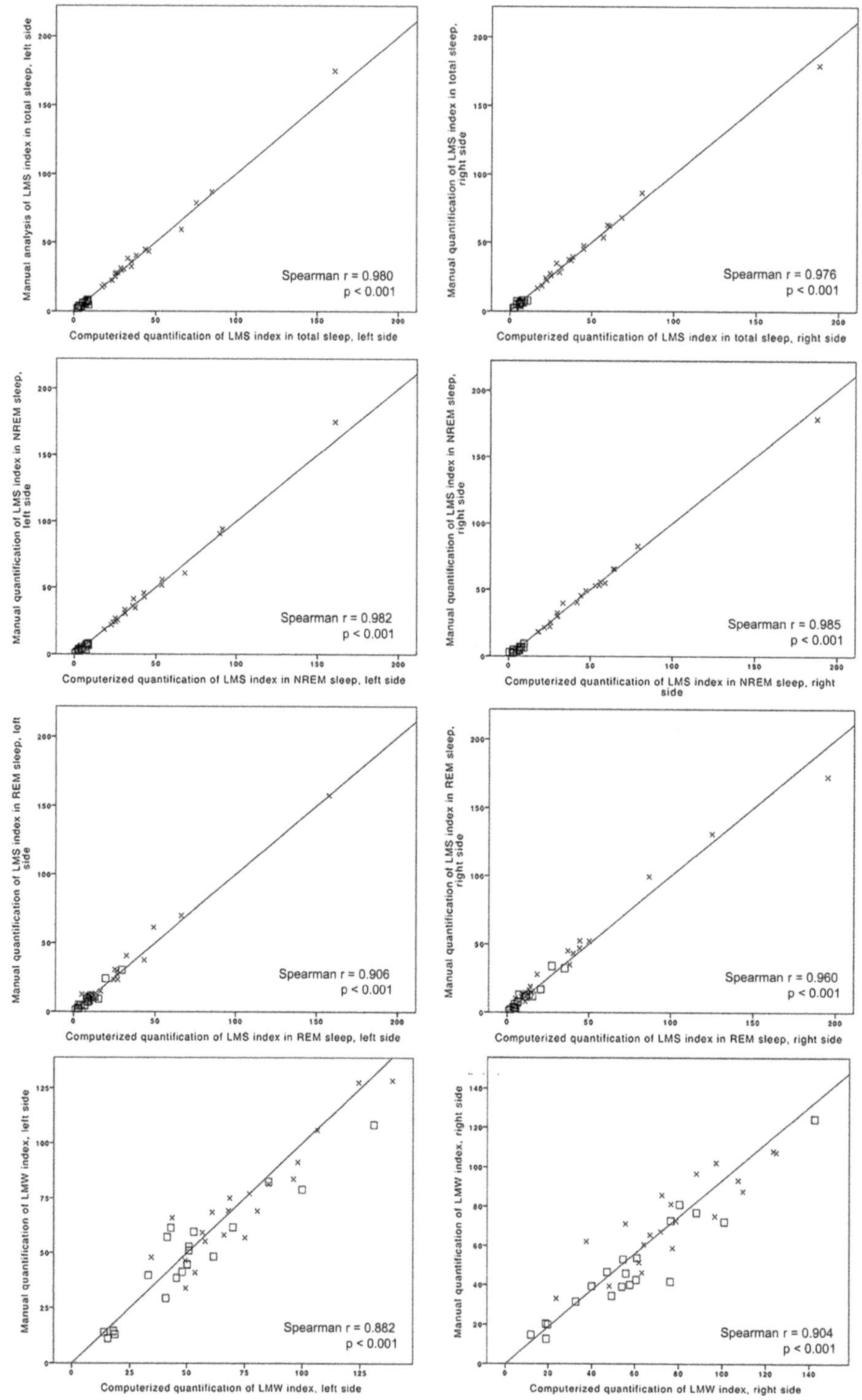

Fig. 1 Correlations between manual and computerized scoring of LM indices. LMS, leg movements during sleep; LMW, leg movements during wakefulness. Single values for patients are represented as *crosses*, for controls as *squares*

sleep analysis. However, this algorithm did not calculate intermovement intervals and periodicity index, and was not evaluated for the detection of PLMW.

Although in this study agreement between manual and automatic analysis was high for all investigated parameters, it was higher for PLM indices than for intermovement

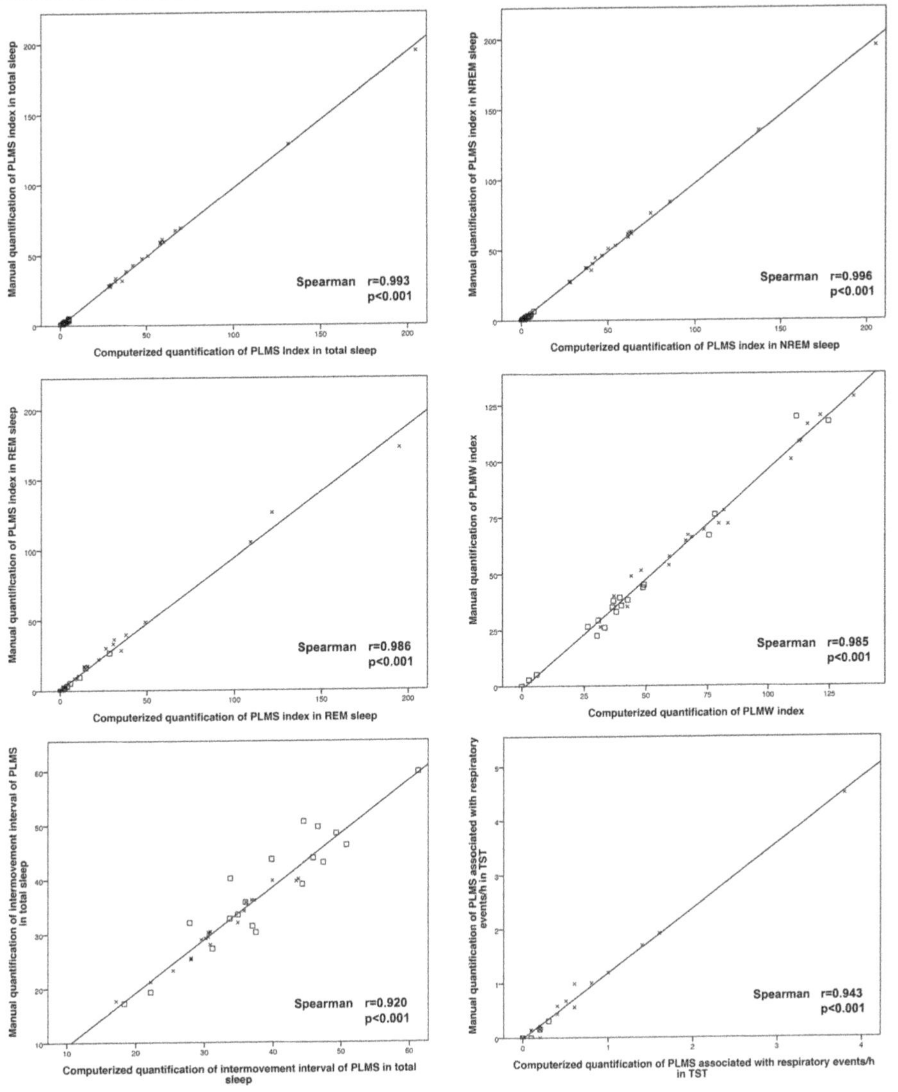

Fig. 2 Correlations between manual and computerized scoring of PLM parameters. PLMS, periodic leg movements during sleep; PLMW, periodic leg movements during wakefulness; TST, total sleep time. Single values for patients are represented as *crosses*, for controls as *squares*

intervals. This is probably due to the fact that scoring or not scoring a few PLM makes little difference in the PLM index but can produce a sizeable difference in the intermovement interval, specifically when overall PLM indices are low. Those differences were more pronounced in REM sleep. A possible explanation is the more difficult quantification of PLM during REM sleep due to fragmentation of movements. The difference in intermovement intervals between manual and computerized scoring was more evident in the control group, which may be attributed to the reason explained above. In fact in such cases, including or not including in the analysis few PLM can produce a relevant change in intermovement intervals. Nevertheless, the software we validated showed high correlations and high agreement between both methods also in subjects with extreme PLM indices, which ranged from 0.2 to 194.6/h. The inclusion and exclusion criteria were specifically designed to validate this software in both subjects without relevant PLM and in subjects with high indices.

Of note, the periodicity indices in the current study were higher than previously reported in both RLS patients and control subjects [11]. In the original study proposing the periodicity index, Ferri and colleagues analyzed PLMS and not PLMW. Although periodicity index is based only on PLMS, including PLMW series occurring during wake after sleep onset (WASO) allows the inclusion of a higher number of PLMS that are part of mixed PLM series containing both PLMS and PLMW but constituted by <4 PLMS, that otherwise would not be counted as PLMS.

The software used for this study is fully implemented in a routine PSG system. This is on the one hand essential

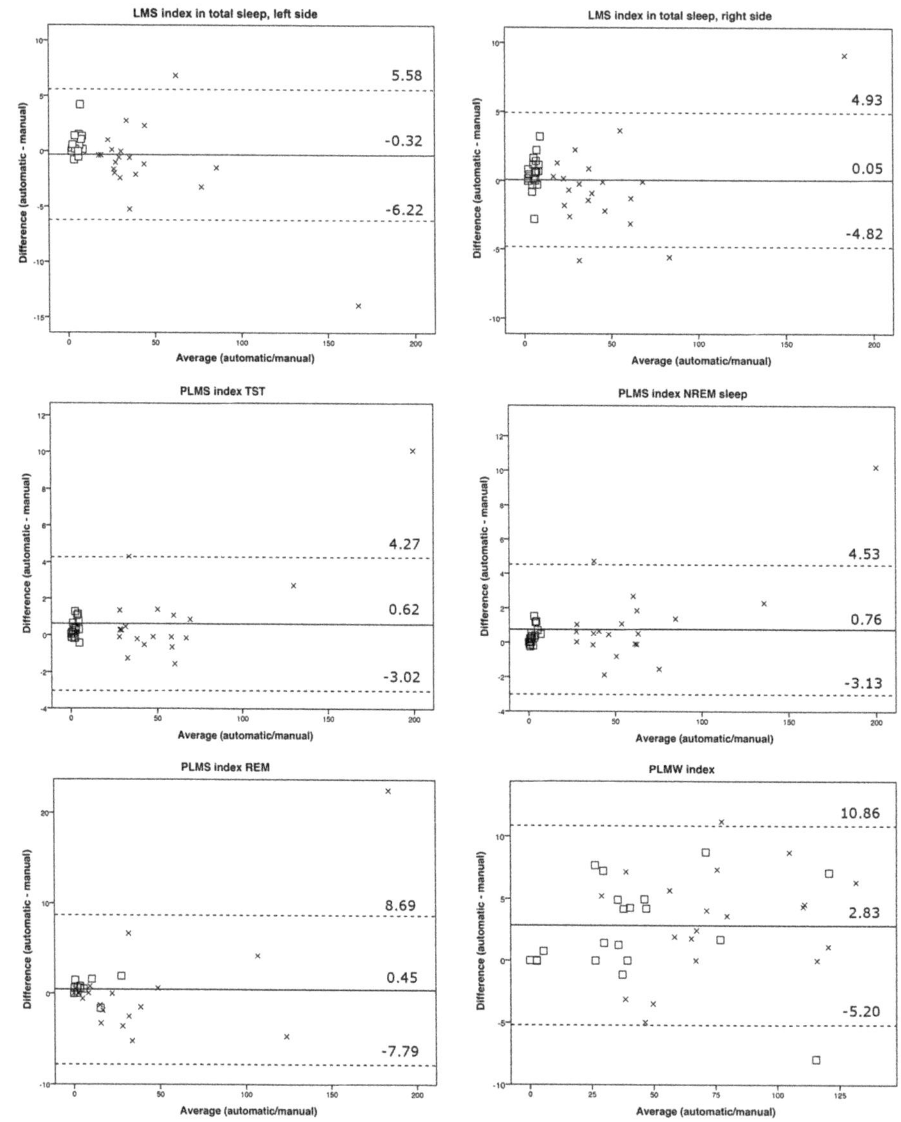

Fig. 3 Bland-Altman plots for the different PLM indices. PLMS, periodic leg movements during sleep; TST, total sleep time; NREM, non-REM sleep; REM, rapid eye movement; PLMW, periodic leg movements during wakefulness. Single values for patients are represented as *crosses*, for controls as *squares*. The *horizontal lines* represent the mean ± 2 standard deviations (SD)

for the clinical routine; on the other hand, it is a time-saving system to obtain good data also for research purposes, as all the LM and PLM indices and variables can be easily calculated. No artifact correction was performed, so that the software can also be used by untrained scorers. However, the validation was done in a study with high recording quality, but manual artifact correction could be needed in recordings with worst signal quality. This software also gives the users the possibility to change several settings, with the result that it can detect and analyze LM also according different criteria.

A limitation of this study is the exclusion of patients with sleep-related breathing disorders, with or without nCPAP therapy. This should be done in further studies. Studies including different age groups, e.g. children, showing more spontaneous activity during the night, would also be of interest. Another aspect that remains to be explored is the importance of movement amplitude [21]. This was not done in this study, but amplitude measurement is possible with the software and this issue should be addressed in future studies.

As this study also validated LM count in addition to PLM analysis, these results will remain of interest also if PLM criteria will change in the future. The algorithm for LM count and PLM analysis is published, so results of the study can be replicated by other groups.

Conclusions

The current study validated a software for the detection and analysis of LM integrated in a PSG system and commercially available against the gold standard visual detection and manual scoring according to AASM criteria, showing high agreement between both methods. The possibility to calculate several indices suggest that time-saving computerized PLM scoring is an excellent tool, useful not only in the clinical practice but also for research purposes.

Additional files

Additional file 1: Figure S1. Settings for computerized detection and analysis of leg movements (LM) and periodic leg movements (PLM).

Additional file 2: Figure S2. Example of computerized detection of periodic leg movements (PLM). Legend: Leg movements are marked with green rectangles, and periodic leg movements with underlining pink bars. An overview of the PLM during the whole night is visible in the upper part of the figure, where PLM are shown as red bars.

Additional file 3: Table S1. Sleep parameters of the study sample. SPT, sleep period time; TST, total sleep time. SPT is defined as the elapsed time from sleep onset through the last epoch of sleep, whereas TST is the duration of time spent in NREM and REM sleep during SPT. * Significant *p*-values are given in bold letters.

Additional file 4: Table S2. Sensitivity and false positive percentages of the computerized LM and PLM analysis, as derived from comparing the automated scoring algorithm to manual scoring on an event-by-event basis. Data are given as median (range) and interquartile range. *P* values are given for the comparison between RLS patients and controls. IQR, interquartile range; LM, leg movements; LMS, leg movements during sleep; LMW, leg movements during wakefulness; NREM, non-REM sleep; PLM, periodic leg movements; PLMS, periodic leg movements during sleep; PLMW, periodic leg movements during wakefulness; REM, rapid eye movement; TST, total sleep time. * Significant *p*-values after correction for multiple comparisons according to Bonferroni are given in bold letters.

Abbreviations

AASM: American Academy of Sleep Medicine; AHI: Apnoea/hypopnea index; CPAP: Continuous positive airway pressure; EMG: Electromyography; IRLSSG: International Restless Legs Syndrome Study Group; LM: Leg movements; LMS: Leg movements during sleep; LMW: Leg movements during wakefulness; PLM: Periodic leg movements; PLMS: Periodic leg movements during sleep; PLMW: Periodic leg movements during wakefulness; PSG: Polysomnography; REM: Rapid eye movement; RLS: Restless legs syndrome; WASO: Wake after sleep onset

Acknowledgments

We are grateful to OSG Belgium for their cooperation, namely to Sabine Wuytens and Guy De Gruyter.

Funding

No funding was obtained for this study.

Authors' contributions

AS study design; acquisition, analysis and interpretation of data; drafting of the manuscript. AH acquisition and interpretation of data, critical revision of the manuscript. HH acquisition and analysis of data, critical revision of the manuscript. BH study conception and design, analysis and interpretation of data, critical revision of the manuscript. All authors read and approved the final manuscript.

Competing interests

The authors declare that they have no competing interests.

References

1. Montplaisir J, Boucher S, Poirier G, Lavigne G, Lapierre O, Lespérance P. Clinical, polysomnographic, and genetic characteristics of restless legs syndrome: a study of 133 patients diagnosed with new standard criteria. Mov Disord. 1997;12:61–5.
2. Moore H, Winkelmann J, Lin L, Peppard P, Mignot E. Periodic leg movements during sleep are associated with polymorphism in BTBD9, TOX3/BC034767, MEIS1, MAP2K5/SKOR1, and PTPRD. Sleep. 2014;37: 1535–42.
3. Baker TL, Guilleminault C, Nino-Murcia G, Dement WC. Comparative polysomnographic study of narcolepsy and idiopathic central nervous system hypersomnia. Sleep. 1986;9:232–42.
4. Ancoli-Israel S, Kripke DF, Mason W, Kaplan OJ. Sleep apnea and periodic movements in an aging sample. J Gerontol. 1985;40:419–25.
5. Wetter TC, Collado-Seidel V, Pollmächer T, Yassouridis A, Trenkwalder C. Sleep and periodic leg movement patterns in drug-free patients with Parkinson's disease and multiple system atrophy. Sleep. 2000;23:361–7.
6. Vetrugno R, Provini F, Cortelli P, et al. Sleep disorders in multiple system atrophy: a correlative video-polysomnographic study. Sleep Med. 2004;5:21–30.
7. Fantini ML, Michaud M, Gosselin N, Lavigne G, Montplaisir J. Periodic leg movements in REM sleep behavior disorder and related autonomic and EEG activation. Neurology. 2002;59:1889–94.
8. Frauscher B, Gabelia D, Mitterling T, et al. Motor events during healthy sleep: a quantitative polysomnographic study. Sleep. 2014;37:763–73.
9. Pennestri MH, Whittom S, Adam B, Petit D, Carrier J, Montplaisir J. PLMS and PLMW in healthy subjects as a function of age: prevalence and interval distribution. Sleep. 2006;29:1183–7.
10. Allen RP, Picchietti DL, Hening WA, Trenkwalder C, Walter AS, Montplaisir J. Restless legs syndrome: diagnostic criteria, special considerations, and epidemiology: A report from the restless legs syndrome diagnosis and epidemiology workshop at the National Institute of Health. Sleep. 2003;4: 101–19.
11. Berry RB, Brooks R, Gamaldo CE, Harding SM, Marcus CL, Vaughn BV for the American Academy of Sleep Medicine. The AASM manual for the scoring of sleep and associated events: rules, terminology and technical specifications, Version 2. Darien, Illinois: American Academy of Sleep Medicine; 2012.
12. Ferri R, Zucconi M, Manconi M, Plazzi G, Bruni O, Ferini-Strambi L. New approaches to the study of periodic leg movements during sleep in restless legs syndrome. Sleep. 2006;29:759–69.
13. Kayed K, Roberts S, Davies WL. Computer detection and analysis of periodic movements in sleep. Sleep. 1990;13:253–61.
14. Tauchmann N, Pollmächer T. Automatic detection of periodic leg movements (PLM). J Sleep Res. 1996;5:273–5.
15. Wetter T, Dirlich G, Streit J, Trenkwalder C, Schuld A, Pollmächer T. An automatic method for scoring leg movements in polygraphic sleep recordings and its validity in comparison to visual scoring. Sleep. 2004;27: 324–8.
16. Sforza E, Mathis J, Bassetti C. The PAM-RL ambulatory device for detection of periodic leg movements: a validation study. Sleep Med. 2005;6:407–13.
17. Gschliesser V, Frauscher B, Brandauer E, et al. PLM detection by actigraphy compared to polysomnography: a validation and comparison of two actigraphs. Sleep Med. 2009;10:306–11.
18. Kemlink D, Pertl M, Sonka K, Nevsimalova S. A comparison of polysomnographic and actigraphic evaluation of periodic limb movements in sleep. Neurol Res. 2008;30:234–8.
19. Huang AS, Skeba P, Yang MS, Sgambati FP, Earley CJ, Allen RP. MATPLM1, a MATLAB script for scoring of periodic limb movements: preliminary validation with visual scoring. Sleep Med. 2015;12:1541–9.
20. Ferri R, Zucconi M, Manconi M, et al. Computer-assisted detection of nocturnal leg motor activity in patients with restless legs syndrome and periodic leg movements during sleep. Sleep. 2005;28:998–1004.
21. Gschliesser V, Brandauer E, Ulmer H, Poewe W, Hogl B. Periodic limb movement counting in polysomnography: effects of amplitude. Sleep Med. 2006;7:249–54.

Clinical features and outcome in patients with osseomuscular type of Wilson's disease

Hao Yu[1], Juan-Juan Xie[1], Yu-Chao Chen[2], Qin-Yun Dong[3], Yi Dong[1], Wang Ni[1] and Zhi-Ying Wu[1,4*]

Abstract

Background: Wilson's disease with osseomuscular type is a rare condition, which often lacks typical hepatic and neurological symptoms and causes misdiagnoses easily. During the past 10 years, eight Chinese patients of osseomuscular type of Wilson's disease were identified in our clinic.

Methods: Clinical information was gathered from medical records and follow-ups. The genetic testing was performed in each patient. Serum ceruloplasmin, Kayser-Fleischer rings, liver function, brain magnetic resonance imaging and abdominal ultrasonography were also evaluated.

Results: The median age of onset is 12 years of age. The patients had their initial musculoskeletal conditions with arthralgia or joint deformity, while the hepatic or neurologic signs were minimal. Most patients (6/8) eventually developed clinical neurological symptoms afterwards with a median interval of 36 months. All of them had normal liver function and low serum ceruloplasmin (<0.1 g/L). Most patients (6/8) present with Kayser-Fleischer rings and abnormal hepatic ultrasonography. The arthralgia was resolved with copper chelation therapy.

Conclusions: Wilson's disease with osseomuscular type occurs without typical hepatic or neurological symptoms, which makes the clinical diagnosis challenging. Serum ceruloplasmin, abdominal ultrasonography, ophthalmic examination and genetic testing help to establish the diagnosis. Early diagnosis can initiate an effective treatment and prevent the further damage.

Keywords: Arthralgia, ATP7B, Copper, Deformity, Osteoarthritis

Background

Wilson's disease (WD), also known as hepatolenticular degeneration, is an autosomal recessive disease (incidence 1/30,000) characterized by Kayser-Fleischer rings of cornea (K-F rings) and multisystem damage, including liver cirrhosis, neurological symptoms and musculoskeletal deformity. The disease is caused by mutations in the *ATP7B* gene, which encodes a copper-transporting ATPase in the liver. The deficiency in the enzyme activity can lead to a toxic copper accumulation in multiple organs, which may be responsible for its wide variety of symptoms [1].

Despite wide varieties of clinical manifestations, WD patients typically present with liver dysfunction or neurological disorders. Musculoskeletal abnormalities, including premature osteoarthritis, skeletal deformity and pathological bone fractures, can be occasionally found in WD patients with hepatic or neurologic type [2, 3], but very rare as initial symptoms (incidence ~2% in Chinese population) [4]. These conditions, also known as "osseomuscular type" of WD, often lack typical hepatic and neurological symptoms and cause misdiagnoses easily [5, 6].

During the past 10 years, we have collected and identified eight Chinese WD patients with osseomuscular type in our clinic. Their genotypes, clinical manifestations, biochemical parameters and outcome of treatment are reported herein, aiming to improve early diagnosis and therapy with this condition.

* Correspondence: zhiyingwu@zju.edu.cn
[1]Department of Neurology and Research Center of Neurology in Second Affiliated Hospital, and the Collaborative Innovation Center for Brain Science, Zhejiang University School of Medicine, 88 Jiefang Rd, Hangzhou 310009, China
[4]Joint Institute for Genetics and Genome Medicine between Zhejiang University and University of Toronto, Zhejiang University, Hangzhou, China
Full list of author information is available at the end of the article

Methods

Subjects

All eight WD patients were diagnosed by genetic testing. The degree of osseomuscular symptoms was based on the published assessment scale (0: Normal. 1: Abnormal skeletal X-ray; asymptomatic.2: Difficulty in ADL but independent. 3: Requires help in ADL. 4: Dependent on others for ADL. 5: Fracture or bedbound) [7]. In addition, ceruloplasmin, K-F rings, liver function, brain magnetic resonance imaging (MRI) and abdominal ultrasonography were also evaluated.

Genotype analysis

Genomic DNA was extracted from peripheral EDTA-treated blood by Blood Genomic Extraction Kit (Qiagen, Hilden, Germany). The Sanger sequencing of *ATP7B* was performed with a procedure described previously [8].

Results

Mutation analysis

All eight patients carried biallelic mutations, and seven of them were compound heterogeneous (Table 1). The most frequent mutation was p.R778L (6/16), which was also the most common mutation of *ATB7B* in Chinese population [9].

Clinical manifestation

All of patients denied WD family histories. The median age of onset is 12 years of age (range 3–17 years). Their complains were all about musculoskeletal problems such as arthralgia and joint deformity (Table 1). The abnormalities include arthralgia of the knees in four patients, genu varum in two patients, arthralgia of hip joints in one patient, genu valgum in one patient and talipse equinovarus in one patient. The median assessment score of osseomuscular symptoms is 3 (range 2–4).

As an example, Patient 8 is a 13-year-old boy with a 10-year history of walking difficulty. After a hernia surgery at 3 years of age, he felt knees and ankles sore after taking a long walk. The condition progressed slowly and he got a hip pain at 12 years of age. The pain was aggravated by walking and rapidly made him unable to walk any more. Physical examination revealed a severely limited movement of bilateral hip joint in lower limbs. The motion range of his hip joint was only about 25° (flexion 45° to 70°). Excessive extension or flexion would elicit intense and sharp pain immediately, so the patient could never straighten his legs. When standing and walking, he had to keep a "crouching" posture with bent hips, and steady himself with hands on knees. His condition had been considered as a rheumatic disease for many years and diagnosed as "arthralgia" or "osteoarthritis" in many hospitals. However, the diagnosis was indefinite and he only received some anti-inflammatory therapy.

Similar to Patient 8, all the other patients also sought for medical attention in orthopedics or rheumatology firstly, due to absence of neurological and hepatic symptoms. Moreover, four patients (Patient 1, 4, 5, 6) with deformities subsequently underwent the orthopedic surgeries. However, the orthopedic surgery did not correct the skeletal abnormalities and neurological deterioration ensued. Patients 1 and 6 showed neurological symptoms shortly after surgeries (<2 months) and the other two developed neurological symptoms after 15 and 36 months respectively (Table 1).

Despite the absence of neurological complaints initially, it is noteworthy that most patients (6/8) eventually developed neurological symptoms afterwards with a median interval of 36 months (range 8–84 months), including

Table 1 Genotype and clinical course in eight cases of WD with osseomuscular type

No	Gender	*ATP7B* mutations	Onset Age (years)	Osseomuscular abnormalities (Degree[a])	Neurological symptoms	Interval from O to N (months)	Orthopedic Surgery	Interval from S to N (months)
1	F	p.A874V + p.P992L	10	Genu valgum (3)	Dysarthria, difficult with writing, musk face	8	Yes	2
2	M	p.M769Hfs*26 + p.R919G	17	Arthralgia in knee joints (2)	Dysarthria, tremor	60	No	-
3	M	p.R778Q + p.I930del	12	Arthralgia in knee joints (2)	Normal	-	No	-
4	F	p.E332* + p.R778L	10	Genu varum (3)	Dysarthria, bradykinesia	18	Yes	15
5	F	p.R778L + p.I1148T	13	Genu varum, femoral head necrosis, dislocation of the left shoulder (3)	Tremor	36	Yes	36
6	F	p.R778L + p.R778L	15	Talipes equinovarus (3)	Tremor writer's cramp	N/A	Yes	<2
7	M	p.R778L + p.G943D	12	Arthralgia in knee joints (4)	Tremor, dysarthria	84	No	-
8	M	p.R778L + p.V1106I	3	Arthralgia in hip and knee joints, dysplasia of thoracic vertebrae (4)	Normal	N/A	No	-

**Translation termination codon*, *O* osseomuscular symptoms, *N* neurological symptom, *S* surgery, *N/A* not available

[a]Based on the published assessment scale for osseomuscular symptoms [7]

tremor, dysarthria, writing difficulty and bradykinesia (Table 1). Then it is the moment when most diagnoses of WD were taken into consideration in these patients. The interval between the onset of osseomuscular symptoms and establishment of the diagnosis was at least 10 months (Patient 1) and could reach as long as 10 years (Patient 8). The neurological symptoms included tremor in four patients, dysarthria in four patients, writing difficulty in two patients and bradykinesia in one patient. Patient 1 also manifested psychiatric symptoms.

Accessory examination

The K-F ring, known as a specific sign in WD [1], was present in most patients (6/8) (Table 2). However, since most patients had developed the neurological symptoms when examining, the initial rate of K-F rings might be lower.

Serum ceruloplasmin concentration was less than 0.1 g/L (reference: 0.2–0.4 g/L) in all patients. No significant abnormalities in liver function were observed, including aminotransferase, bilirubin and albumin parameters. However, the ultrasonography showed features of chronic hepatic diseases in most patients (6/8) (Table 2). All the patients were evaluated as Class A based on Child-Pugh score.

Among the five patients taking the brain MRI, four showed different degree of abnormal MRI signals. Abnormal T2 signals were discovered in three cases in basal ganglia, and two cases in the brain stem (Table 2).

For Patient 8, despite a decreased serum ceruloplasmin (0.05 g/L), he had no K-F rings, no abnormalities in brain MRI or hepatic ultrasonography. His X-rays films showed bilateral hip osteoarthritis (Fig. 1) and knee degenerative changes (Fig. 2). Notably, the thoracic MRI incidentally found the dysplasia of thoracic vertebrae (Fig. 3). Due to the absence of hepatic, neurologic symptoms and K-F ring, his diagnosis of WD was confirmed by genetic testing (Table 1).

Outcome of treatment

After the establishment of diagnosis, all patients received a copper chelator treatment with D-penicillamine, dimercaptosuccinic acid (DMSA) or dimercaptopropane sulfonate (DMPS). No serious related adverse reaction was observed in these patients. The patients responded generally well to the therapy. The arthralgia was all resolved and neurological symptoms showed different degrees of improvement (Table 2). However, the improvements in bone deformity were minimal.

The Patient 8 improved remarkably by treatment. After one course of intravenous DMPS (0.25 g q.d. for 6 days) and 3 months of oral DMSA (0.5 g b.i.d.), the patient felt less painful to move his legs and easier to stand up from a chair. The physical examination confirmed an improved movement of his hip joint. The range of motion was able to reach a degree of 35°, which increased by 40% compared with the condition 3 months ago. After 6 month of treatment, the range increased to a

Table 2 Clinical findings and treatment outcomes in eight cases of WD with osseomuscular type

No	K-F ring	Neurologic Examination			CP (g/L)	Involvement on brain MRI	Abdominal ultrasonography	Outcomes of Chelation Therapy (Degree[a])
		Strength	Tone	Reflex				
1	+	UE & LE 5	UE ↑	(++)	<0.02	Basal ganglia	Hepatic diffuse disease	(9 months after treatment) Dystonia in the right hand partially relieved; blurred speech persist; walking better (2)
2	+	UE & LE 5	Normal	(++)	0.02	Basal ganglia and brain stem	Hepatic diffuse disease, splenomegaly	(3 months after the treatment) Pain relieved with improved speech (0)
3	+	UE & LE 5	Normal	(++)	<0.02	Normal	Hepatic diffuse disease, splenomegaly	(14 months after treatment) Pain relieved (0)
4	+	UE & LE 5	UE & LE ↑	(++)	0.07	N/A	Hepatic diffuse disease	(after 23 months of inconsecutive treatment) No obvious improvement (3)
5	N/A	UE & LE 5	UE ↑	UE & LE (+++)	0.03	Basal ganglia and brain stem	Hepatic diffuse disease, splenomegaly	N/A
6	+	UE & LE 5	UE & LE ↓	(++)	0.03	N/A	Normal	N/A
7	+	UE 5; pLE 4; dLE 4-	UE & LE ↓	Knee (+++)	0.02	N/A	Hepatic diffuse disease, splenomegaly	N/A
8	-	UE 4; LE 4-	LE ↑	Knee (+++)	0.05	Normal	Increased echogenicity	(6 months after treatment) Pain relieved with improved joint motion (2)

UE upper extremity, *LE* lower extremity, *dLE* distal lower extremity, *pLE* proximal lower extremity, *CP* ceruloplasmin, *N/A* not available
[a]Based on the published assessment scale for osseomuscular symptoms [7]

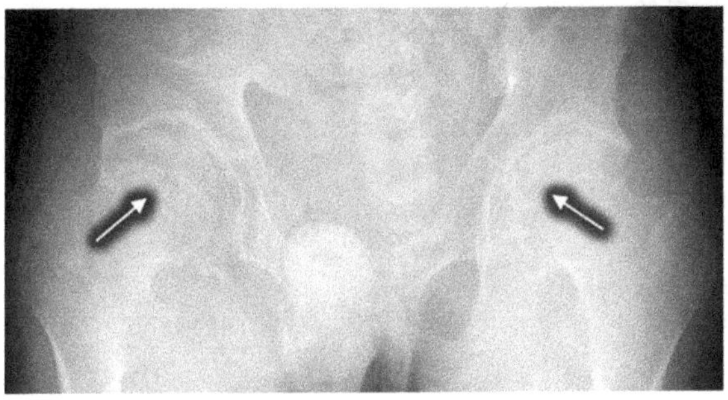

Fig. 1 The plain film showed hip osteoarthritis with narrowing joint space, incomplete articular surface and swelling joint capsule (*Arrows*)

degree of 80° and the patient can stand and walk without the assistance of his hand.

Discussion

WD is one of the limited genetic diseases that can be clinically cured by timely treatment. The osseomuscular type of WD begins without typical hepatic and neurological symptoms, which makes the diagnosis challenging. Most patients are never considered WD until the neurological symptoms emerged. However, some typical signs were present in our patients, such as K-F rings or abnormal liver ultrasonography. Moreover, serum ceruloplasmin is a sensitive test in WD patients even without any hepatic and neurological signs. WD should be highly suspected when ceruloplasmin is below 0.1 g/L, but lower levels can also occur with aceruloplasminemia, renal or enteric protein loss, liver disease and heterozygotes for WD [10]. Therefore, if the patient has a low serum ceruloplasmin without K-F rings, the diagnosis should be based on combination of other tests. Genetic testing is confirmatory and non-invasive, and also convenient for screening family members.

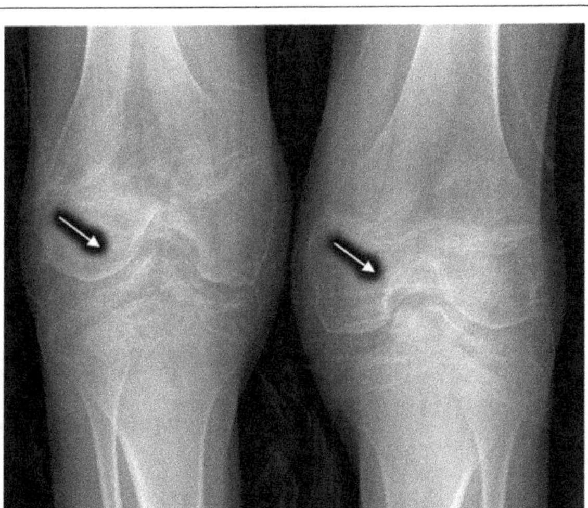

Fig. 2 The knee plain film of knee joints showed degenerative changes with articular surface hyperosteogeny and swelling joint capsule (*Arrows*)

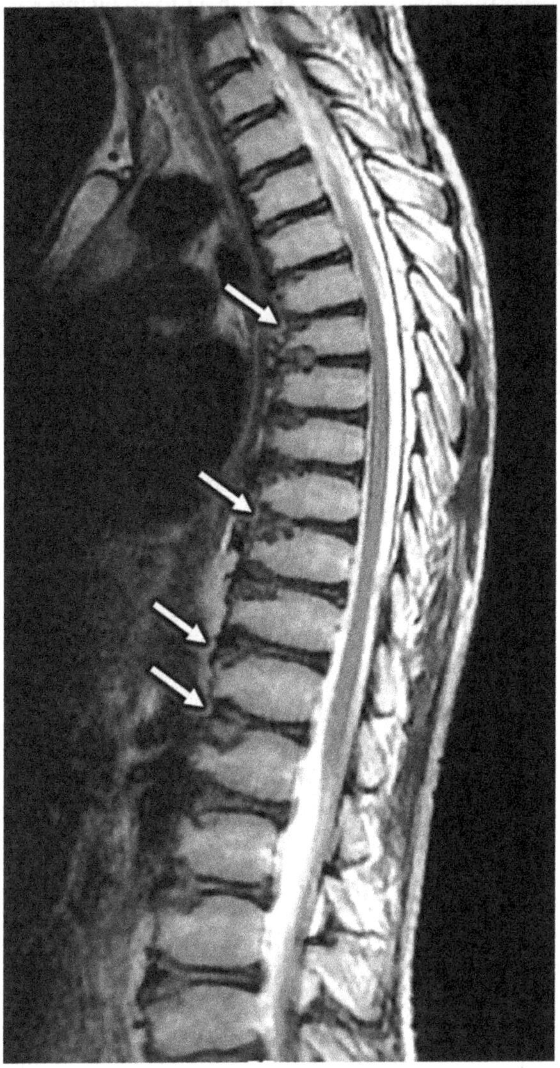

Fig. 3 The thoracic MRI showed the dysplasia of thoracic vertebrae, which had bullet-like shapes with focal cartilage defects at the front edge (*Arrows*)

The pathogenic mechanisms underlying the musculoskeletal damage are not clear. However, it may be a result of abnormal bone metabolism. Abnormal copper deposit are found in multiple organs and structures of WD patients, including the bone, in which the copper concentration increases about four times [11]. The radiological changes of arthropathy have been frequently encountered among WD patients [11–13]. Moreover, the pathological findings suggested a chronic inflammatory process or degradation of collagen and protein secondary to a deposition of copper [14]. Besides, the calcium regulation disorder also makes the bone more vulnerable to other stimuli, which can result from vitamin D insufficiency. The hepatic damage in WD can impede the conversion of vitamin D to its active form, thus impaired absorption of calcium and led to osteoporosis and bone deformity [15]. The similar effects caused by the damage of kidney and parathyroid gland in WD patients are also reported [16, 17]. These pathological conditions may be corrected by timely chelation therapy and hormone supplement.

Dystonia, which is characterized by "sustained or intermittent muscle contractions causing abnormal, often repetitive, movements, postures or both", can develop into contracture and joint deformity in severe cases [18]. These conditions usually demonstrate spasticity with markedly increased muscle tone. In our patients, half of them (Patient 1, 4, 5, 8) had focal or general increase tones. However, they took 8–36 months to develop the other neurological symptoms, such as dysarthria, which usually arose with dystonia in other WD patients. In addition, Patient 8 never developed any other neurological signs in his 10-year course, which made it. Therefore, it remains obscure whether the osseomuscular type of WD is a result of long-term dystonia or a natural course of osteopathy.

Conclusions

Although most WD patients with osseomuscular type will develop neurological symptoms, it is easily misdiagnosed when it only manifests as joint pain or bone deformity. A long-term misdiagnosis may lead to irreversible damage to the musculoskeletal system, such as a permanent deformity, which often requires surgical intervention and has a poor response to the drug. Therefore, if a child or adolescent presents with unexplained musculoskeletal problems, the possibility of WD should be considered. Serum ceruloplasmin, abdominal ultrasonography, ophthalmic examinations and genetic testing will help to establish the diagnosis. Early diagnosis can initiate an effective treatment and prevent the further damage.

Abbreviations

DMPS: Dimercaptopropane sulfonate; DMSA: Dimercaptosuccinic acid; K-F ring: Kayser-Fleischer ring; MRI: Magnetic resonance imaging; WD: Wilson's disease

Acknowledgments

We gratefully acknowledge all participants for their help and willingness to participate this study.

Funding

This work was supported by a grant from the National Natural Science Foundation of China to Zhi-Ying Wu (81125009) and the research foundation for distinguished scholar of Zhejiang University to Zhi-Ying Wu (188020-193810101/089).

Authors' contributions

Z-YW designed the project. HY, J-J X and Q-Y D initiated the project. HY, J-J X, Y-C C, Q-Y D, Y D, WN and Z-YW collected the medical information. J-JX, Y-C C and WN performed the sequencing and analyzed the data. HY wrote the manuscript. Z-YW commented and revised on the manuscript. Z-YW supervised all aspects of the project. All authors read and approved the final manuscript.

Competing interests

The authors declare that they have no competing interests.

Author details

[1]Department of Neurology and Research Center of Neurology in Second Affiliated Hospital, and the Collaborative Innovation Center for Brain Science, Zhejiang University School of Medicine, 88 Jiefang Rd, Hangzhou 310009, China. [2]Department of Neurology and Institute of Neurology, First Affiliated Hospital, Fujian Medical University, Fuzhou, China. [3]Department of Neurology and Institute of Neurology, Huashan Hospital, Shanghai Medical College, Fudan University, Shanghai, China. [4]Joint Institute for Genetics and Genome Medicine between Zhejiang University and University of Toronto, Zhejiang University, Hangzhou, China.

References

1. Huster D. Wilson disease. Best Pract Res Clin Gastroenterol. 2010;24(5):531–9.
2. Balint G, Szebenyi B. Hereditary disorders mimicking and/or causing premature osteoarthritis. Baillieres Best Pract Res Clin Rheumatol. 2000;14(2):219–50.
3. Quemeneur AS, Trocello JM, Ea HK, Woimant F, Liote F. Miscellaneous non-inflammatory musculoskeletal conditions. Musculoskeletal conditions associated with Wilson's disease. Best Pract Res Clin Rheumatol. 2011;25(5):627–36.
4. Cai YZ, Jiang TZ, Yang RM. Osseomuscular type of hepatolenticular degeneration: Report of 11 cases. Lin Chuang Shen Jing Bing Xue Za Zhi. 1994;7(3):142–4.
5. Dastur DK, Manghani DK, Wadia NH. Wilson's disease in India. I. Geographic, genetic, and clinical aspects in 16 families. Neurology. 1968;18(1 Pt 1):21–31.
6. Wu ZY, Wang N, Murong SX. Analysis of misdiagnosis of 5 cases of osseomuscular type of hepatolenticular degeneration. Chin J Pract Intern Med. 1995;15(11):669.
7. Aggarwal A, Aggarwal N, Nagral A, Jankharia G, Bhatt M. A novel Global Assessment Scale for Wilson's Disease (GAS for WD). Mov Disord. 2009;24(4): 509–18.
8. Wu ZY, Zhao GX, Chen WJ, Wang N, Wan B, Lin MT, Murong SX, Yu L. Mutation analysis of 218 Chinese patients with Wilson disease revealed no correlation between the canine copper toxicosis gene MURR1 and Wilson disease. J Mol Med (Berl). 2006;84(5):438–42.
9. Wu ZY, Wang N, Lin MT, Fang L, Murong SX, Yu L. Mutation analysis and the correlation between genotype and phenotype of Arg778Leu mutation in chinese patients with Wilson disease. Arch Neurol. 2001;58(6):971–6.
10. European Association for Study of L. EASL clinical practice guidelines: Wilson's disease. J Hepatol. 2012;56(3):671–85.
11. Xie YZ, Zhang XZ, Xu XH, Zhang ZX, Feng YK. Radiologic study of 42 cases of Wilson disease. Skeletal Radiol. 1985;13(2):114–9.
12. Golding DN, Walshe JM. Arthropathy of Wilson's disease. Study of clinical and radiological features in 32 patients. Ann Rheum Dis. 1977;36(2):99–111.
13. Taly AB, Meenakshi-Sundaram S, Sinha S, Swamy HS, Arunodaya GR. Wilson disease: description of 282 patients evaluated over 3 decades. Medicine (Baltimore). 2007;86(2):112–21.
14. Kaklamanis P, Spengos M. Osteoarticular changes and synovial biopsy findings in Wilson's disease. Ann Rheum Dis. 1973;32(5):422–7.
15. Cavallino R, Grossman H. Wilson's disease presenting with rickets. Radiology. 1968;90(3):493–4.
16. Carpenter TO, Carnes Jr DL, Anast CS. Hypoparathyroidism in Wilson's disease. N Engl J Med. 1983;309(15):873–7.
17. Monro P. Effect of treatment on renal function in severe osteomalacia due to Wilson's disease. J Clin Pathol. 1970;23(6):487–91.
18. Chin TY, Duncan JA, Johnstone BR, Graham HK. Management of the upper limb in cerebral palsy. J Pediatr Orthop B. 2005;14(6):389–404.

A rare case of bilateral cervical vagal neurofibromas: role of high-resolution ultrasound

Bin Liu[1†], Yuanding Zhang[2†], Lili Zhang[3], Fan Zhang[4], Hongyu Li[3], Shuang Li[3], Yafang Liu[5], Jie Du[3] and Lirong Zhao[3*]

Abstract

Background: Neurofibromas originating from vagus nerves are rarely reported in the literature. In particular, plexiform neurofibromas of the bilateral cervical vagus nerve are extremely rare.

Case presentation: A 21-year-old female presented with a 2-year history of swelling on the right side of her neck. Physical examination revealed a soft-tissue mass on the right side of her neck. Ultrasonography (US) and magnetic resonance (MR) imaging showed a tumor centered in the right carotid sheath between the internal jugular vein and the common carotid artery. In addition, a similar nodular mass in the left carotid sheath was detected on US. The right mass was surgically resected; histopathological examination revealed a neurofibroma.

Conclusions: US can be a valuable method for preoperative evaluation of cervical mass, as it is capable of displaying the vagus nerve and provides sufficient diagnostic information. The cervical vagal neurofibroma can manifest as solitary or multifocal lesion. Bilateral neurofibromas are usually associated with neurofibromatosis type 1 (NF1). Early diagnosis and prompt surgical treatment should be considered.

Keywords: Vagal neurofibroma, High-resolution ultrasonography, Neurofibromatosis Type 1

Background

Neurofibromatosis type 1 (NF-1) is an autosomal dominant genetic disease, caused by NF1 gene mutations at chromosome 17q11.2 [1]. The condition is characterized by multiple skin lesions such as café-au-lait macules and neurofibromas growing along the parent nerves. Bilateral cervical vagal neurofibromas are extremely rare among patients with neurofibromatosis type 1. To our knowledge, this is the first report of bilateral cervical neurofibromas originating from the vagal nerves. Plexiform neurofibromas represent a special variant of NF-1 in which neurofibromas can arise from multiple nerves as bulging and deforming masses. Herein, we report a rare case of NF-1 with bilateral plexiform neurofibromas arising from cervical vagus nerves.

* Correspondence: liubinzhlr@aliyun.com
†Equal contributors
[3]Department of Electrical Diagnosis, the First Bethune Hospital of Jilin University, No. 3302, Jilin Road, Changchun 130021, China
Full list of author information is available at the end of the article

Case presentation

A 21-year-old woman presented with a 2-year history of focal swelling on the right side of her neck. She did not have any other significant symptoms. Past medical history was unremarkable and she denied any family history of similar lesions or other skin lesions. Physical examination revealed a 7 cm × 5 cm soft-tissue mass on the right side of her neck, and widespread cafe-au-lait spots on her body (Fig. 1c). The mass had smooth surface and was non-pulsatile; it had mobility in lateral direction but not in vertical direction. No hoarseness of voice or change in heart rate was observed on compression of the mass.

Her neurological examinations were otherwise normal. Magnetic resonance (MR) imaging with a 1.5 TMR scanner (Skyra, Siemens Medical Solutions, Erlangen, Germany) showed a 7.7 cm × 4.1 cm × 3.0 cm well-defined mass adjacent to the right internal carotid artery (Fig. 2c and d). Ultrasonography (US) performed with a linear probe (Philips Healthcare IU22, Bothell, WA,

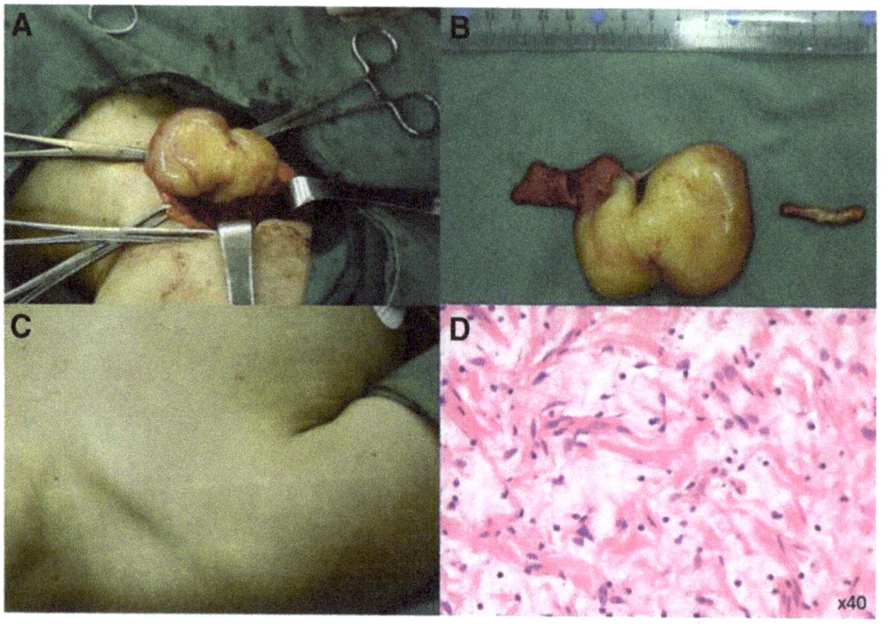

Fig. 1 **a** Intraoperative findings demonstrating that the tumor originates from the vagus nerve. **b** After the mass was removed, we cut the affected distal vagus nerve. **c** Physical examination revealing "cafe-au-lait" spots. **d** Histopathological examination showing spindle-shaped cells with narrow nucleus interspersed with thick bands of collagen (hematoxylin and eosin staining; magnification × 40)

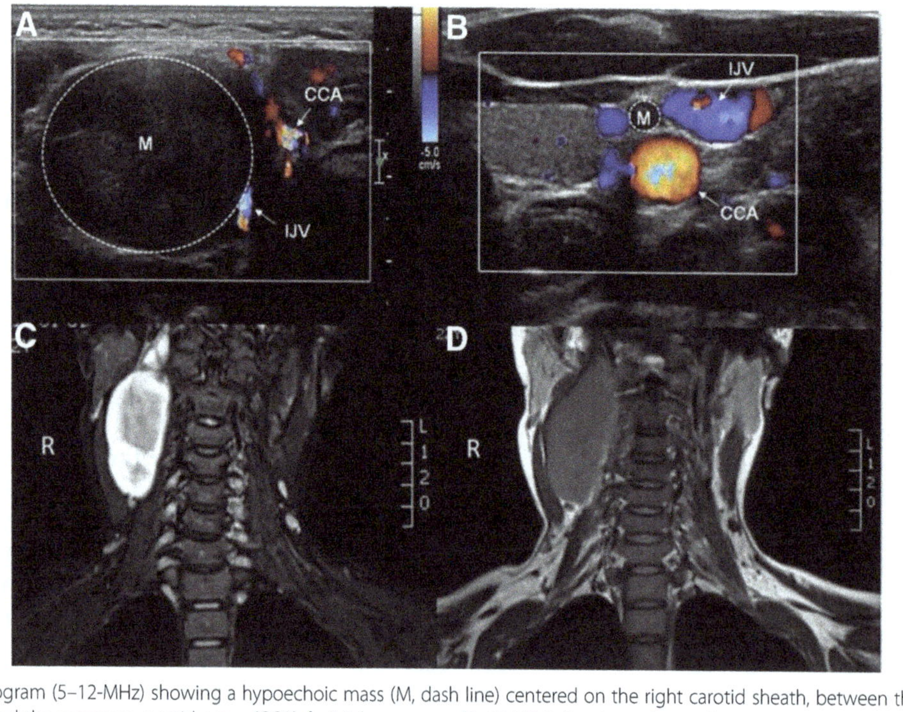

Fig. 2 **a** Axial sonogram (5–12-MHz) showing a hypoechoic mass (M, dash line) centered on the right carotid sheath, between the internal jugular vein (IJA) and the common carotid artery (CCA). **b** Axial sonogram (5–12-MHz) showing a hypoechoic mass (M, dash line), vagus nerve (arrow) and common carotid artery (CCA). **c** The coronal T2-weighted MR imaging shows a 7.7 cm × 4.1 cm × 3.0 cm well-defined hyperintense mass adjacent to the right internal carotid artery. **d** The right tumor appeared hypointense on coronal T1-weighted MR imaging

USA), revealed an almost elliptical, well-circumscribed heterogeneously hypoechoic mass centered on the right carotid sheath between the internal jugular vein and the common carotid artery (Fig. 2a). On grayscale images, the mass appeared heterogeneously hypoechoic with no evidence of calcification, cystic change or internal necrosis. Color Doppler US showed strip-like low-velocity arterial flows within the mass. Furthermore, both the proximal and distal ends of the mass were in continuity with a thick cord like structure which possibly represented the vagus nerve. The left carotid sheath also showed an elongated homogenously hypoechoic nodular mass, and both the proximal and distal ends of the mass were seen in continuity with vagus nerve (Fig. 2b). Homogeneous mass lesions from right thigh intermuscular space and surface of left gastrocnemius also were detected on US. Flexible laryngoscopy showed no evidence of vocal cord paralysis.

A right radical neck dissection was performed. Intraoperatively, the tumor was confirmed to originate from the vagus nerve (Fig. 1a); no adhesions to the adjacent common carotid artery or internal jugular vein were noted. Stimulation of the mass did not induce any obvious electrocardiogram abnormalities. The tumor extended up to the jugular foramen and down to the thyroid cartilage. The gross tumor was totally resected from the proximal and distal vagus nerve. After the mass was removed, we found that the distal vagus nerve was also infiltrated, and therefore we cut the affected distal vagus nerve further (Fig. 1b).

The pathological examination was consistent with the diagnosis of neurofibroma (Fig. 1d). Immunohistochemical staining showed positivity for S-100 protein, while glial fibrillary acidic portein (GFAP) and oligodendrocyte transcription factor-2 (Olig-2) were negative. The Ki-67 labeling index was low (<2%) (Fig. 3a, b, c and d). Considering that the mass on the left side of her neck was still small, no surgery was performed. However, both the proximal and distal ends of the mass were in continuity with the left vagus nerve, and the peritumoral fibers in the left vagus nerve were also thickened. Combined with the cafe-au-lait spots and multifocal tumors, a diagnosis of NF-1 was established [2]. Postoperatively, there were no cardiac complications, nevertheless a laryngoscopy revealed the right vocal cord palsy. A regular ultrasonographic follow-up was scheduled. During a follow-up period of 8 months, no recurrence or progression of the tumors was observed.

Discussion

Bilateral vagal nerve schwannomas are more generally found in the context of NF-2. Neurofibromas that arise from the vagus nerve in NF-1 patients are rare [3, 4]. Plexiform neurofibroma of the bilateral cervical vagus nerve is extremely rare. The clinical presentation of these entities is usually not related to the tumor size. Dysphagia, vocal cord paralysis, hoarseness of voice, and heart rate

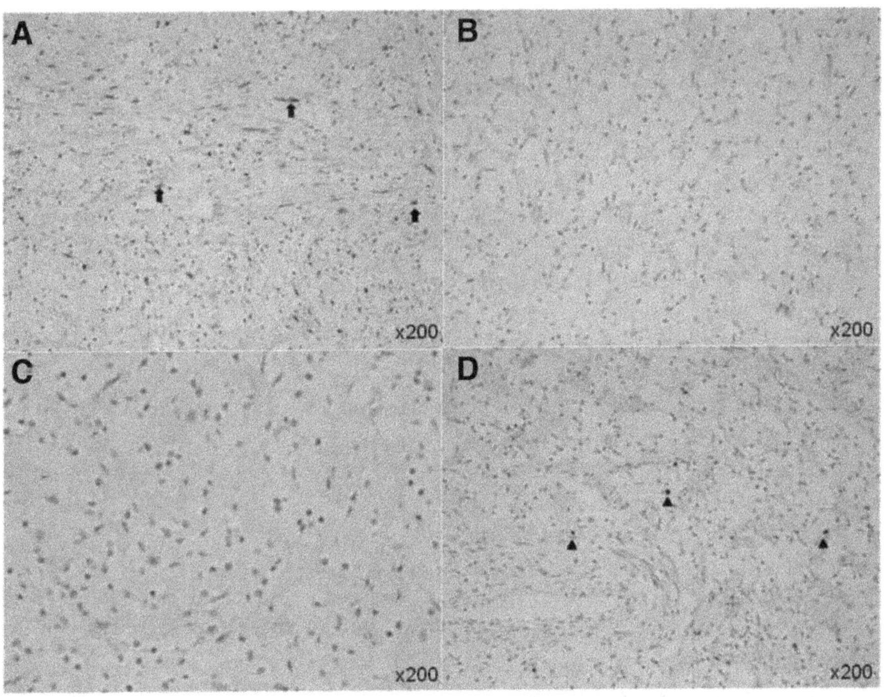

Fig. 3 Immunohistochemical staining (original magnification × 200) of NF1-associated neurofibroma showed positivity for S-100 protein (**a**, arrows), while GFAP (**b**) and Olig-2 (**c**) were negative. The Ki-67 labeling index (**d**, arrowheads) was low (<2%)

changes are the most common manifestations; however, none of these symptoms existed in the current case.

Preoperative diagnosis of a neurofibroma arising from cervical vagus nerve is challenging. The differential diagnosis includes enlarged lymph node and other neurogenic tumors. Echogenic hilum of a lymph node can serve as an important clue to differentiate it from neurogenic tumors. Only tumors arising from the vagus nerve can splay the internal jugular vein and the carotid artery, and the tumors arising from the carotid body will push the vascular structures to lateral or medial position. Lymph nodes and carotid body tumors would not demonstrate continuity with vagus nerve.

A preoperative diagnosis is critical to surgical planning. The internal carotid artery or internal jugular vein splaying, together with the specific clinical symptoms facilitate the preoperative identification of the involved nerve [5]. Schwannomas are common isolated, unilateral tumors. Internal cystic changes are more common in schwannomas. In addition, isolated schwannomas can be completely resected from the parent nerves. On the contrary, neurofibromas tend to intertwine themselves with several fascicles of nerve of origin. The adjacent nerves may show irregular thickening. Therefore it is often impossible to completely remove the neurofibroma whilst ensuring preservation of the parent nerve. Surgical resection of neurofibromas is therefore more difficult than that of schwannomas.

Neurofibromas typically exhibit intermediate signal intensity on T1-weighted images, and in T2-weighted images these exhibit a moderate to marked high signal intensity, as was seen in the current case. MR imaging can clearly observe the relationship between large tumors and the adjacent structures, but this modality may not delineate a small mass like the neurofibroma of the left vagus nerve in our patient. In such cases, high-resolution US can overcome the shortcomings of MRI. Color Doppler US can detect low-velocity arterial flows within the mass, and explicit the anatomical relationship between the mass and its peripheral vascular. Additionally, it makes it feasible to evaluate adherence of the tumor to vessels by applying gentle pressure on the probe. Moreover, the high-resolution images on US can help to identify the origin of tumors. In the present case, US revealed a hypoechoic tumor centered on the carotid sheath; both the proximal and distal ends of the tumor were in continuity with the vagus nerve; these radiological features were important diagnostic clues to its vagal nerve origin. Once a diagnosis of neurofibroma of the vagus nerve is made on one side, the possibility of bilateral tumors should be considered. This prompted us to scan the other side of the neck as well, which revealed a fusiform mass involving the left vagus nerve. Additionally, we scanned the extremities, and found the sural nerve was also affected. Together with the widespread cafe-au-lait spots, this patient met the diagnostic criteria for NF-1 [2]. That would truly be a lesson learned from the paper - I would have relied on the MR imaging alone for surgery!

In the current case, the right tumor was completely resected from the proximal and distal vagus nerve, and we cut the distal affected vagus nerve as well. Since both vagus nerves were affected; considering the potential risk of bilateral vagal resection such as dysphonia, dysphagia, cough, tongue weakness, hoarseness, cranial nerve palsy, and cardiac events [6], we recommended monitoring of the smaller left-sided neck mass.

Conclusions

Our experience suggests that US can be a valuable method for preoperative evaluation of a cervical mass, as it is capable of displaying the vagus nerve and provides sufficient diagnostic information. Therefore, high-resolution US could be an alternative diagnostic imaging modality to MR imaging for patients with suspected neurogenic tumors of the cervical vagus nerve, especially in patients for whom MR imaging is contraindicated.

Abbreviations

MR: Magnetic resonance; NF-1: Neurofibromatosis type 1; US: Ultrasonography

Acknowledgements

None declared.

Funding

None.

Authors' contributions

LB and ZYD designed the study, conducted all searches, appraised all potential studies and wrote and revised the draft manuscript and subsequent manuscripts. ZLL, ZF and LHY revised the draft manuscript and subsequent manuscripts. LS, LYF and DJ assisted with the presentation of findings and assisted with drafting and revising the manuscript. ZLR conceived and designed the study, assisted with searches, appraised relevant studies and assisted with drafting and revising the manuscript. All authors read and approved the final manuscript.

Competing interests

We declare that we have no conflict of interest.

Author details

[1]Department of Hand Surgery, the First Bethune Hospital of Jilin University, Changchun 130021, China. [2]Department of Otolaryngology, the First Bethune Hospital of Jilin University, Changchun 130021, China. [3]Department of Electrical Diagnosis, the First Bethune Hospital of Jilin University, No. 3302, Jilin Road, Changchun 130021, China. [4]Department of Hand Surgery, China-Japan Union Hospital of Jilin University, Changchun 130033, China. [5]Department of Pathology, the First Bethune Hospital of Jilin University, Changchun 130021, China.

References

1. Ledbetter DH, Rich DC, O'Connell P, Leppert M, Carey JC. Precise localization of NF1 to 17q11.2 by balanced translocation. Am J Hum Gene. 1989;44(1):20–4.
2. National Institutes of Health Consensus Development Conference Statement. neurofibromatosis. Bethesda, Md., USA, July 13–15, 1987. Neurofibromatosis . 1988;1(3):172–8.
3. Heitmiller RF, Labs JD, Lipsett PA. Vagal schwannoma. Ann Thorac Surg. 1990;50(5):811–3.
4. Dabir RR, Piccione Jr W, Kittle CF. Intrathoracic tumors of the vagus nerve. Ann Thorac Surg. 1990;50(3):494–7.
5. Graffeo CS, Van Abel KM, Morris JM, Carlson ML, Van Gompel JJ, Moore EJ, Price DL, Kasperbauer JL, Janus JR, Olsen KD, et al. Preoperative diagnosis of vagal and sympathetic cervical schwannomas based on radiographic findings. J Neurosurg. 2016;2016:1–8.
6. Shintani Y, Ohta M, Hazama K, Minami M, Okumura M, Hirabayashi H, Matsuda H. Bilateral cervicomediastinal neurofibroma originating from the vagal nerve in a patient with von Recklinghausen's disease: report of a case. Surg Today. 2002;32(12):1068–71.

32

Why use a mirror to assess visual pursuit in prolonged disorders of consciousness? Evidence from healthy control participants

Damian Cruse[1*], Marco Fattizzo[2], Adrian M. Owen[3] and Davinia Fernández-Espejo[1]

Abstract

Background: Evidence of reliable smooth visual pursuit is crucial for both diagnosis and prognosis in prolonged disorders of consciousness (PDOC). However, a mirror is more likely than an object to elicit evidence of smooth pursuit. Our objective was to identify the physiological and/or cognitive mechanism underlying the mirror benefit.

Methods: We recorded eye-movements while healthy participants simultaneously completed a visual pursuit task and a cognitively demanding two-back task. We manipulated the stimulus to be pursued (two levels: mirror, ball) and the simultaneous cognitive load (pursuit only, pursuit plus two-back task) within subjects.

Results: Pursuit of the reflected-own-face in the mirror was associated with briefer fixations that occurred less uniformly across the horizontal plane relative to object pursuit. Secondary task performance did not differ between pursuit stimuli. The secondary task also did not affect eye movement measures, nor did it interact with pursuit stimulus.

Conclusions: Reflected-own-face pursuit is no less cognitively demanding than object pursuit, but it naturally elicits smoother eye movements (i.e. briefer pauses to fixate). A mirror therefore provides greater sensitivity to detect smooth visual pursuit in PDOC because the naturally smoother eye movements may be identified more confidently by the assessor.

Keywords: Brain injuries, Consciousness disorders, Diagnosis, Smooth pursuit

Background

Visual pursuit of a moving object signifies the transition from unawareness to awareness in prolonged disorders of consciousness (PDOC) – i.e. from vegetative state to minimally conscious state [1]. Accurate differential diagnosis is crucial in PDOC because treatment decisions may be influenced by differences in likelihood of functional recovery that are associated with each diagnostic group [2, 3].

Two recent studies found that visual pursuit is significantly more likely to be observed in PDOC when the stimulus to be pursued is the patient's own face reflected in a mirror, relative to when the stimulus is an object or person. [4, 5]. The cause of this effect is unclear, although it has been hypothesised that the patient's own face is more likely to attract the gaze as it is a salient and auto-referential stimulus [4, 5]. This hypothesis, however, presumes that reflected-own-face pursuit indexes consciousness to the same extent as object pursuit. In other words, a patient who only pursues their reflected-own-face, and not an object, is considered to be conscious to the same clinical level as a patient who pursues both. Any difference in pursuit behaviour between these two patients is considered to stem from an attention deficit that can be overcome with a sufficiently salient stimulus [4, 5].

However, extremely highly learned stimuli, such as one's own name or own face, can elicit complex responses in the absence of awareness. For example, one's own name is subjected to complex neural processing even during non-REM sleep — a period in which an individual is demonstrably unaware [6]. Furthermore, the brain's electrophysiological response differentiates one's own-face from faces of others even when the individual is unaware of having seen a face at all [7]. An alternate interpretation, therefore, is that processing of high relevance stimuli, such

* Correspondence: d.cruse@bham.ac.uk
[1]School of Psychology, University of Birmingham, Birmingham B15 2TT, England
Full list of author information is available at the end of the article

as pursuit of one's own reflected face, may be less reliant on overt consciousness than processing of less salient stimuli, such as pursuit of an object. In other words, is reflected-own-face pursuit less demanding than object pursuit, thus allowing patients with lower cognitive abilities, or even lower levels of consciousness, to exhibit reliable pursuit? This interpretation has important implications for diagnoses achieved through responses to high relevance stimuli, such as own-face and own-name [8–10]. A further alternative physiological interpretation for the difference in pursuit behaviour is that conscious patients are actively attempting to pursue both stimuli, but that the eye movements during reflected-own-face pursuit are naturally smoother and therefore easier for an assessor to identify confidently.

To test these hypotheses, we asked a group of healthy participants to separately pursue an object and their reflection in a mirror while completing a challenging secondary task designed to reduce the cognitive resources available for smooth pursuit. If reflected-own-face pursuit does not draw on conscious resources to the same extent as object pursuit, we would predict differential performance on the secondary task and on measures of smooth pursuit, quantified via a head-mounted eye-tracker.

Methods

Participants

We recruited 25 participants from the research pool of the University of Western Ontario (UWO). All participants reported normal vision and were compensated with course credit. We excluded data from 8 participants due to hardware malfunction ($n = 3$) or chance-level task performance ($n = 5$), leaving 17 participants (median age: 18-years, range 18–23). The Research Ethics Board of UWO approved this study.

Equipment

A robot arm repeatedly moved objects through 90° on the horizontal plane ~30-cm in front of the participant's eyes (45° either side of forward-facing; manufactured by Bonneville Scientific Inc., Salt Lake City, Utah, USA). One full oscillation lasted 10-s. An Eyelink II (SR Research Ltd, Mississauga, Ontario, Canada) tracked the movements of the left-eye (sample rate: 500-Hz; Fig. 1). The experimenter recalibrated the eye-tracker prior to each trial. The object stimulus (a ball) was mounted to the back of the mirror at the end of the robot arm, and the appropriate stimulus turned to face the participant on each trial. This ensured that the size of the moving portion of the arm was consistent across stimulus conditions. Prior to completion of mirror trials, the experimenter ensured that the mirror was placed in such a way that the participant could see the reflection of their face throughout the robot arm's range of movement.

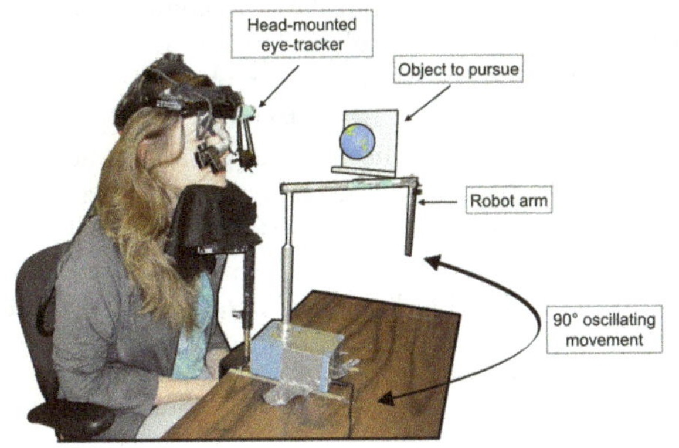

Fig. 1 Experimental setup including eye-tracker, robot arm, and object to be pursued

Cognitive task

To increase cognitive load while participants pursued the stimuli, we developed a two-back category-matching task. Participants heard a series of spoken letters (3-s onset asynchrony) and indicated via button press whether or not each item was from the same category as that two items previously. Five letters that contain horizontal lines when written in their capital form comprised one category (E, F, H, L, T) and five that did not (V, W, X, Q, S) comprised the other. Such an orthographic comparison task was hypothesised to tax visual processing and interfere with pursuit demands. A pseudo-random series of 90 letters (22 matches) was created per trial.

Design and procedure

Participants completed four trials from a two-by-two design — two stimuli (mirror, ball) x two levels of cognitive load (pursuit only, pursuit plus two-back) – in counterbalanced order. Prior to the experiment, participants completed a practice two-back task until they understood the procedure. Participants were instructed to smoothly pursue the moving stimuli with their eyes without moving their head. Each trial lasted 4.5-min followed by a brief rest.

Analyses

To rule out potential task non-compliance, we excluded those participants with chance performance on either trial. Specifically, we shuffled the recorded button presses within trials and calculated the corresponding discrimination value (p[hit] minus p[false alarm] [11]), thus controlling for response biases. We performed this procedure 1000 times, creating a distribution under the null hypothesis that discrimination was not different from chance. Participants with discrimination within the lower 95% of the surrogate distribution (i.e. $p > .05$) were excluded from analyses (conducted with MATLAB).

Frequentist and equivalent Bayesian comparisons with default priors were conducted with JASP Version 0.7.1.12 [12, 13]. Specifically, to complement the t-tests, the Jeffrey-Zellner-Siow Bayes factor (JZS-BF_{10}) tested the strength of the evidence for each observed effect size [14]. A JZS-BF_{10} ANOVA approach contrasted the strength of evidence for models reflecting the null, main effects, and interaction [15]. A JZS-BF_{10} between 1/3 and 3 is considered to be only weak/anecdotal evidence for an effect; 3–10: substantial evidence; 10–100: strong evidence; >100: very strong evidence [16]. The same category descriptions hold for the inverse.

Results

Cognitive task

Discrimination did not significantly differ between pursuit stimuli in a paired samples *t*-test ($t(16) = .330$, $p = .746$). A Bayesian equivalent indicated substantial evidence in favour of the null hypothesis (JZS-$BF_{10} = .261$). Mean reaction time did not significantly differ between pursuit stimuli in a paired samples *t*-test ($t(16) = .866$, $p = .399$). A Bayesian equivalent indicated marginally more evidence for the null hypothesis (JZS-$BF_{10} = .346$).

Fixations

A two-way repeated measures ANOVA on numbers of fixations with factors of stimulus (ball, mirror) and cognitive load (pursuit only, pursuit plus two-back) revealed a marginal effect of load only ($F(1,16) = 4.486$, $p = .050$; stimulus: $F(1,16) = .053$, $p = .821$; interaction: $F(1,16) = .004$, $p = .948$). A Bayesian equivalent indicated that no model was preferred relative to the null model (all JZS-$BF_{10} < .506$).

A further ANOVA on average durations of fixation with the same factors revealed a significant effect of stimulus ($F(1,16) = 15.763$, $p = .001$), a marginal effect of load ($F(1,16) = 3.294$, $p = .088$), and no significant interaction ($F(1,16) = .718$, $p = .409$). A Bayesian equivalent indicated greater evidence for an effect of stimulus only, relative to all other models (JZS-$BF_{10} = 121.430$ relative to null). See Fig. 2a.

Post-hoc analyses

During data quality checks, we noticed a qualitative difference in the spatial distribution of fixations (Fig. 2b). Specifically, fixations during object pursuit occurred relatively uniformly across the tracking space, while fixations during reflected-own-face pursuit occurred mostly when the mirror changed direction. To quantify this difference, we conducted the following post-hoc analysis. First, we removed outlier fixations (>2 standard deviations from mean horizontal or vertical coordinates). Next, we scaled the X-coordinates of fixations to be between 0 and 1, and tested this distribution against a uniform distribution (Chi-square goodness of fit, 10-bins). An ANOVA on the log-normalised Chi-square statistics with the same factors as above revealed a significant effect of stimulus only ($F(1,16) = 14.299$, $p = .002$; load: $F(1,16) = .310$, $p = .585$; interaction: $F(1,16) < .001$, $p = .982$). A Bayesian equivalent revealed substantial evidence for the model containing only the factor of stimulus relative to all other models (all JZS-BF10 > 3.735).

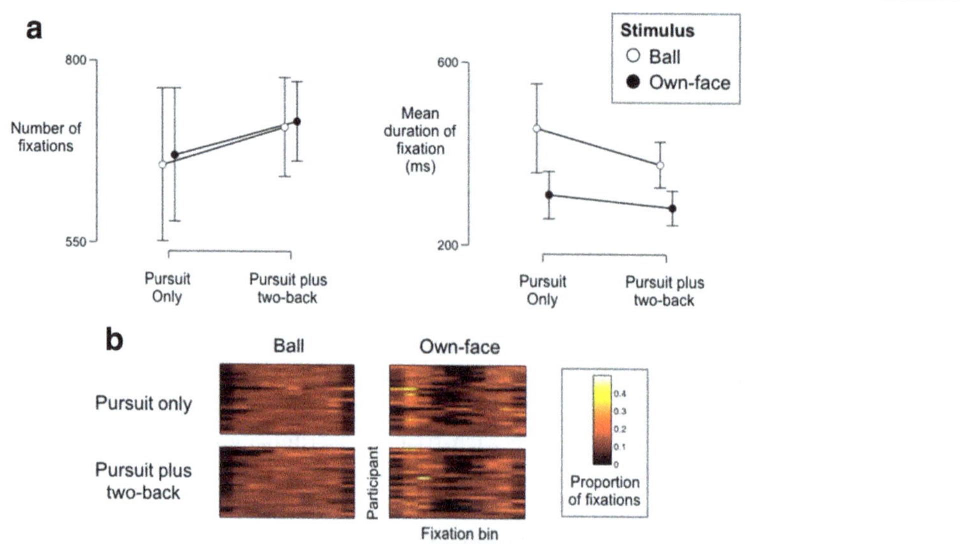

Fig. 2 a Fixation behaviour across trials. Bars show 95% confidence intervals. **b** Single-subject distributions of fixations across trials. Each row of each panel shows data from one participant separated into ten bins across the horizontal plane of pursuit. Right-hand images highlight greater foci of fixations at the tails during reflected-own-face pursuit

Discussion

Our data indicate that pursuit of one's own face reflected in a mirror is no less cognitively demanding than pursuit of an object, and therefore that both stimuli tap similar diagnostically important abilities in PDOC. Indeed, a Bayesian analysis indicates substantial evidence in favour of no differences in secondary task performance during reflected-own-face or object-pursuit.

Eye-tracking indicates that reflected-own-face pursuit is naturally smoother than object pursuit, and may therefore be less likely to be missed or confused with irrelevant staccato eye movements (e.g. nystagmus). Indeed, the data provide very strong evidence for significantly shorter mean eye fixations during reflected-own-face pursuit, which we interpret as a sign of smoother pursuit because the eyes do not take long pauses to fixate. Fixations also occur more uniformly across the space of object pursuit, consistent with less smooth pursuit.

While it is possible that the eye movements of healthy participants reported here do not generalise to PDOC, recent eye-tracking evidence suggests generalisability between patients and healthy controls [17]. We cannot rule out the possibility that a more demanding secondary task will have an effect on our measures of smooth pursuit, unlike the two-back task we employed here. However, even if this were the case, it is unlikely that the interaction between task performance and pursuit stimulus would be borne out, as indicated by the strong evidence against interaction models in our data (number of fixations: interaction JZS-$BF_{10} = .040$; duration of fixations: interaction JZS-$BF_{10} = .404$; relative to model with highest evidence). We therefore conclude that the cognitive demands of reflected-own-face pursuit and object pursuit are comparable.

These data provide further support for the use of a mirror in clinical assessments of awareness [4, 10]. It has been suggested that the greater sensitivity of the reflected-own-face stimulus stems from its higher salience and subsequent auto-referential processing – i.e. self-awareness [4, 5]. Indeed, there is evidence that autonomic responses to own-face photographs in the minimally conscious state are more similar to healthy individuals, while the autonomic response of patients in the vegetative state fails to differentiate between own-face and control stimuli [18]. Nevertheless, open questions remain regarding the subjective experience of patients who pursue their reflected own-face: does reflected-own-face pursuit index a simultaneous subjective experience of self-awareness on the part of the patient? Contemporary advances in brain imaging and physiological recordings may provide some insight into this question. Regardless, our data are consistent with the view that visual pursuit of reflected-own-face in PDOC is evidence of a similar level of consciousness and cognition to that identified by object pursuit, and therefore is a more appropriate method in clinical assessment.

Conclusions

Our data provide substantial evidence that a mirror provides greater sensitivity to detect visual pursuit in patients with PDOC not because reflected-own-face pursuit is a less complex ability, but because the mirror naturally elicits smoother eye movements that can be identified more confidently by the assessor. These smoother and more reliable eye movements may be driven by the self-referential nature of the reflected-own-face stimulus, although further research is needed to appropriately characterise the relationship with subjective self-awareness.

Abbreviations

ANOVA: Analysis of variance; JZS-BF: Jeffrey-Zellner-Siow Bayes factor; PDOC: Prolonged disorder of consciousness; REM: Rapid eye movement

Acknowledgements

We thank Finola D'Souza and Natalie Osborne for their assistance in data collection.

Funding

We thank the Canada Excellence Research Chairs Programme (CERC; 215063) and the Canadian Institutes for Health Research (MFE 123754) for funding this study.

Authors' contributions

MF contributed to data collection. DC analysed the data and drafted the manuscript. DC, MF, AMO, & DFE designed the study, contributed to interpretation of data, and the final manuscript. All authors read and approved the final manuscript.

Competing interests

The authors declare that they have no competing interests.

Author details

[1]School of Psychology, University of Birmingham, Birmingham B15 2TT, England. [2]Department of Neurorehabilitation, University Hospital of Ghent, Ghent 9000, Belgium. [3]The Brain and Mind Institute, University of Western Ontario, London, Ontario N6A 5B7, Canada.

References

1. The Royal College of Physicians. Prolonged disorders of consciousness: national clinical guidelines. London: Royal College of Physicians; 2013. p. 1–130.
2. Giacino JT, Kalmar K. The vegetative and minimally conscious states: a comparison of clinical features and functional outcome. J Head Trauma Rehabil. 1997;12:36.
3. Luaute J, Maucort-Boulch D, Tell L, Quelard F, Sarraf T, Iwaz J, et al. Long-term outcomes of chronic minimally conscious and vegetative states. Neurology. 2010;75:246–52.
4. Thonnard M, Wannez S, Keen S, Bredart S, Bruno M-A, Gosseries O, et al. Detection of visual pursuit in patients in minimally conscious state: a matter of stimuli and visual plane? Brain Inj. 2014;28:1164–70.

5. Vanhaudenhuyse A, Schnakers C, Bredart S, Laureys S. Assessment of visual pursuit in post-comatose states: use a mirror. J Neurol Neurosurg Psychiatry. 2008;79:223–3.
6. Perrin F. A differential brain response to the subject's own name persists during sleep. Clin Neurophysiol. 1999;110:2153–64.
7. Geng H, Zhang S, Li Q, Tao R, Xu S. Dissociations of subliminal and supraliminal self-face from other-face processing: Behavioral and ERP evidence. Neuropsychologia. 2012;50:2933–42.
8. Perrin F, Castro M, Tillmann B, Luaute J. Promoting the use of personally relevant stimuli for investigating patients with disorders of consciousness. Front Psychol. 2015;6:345.
9. Cheng L, Gosseries O, Ying L, Hu X, Yu D, Gao H, et al. Assessment of localisation to auditory stimulation in post-comatose states: use the patient's own name. BMC Neurol. 2013;13:27.
10. Di H, Nie Y, Hu X, Tong Y, Heine L, Wannez S, et al. Assessment of visual fixation in vegetative and minimally conscious states. BMC Neurol. 2014;14:147.
11. Green DM, Swets JA. Signal detection theory and psychophysics. New York: Wiley; 1966.
12. Love J, Selker R, Marsman M, Jamil T, Dropmann D, Verhagen AJ, et al. JASP (Version 0.7.1) [Computer Software].
13. Morey RD, Rouder JN. BayesFactor (Version 0.9.11-3) [Computer Software].
14. Rouder JN, Speckman PL, Sun D, Morey RD, Iverson G. Bayesian t tests for accepting and rejecting the null hypothesis. Psychon Bull Rev. 2009;16:225–37.
15. Rouder JN, Morey RD, Speckman PL, Province JM. Default Bayes factors for ANOVA designs. J Math Psychol. 2012;56:356–74.
16. Jeffreys H. Theory of probability. Oxford: Oxford University Press; 1961.
17. Hoyoux T, Wannez S, Langohr T, Wertz J, Laureys S, Verly JG. A new computer vision-based system to help clinicians objectively assess visual pursuit with the moving mirror stimulus for the diagnosis of minimally conscious state. 2016 IEEE Winter Conference on Applications of Computer Vision (WACV). IEEE; p. 1–8. doi:10.1109/WACV.2016.7477604.
18. Bagnato S, Boccagni C, Prestandrea C, Galardi G. Autonomic correlates of seeing one's own face in patients with disorders of consciousness. Neuroscience of Consciousness. The Oxford University Press; 2015; 2015:niv005. doi:10.1093/nc/niv005.

Permissions

All chapters in this book were first published in NEUROLOGY, by BioMed Central; hereby published with permission under the Creative Commons Attribution License or equivalent. Every chapter published in this book has been scrutinized by our experts. Their significance has been extensively debated. The topics covered herein carry significant findings which will fuel the growth of the discipline. They may even be implemented as practical applications or may be referred to as a beginning point for another development.

The contributors of this book come from diverse backgrounds, making this book a truly international effort. This book will bring forth new frontiers with its revolutionizing research information and detailed analysis of the nascent developments around the world.

We would like to thank all the contributing authors for lending their expertise to make the book truly unique. They have played a crucial role in the development of this book. Without their invaluable contributions this book wouldn't have been possible. They have made vital efforts to compile up to date information on the varied aspects of this subject to make this book a valuable addition to the collection of many professionals and students.

This book was conceptualized with the vision of imparting up-to-date information and advanced data in this field. To ensure the same, a matchless editorial board was set up. Every individual on the board went through rigorous rounds of assessment to prove their worth. After which they invested a large part of their time researching and compiling the most relevant data for our readers.

The editorial board has been involved in producing this book since its inception. They have spent rigorous hours researching and exploring the diverse topics which have resulted in the successful publishing of this book. They have passed on their knowledge of decades through this book. To expedite this challenging task, the publisher supported the team at every step. A small team of assistant editors was also appointed to further simplify the editing procedure and attain best results for the readers.

Apart from the editorial board, the designing team has also invested a significant amount of their time in understanding the subject and creating the most relevant covers. They scrutinized every image to scout for the most suitable representation of the subject and create an appropriate cover for the book.

The publishing team has been an ardent support to the editorial, designing and production team. Their endless efforts to recruit the best for this project, has resulted in the accomplishment of this book. They are a veteran in the field of academics and their pool of knowledge is as vast as their experience in printing. Their expertise and guidance has proved useful at every step. Their uncompromising quality standards have made this book an exceptional effort. Their encouragement from time to time has been an inspiration for everyone.

The publisher and the editorial board hope that this book will prove to be a valuable piece of knowledge for researchers, students, practitioners and scholars across the globe.

List of Contributors

Bin Han, Chao Zhang and Junwei Hao
Department of Neurology, Tianjin Neurological Institute, Tianjin Medical University General Hospital, Tianjin 300052, China

Shoufeng Liu
Department of Neurology, Tianjin HuanHu Hospital, Tianjin 300060, China

Yiping Xia
Laboratory of Physical and Chemical Research, Tianjin Centers for Disease Control and Prevention, Tianjin 300011, China

Hao Sun
Department of Neurology, Shandong Provincial Hospital Affiliated to Shandong University, Jinan, Shandong 250021, China

Zhongying Gong
Department of Neurology, Tianjin First Center Hospital, Tianjin Medical University, Tianjin 300192, China

Alain R. Simard
Département de chimie et biochimie, Université de Moncton, Moncton, New Brunswick E1A 3E9, Canada

Qiang Liu
Department of Neurology, Tianjin Neurological Institute, Tianjin Medical University General Hospital, Tianjin 300052, China
Department of Neurology, Barrow Neurological Institute, St. Joseph's Hospital and Medical Center, Phoenix, AZ 85013, USA

J. D. Rollnik
Institute for Neurorehabilitation Research (InFo), BDH-Klinik Hessisch Oldendorf, Hannover Medical School (MHH), Greitstr. 18-28, 31840 Hess. Oldendorf, Germany

M. Bertram and G. Ketter
Kliniken Schmieder Heidelberg, Heidelberg, Germany

C. Bucka
Neurologische Klinik Westend, Bad Wildungen, Germany

M. Hartwich
Asklepios Schlossberg Klinik Bad König, Bad König, Germany

M. Jöbges
Brandenburg Klinik Bernau, Berlin, Germany

W. Wallesch
BDH-Klinik Elzach, Elzach, Germany

C H. Woldag
Neurologisches Rehabilitationszentrum Leipzig, Bennewitz, Germany

P. Peschel
Department of Public Health, University of Dresden, Dresden, Germany

J. Mehrholz
Department of Public Health, University of Dresden, Dresden, Germany

M. Pohl
Klinik Schloss Pulsnitz, Pulsnitz, Germany

Bontle G. Malatji, Shayne Mason, Mari van Reenen and Carolus J. Reinecke
Centre for Human Metabolomics, Faculty of Natural Sciences, North-West University (Potchefstroom Campus), Private Bag X6001, Potchefstroom, South Africa

Helgard Meyer
Department of Family Medicine, Kalafong Hospital, University of Pretoria, Pretoria, South Africa

Udo F.H. Engelke and Ron A. Wevers
Translational Metabolic Laboratory, Department of Laboratory Medicine, Radboud University Nijmegen Medical Centre, Nijmegen, The Netherlands

Isaäc Bos, Jan B.M. Kuks and Hubertus P.H. Kremer
Department of Neurology, University Medical Center Groningen, University of Groningen, The Netherlands

Klaske Wynia
Department of Neurology, University Medical Center Groningen, University of Groningen, The Netherlands
Department of Health Sciences, Community and Occupational Health, University Medical Center Groningen, University of Groningen, Groningen, the Netherlands

Josué Almansa
Department of Health Sciences, Community and Occupational Health, University Medical Center Groningen, University of Groningen, Groningen, the Netherlands

Masahiko Fukatsu, Takenobu Murakami, Suguru Kadowaki, Itaru Sasaki, Mari Segawa, Tomoko Soeda, Akihiko Hoshi and Yoshihiro Sugiura
Department of Neurology, Fukushima Medical University, 1 Hikariga-oka, Fukushima, Fukushima 960-1295, Japan

Hiroshi Ohkawara, Hiroshi Takahashi, Akiko Shichishima-Nakamura, Kazuei Ogawa and Takayuki Ikezoe
Department of Hematology, Fukushima Medical University, Fukushima, Japan

Kazuhiko Ikeda
Department of Hematology, Fukushima Medical University, Fukushima, Japan
Department of Blood Transfusion and Transplantation Immunology, Fukushima Medical University, Fukushima, Japan

Shunichi Saito and Hitoshi Ohto
Department of Blood Transfusion and Transplantation Immunology, Fukushima Medical University, Fukushima, Japan

Yasuchika Takeishi
Department of Cardiovascular Medicine, Fukushima Medical University, Fukushima, Japan

Yoshikazu Ugawa
Department of Neurology, Fukushima Medical University, 1 Hikariga-oka, Fukushima, Fukushima 960-1295, Japan
Fukushima Global Medical Science Center, Advanced Clinical Research Center, Fukushima Medical University, Fukushima, Japan

Laura Kytövuori, Mikko Kärppä and Kari Majamaa
Research Unit of Clinical Neuroscience, University of Oulu, FI-90014 Oulu, Finland
Medical Research Center Oulu, Oulu University Hospital and University of Oulu, Oulu, Finland
Department of Neurology, Oulu University Hospital, FI-90029 Oulu, Finland

Hannu Tuominen
Department of Pathology, Cancer and Translational Medicine Research Unit, University of Oulu and Department of Pathology, Oulu University Hospital, Oulu, Finland

Johanna Uusimaa and Reetta Hinttala
Medical Research Center Oulu, Oulu University Hospital and University of Oulu, Oulu, Finland
PEDEGO Research Unit, University of Oulu,Finland
Department of Children and Adolescents, Division of Pediatric Neurology, Oulu University Hospital, Oulu, Finland
Biocenter Oulu, University of Oulu, Finland

Markku Saari
Turku Centre for Biotechnology, Cell Imaging Core, University of Turku, FI-20520 Turku, Finland

Goran Rakocevic
Department of Neurology, Thomas Jefferson University, 901 Walnut Street, Room 408, Philadelphia, PA 19107, USA

Mark Moster
Wills Eye Hospital, Thomas Jefferson University, Philadelphia, PA, USA

Mary Kay Floeter
EMG Section, National Institute of Neurological Disorders and Stroke, National Institutes of Health, Bethesda, MD, USA

Yong S. Shim
Department of Neurology, Bucheon St. Mary's Hospital, College of Medicine, The Catholic University of Korea, Seoul, Republic of Korea
327 Sosa-ro, Wonmi-gu, Bucheon-si, Gyeonggi-do 14647, South Korea

Dong Won Yang
Department of Neurology, Seoul St. Mary's Hospital, College of Medicine, The Catholic University of Korea, Seoul, Republic of Korea

Hee-Jin Kim
Department of Neurology, College of Medicine, Hanyang University, Seoul, Republic of Korea

Young Ho Park
Department of Neurology, Seoul National University College of Medicine & Clinical Neuroscience Center, Seoul National University Bundang Hospital, Seoul, Republic of Korea

SangYun Kim
Department of Neurology, Seoul National University College of Medicine & Clinical Neuroscience Center, Seoul National University Bundang Hospital, Seoul, Republic of Korea 82, Gumi-ro 173 beon-gil, Bundang-gu, Seongnam-si, Gyeonggi-do 13620, South Korea

Ming-Feng Liao, Jung-Lung Hsu, Ai-Lun Lo, Hung-Chou Kuo, Rong-Kuo Lyu and Long-Sun Ro
Department of Neurology, Chang Gung Memorial Hospital Linkou Medical Center and Chang Gung University College of Medicine, No.199, Tung Hwa N. Rd., Songshan Dist, Taipei City 105, Taiwan, Republic of China

Hui-Ching Hsu
Department of Traditional Chinese Medicine, Division of Chinese Acupuncture and Traumatology, Chang Gung Memorial Hospital Linkou Medical Center and Chang Gung University College of Medicine, No.5, Fuxing St., Guishan Dist, Taoyuan City 333, Taiwan, Republic of China

Victor Chien-Chia Wu
Department of Cardiology, Chang Gung Memorial Hospital Linkou Medical Center and Chang Gung University College of Medicine, No.5, Fuxing St., Guishan Dist, Taoyuan City 333, Taiwan, Republic of China

Chih-Wei Wang
Department of Anatomic Pathology, Chang Gung Memorial Hospital Linkou Medical Center and Chang Gung University College of Medicine, No.5, Fuxing St., Guishan Dist, Taoyuan City 333, Taiwan, Republic of China

Volker Limmroth and Kathrin Gerbershagen
Department of Neurology, Cologne General Hospitals, University of Cologne, Cologne, Germany

Tjalf Ziemssen
Center of Clinical Neuroscience, University Clinic Carl Gustav Carus Dresden, Dresden, Germany

Michael Lang
NTD Study Group, Neurologische Praxis, Ulm, Germany

Stephan Richter and Bert Wagner
NeuroMVZ, Stuttgart, Germany

Judith Haas
Jewish Hospital Berlin, Berlin, Germany

Stephan Schmidt
NTD Study Group, Neurologische Gemeinschaftspraxis, Bonn, Germany

Christoph Lassek
Neurologische Gemeinschaftspraxis Kassel und Vellmar, Kassel, Germany

Luisa Klotz
Department of Neurology, University of Muenster, Muenster, Germany

Olaf Hoffmann and Christian Albert
St. Josefs-Krankenhaus Potsdam-Sanssouci, Potsdam, Germany

Katrin Schuh, Monika Baier-Ebert, Guillaume Wendt, Heinke Schieb and Susanne Hoyer
Novartis Pharma GmbH, Nuremberg, Germany

Ralf Dechend
Experimental and Clinical Research Center, Charité-Campus Buch, Berlin, Germany

Wilhelm Haverkamp
Charité Universitaetsmedizin Berlin, Campus Virchow Klinikum, Augustenburger Platz 1, Berlin 13353, Germany

Jie Cao and Min Zhang
Department of Neurology, Tongji Hospital, Tongji Medical College, Huazhong
University of Science and Technology, No. 1095 Jiefang Avenue, Wuhan 430030, China

Kathrin Habig, Wolfgang Schirner, Gothje Lautenschläger and Heidrun H. Krämer
Department of Neurology, Justus Liebig University, Klinikstr. 33, 35392 Giessen, Germany

Anne Schänzer
Institute of Neuropathology, Justus Liebig University, Arndtstr. 16, 35392 Giessen, Germany

Benjamin Dassinger
Department of Radiology, Justus Liebig University, Klinikstr.33, 35392 Giessen, Germany

Håkan Olausson
Center for Social and Affective Neuroscience, Linköping University, Linköpings Universitet, 58183 Linköping, Sweden

Frank Birklein
Department of Neurology, University Medical Center, Johannes Gutenberg-University, Langenbeckstr. 1, 56101 Mainz, Germany

Elke R. Gizewski
Department of Neuroradiology, Medical University Innsbruck, Innrain 52, 6020 Innsbruck, Austria

Anne K. Braczynski, Jan-Philipp Bach, Jörg B. Schulz and Simone C. Tauber
Department of Neurology, RWTH University Hospital, Pauwelsstr. 30, 52074 Aachen, Germany

Marc A. Brockmann
Department of Diagnostic and Interventional Neuroradiology, RWTH University Hospital, Aachen, Germany

Torben Scholz
Department of Neurosurgery, RWTH University Hospital, Aachen, Germany

Benedikt Schoser
Friedrich-Baur-Institut, Neurologische Klinik und Poliklinik, Klinikum der Universität München, Ludwig-Maximilians-Universität München, Ziemssenstr, D-80336 Munich, Germany

Deborah A. Bilder
Department of Psychiatry, Division of Child and Adolescent Psychiatry, University of Utah School of Medicine, Salt Lake City, UT, USA

David Dimmock
Rady Children's Institute for Genomic Medicine, San Diego, CA 92123, USA

Digant Gupta
Bridge Medical Consulting Ltd, Gainsborough House, 2 Sheen Road, Richmond, London TW9 1AE, UK

Emma S. James and Suyash Prasad
Audentes Therapeutics, 600 California Street, Floor 17, San Francisco, CA 94104, USA

Chahra Chbili, Neila Fathallah, Manel Nouira and Saad Saguem
Metabolic Biophysics, Professional Toxicology and Applied Environmental Laboratory, Department of Biophysics, Medicine Faculty of Sousse, Sousse University, Avenue Mohamed Karoui, 4002 Sousse, Tunisia

Anis Hassine
Metabolic Biophysics, Professional Toxicology and Applied Environmental Laboratory, Department of Biophysics, Medicine Faculty of Sousse, Sousse University, Avenue Mohamed Karoui, 4002 Sousse, Tunisia
Neurology Department of Central Hospital University (CHU), Sousse University, 4002 Sousse, Tunisia

Salma Naija and Sofiene Ben Ammou
Neurology Department of Central Hospital University (CHU), Sousse University, 4002 Sousse, Tunisia

James E. Peters
Cardiovascular Epidemiology Unit, Department of Public Health and Primary Care, Worts Causeway, University of Cambridge, Cambridge CB1 8RN, UK
Department of Rheumatology, The Royal London and Mile End Hospitals, Barts Health NHS Trust, Bancroft Road, London E1 4DG, UK

Vivek Gupta and Ali S. M. Jawad
Department of Rheumatology, The Royal London and Mile End Hospitals, Barts Health NHS Trust, Bancroft Road, London E1 4DG, UK

Ibtisam T. Saeed
Department of Histopathology, Queen's Hospital, Rom Valley Road, Romford RM7 0AG, UK

Curtis Offiah
Department of Radiology, The Royal London Hospital, Barts Health NHS Trust, Whitechapel Road, London E1 1BB, UK

Yuxiao Sun, Jianan Wang, Wangshan Huang, Jing Wang, Nantu Hu, Xiaohui Fang, Supeng Huang and Haibo Di
International Vegetative State and Consciousness Science Institute, Hangzhou Normal University, Hangzhou, China

Steven Laureys
GIGA, GIGA-Consciousness, Coma Science Group, University & Neurology Department, Hospital of Liege, Liege, Belgium

Lizette Heine
GIGA, GIGA-Consciousness, Coma Science Group, University & Neurology Department, Hospital of Liege, Liege, Belgium
Audition Cognition and Psychoacoustics Team, Lyon Neuroscience Research Center, Lyon, France

Xiaohua Hu
Rehabilitation Center for Brain Damage, Wujing Hospital of Hangzhou City, Hangzhou, China

Hiroto Ito, Yumiko Harada, Rei Kobayashi, Hisashi Okada and Satoshi Okuda
Department of Neurology, National Hospital Organization Nagoya Medical Center, 4-1-1 Sannomaru, Naka-ku, Nagoya, Japan

Ayumi Uchibori and Atsuro Chiba
Department of Neurology, Kyorin University, 6-20-2 Shinkawa, Mitakai, Tokyo, Japan

Yuki Hatanaka
Department of Neurology, Teikyo University, 2-11-1 Kaga, Itabashi-ku, Tokyo 173-8605, Japan

Yuki Fukami
Department of Neurology, Nagoya University Hospital, 65 Tsurumai-cho, Showa-ku, Nagoya, Aichi, Japan

Yun Zhang and Xuejun Zeng
Department of General Internal Medicine, Peking Union Medical College Hospital (PUMCH), Chinese Academy of Medical Science (CAMS) and Peking Union Medical College (PUMC), Beijing 100730, China

Dongmei Wang
Department of Neurology, Nanfang Hospital, Southern Medical University, Guangzhou 510515, China

Wei Wei
Department of Internal Medicine, Peking Union Medical College Hospital (PUMCH), Chinese Academy of Medical Science (CAMS) and Peking Union Medical College (PUMC), Beijing 100730, China

Bruno Eymard and Jean-Yves Hogrel
Institute of Myology, GH Pitié-Salpêtrière (AP-HP), Bd de l'Hôpital, 75651 Paris Cedex 13, France

Pierre Portero
Bioingénierie, Tissus et Neuroplasticité, EA 7377 Université Paris-Est Créteil Faculté de Médecine, 8 rue Jean Sarrail, 94010 Créteil, France

Simone Birnbaum
Institute of Myology, GH Pitié-Salpêtrière (AP-HP), Bd de l'Hôpital, 75651 Paris Cedex 13, France
Bioingénierie, Tissus et Neuroplasticité, EA 7377 Université Paris-Est Créteil Faculté de Médecine, 8 rue Jean Sarrail, 94010 Créteil, France
Unité de Recherche Clinique Paris Île- de- France Ouest (URC PIFO), Raymond Poincaré Hospital, AP-HP, Garches, France

Tarek Sharshar
Medical and Surgical Neurointensive Care Centre, Hospital Sainte Anne, Paris, France
Laboratory of human histopathology and animal models, Institute Pasteur, Paris, France
Université Paris Descartes, Paris, France

Marie Theaudin
Department of Neurology, CHUV, Rue du Bugnon, 46 1011 Lausanne, Switzerland

Jing Miao, Xiao-jing Wei, Xue-mei Liu, Zhi-xia Kang, Yan-lu Gao and Xue-fan Yu
Department of Neurology and Neuroscience Center, the First Affiliated Hospital of Jilin University, Changchun 130021, Jilin, People's Republic of China

Chien-Heng Lin
Division of Pediatrics Pulmonology, China Medical University, Children's Hospital, Taichung, Taiwan

Wei-De Lin
Department of Medical Research, China Medical University Hospital, Taichung, Taiwan

I-Ching Chou
Division of Pediatrics Neurology, China Medical University, Children's Hospital, Taichung, Taiwan
Graduate Institute of Integrated Medicine, College of Chinese Medicine, China Medical University, Taichung, Taiwan

Inn-Chi Lee
Department of Pediatrics, Chung Shan Medical University Hospital and Institute of Medicine, School of Medicine, Chung Shan Medical University, Taichung, Taiwan

Hueng-Chuen Fan
Department of Pediatrics, Tungs' Taichung Metroharbor Hospital, Wuchi, 435 Taichung, Taiwan
Department of Nursing, Jen-Teh Junior College of Medicine, Nursing and Management, 356 Miaoli, Taiwan

Syuan-Yu Hong
Division of Pediatrics Neurology, China Medical University, Children's Hospital, Taichung, Taiwan
Department of Pediatrics, China Medical University Hospital, 2 Yuh-Der Road, Taichung 404, Taiwan

Xue-qian Zhang, Yu-juan Tian and Ying Wang
Department of Neurology, The Second Hospital of Hebei Medical University, Hebei, Shijiazhuang 050000, People's Republic of China

Li-jing Jia and Zhen-zhen Qu
Department of Neurology, The Second Hospital of Hebei Medical University, Hebei, Shijiazhuang 050000, People's Republic of China
Institution of Cardiocerebrovascular Disease, Hebei, West Heping Road 215, Shijiazhuang 050000, People's Republic of China
Neurological Laboratory of Hebei Province, Hebei, Shijiazhuang 050000, People's Republic of China

Aurélie Degeneffe, Marie Dagonnier and Jose Antonio Elosegi
Department of Neurology, CHU Ambroise Paré Hospital, Boulevard John Fitzgerald Kennedy 2, 7000 Mons, Belgium

Alain D'hondt
Intensive Care Unit, CHU Ambroise Paré Hospital, Mons, Belgium

Melissa A. Elafros
Department of Neurology, Johns Hopkins Hospital, Sheik Zayed Tower, Room 6005, 1800 Orleans Street, Baltimore, MD 21287, USA Brent

A. Johnson
Department of Biostatistics and Computational Biology, University of Rochester, 265 Crittenden Boulevard, CU 420-630, Rochester, NY 14642-0630, USA

Omar K. Siddiqi
Global Neurology Program, Division of Neuroimmunology, Department of Neurology, E/CLS 1017B Beth Israel Deaconess Medical Center, 330 Brookline Avenue, Boston, MA 02215, USA
Department of Internal Medicine, University of Zambia School of Medicine, Lusaka, Zambia

Michael J. Potchen
Neuroradiology Division, Department of Imaging Sciences, University of Rochester Medical Center, 601 Elmwood Ave,, Rochester, NY 14642, USA

Igor J. Koralnik
Department of Neurological Sciences, Rush University Medical Center, 1725 W. Harrison Street, Suite 1106, Chicago, IL 60612, USA

William H. Theodore
Clinical Epilepsy Section, National Institute of Neurological Disorders and Stroke, NINDS NIH Building 10 Room 7D-43, Bethesda, MD 20892, USA

Lisa Kalungwana
Department of Psychology, University of Zambia,10101 Lusaka, Zambia

Gretchen L. Birbeck
Epilepsy Division, Department of Neurology, University of Rochester School of Medicine & Dentistry, 265 Crittenden Blvd, CU420694, Rochester, NY 14642–0694, USA
Epilepsy Care Team, Chikankata Hospital, Private Bag S2, Mazabuka, Zambia

Burcu Balci-Hayta and Pervin Dincer
Department of Medical Biology, Hacettepe University Faculty of Medicine, 06100 Sihhiye, Ankara, Turkey

Beril Talim and Gulsev Kale
Department of Pediatrics, Pathology Unit, Hacettepe University Faculty of Medicine, 06100 Sihhiye, Ankara, Turkey

Ji Yeon Chung
Department of Neurology, Chosun University School of Medicine, Gwangju 61453, Republic of Korea

Seung Jae Lee
Institute for Molecular Biology and Genetics and Department of Chemistry, Chonbuk National University, Jeonju 54896, Republic of Korea

Byoung-Soo Shin and Hyun Goo Kang
Department of Neurology, Chonbuk National University School of Medicine, Jeonju 54896, Republic of Korea
Department of Neurology & Research Institute of Clinical Medicine of Chonbuk National University - Biomedical Research Institute of Chonbuk National University Hospital, 20 Geonji-ro, Deokjin-gu, Jeonju-si, Jeonbuk-do 54907, South Korea

Mikko Kärppä, Laura Kytövuori and Kari Majamaa
Research Unit of Clinical Neuroscience, University of Oulu, FI-90014 Oulu, Finland
Medical Research Center Oulu, Oulu University Hospital and University of Oulu, Oulu, Finland
Department of Neurology, Oulu University Hospital, FI-90029 OYS Oulu, Finland

Markku Saari
Turku Centre for Biotechnology, Cell Imaging Core, University of Turku, FI-20520 Turku, Finland

Ambra Stefani, Anna Heidbreder, Heinz Hackner and Birgit Högl
Department of Neurology, Medical University of Innsbruck, Anichstrasse 35, Innsbruck A-6020, Austria

Hao Yu, Juan-Juan Xie, Yi Dong and Wang Ni
Department of Neurology and Research Center of Neurology in Second Affiliated Hospital, and the Collaborative Innovation Center for Brain Science, Zhejiang University School of Medicine, 88 Jiefang Rd, Hangzhou 310009, China

Yu-Chao Chen
Department of Neurology and Institute of Neurology, First Affiliated Hospital, Fujian Medical University, Fuzhou, China

Qin-Yun Dong
Department of Neurology and Institute of Neurology, Huashan Hospital, Shanghai Medical College, Fudan University, Shanghai, China

Zhi-Ying Wu
Department of Neurology and Research Center of Neurology in Second Affiliated Hospital, and the Collaborative Innovation Center for Brain Science, Zhejiang University School of Medicine, 88 Jiefang Rd, Hangzhou 310009, China
Joint Institute for Genetics and Genome Medicine between Zhejiang University and University of Toronto, Zhejiang University, Hangzhou, China

Bin Liu
Department of Hand Surgery, the First Bethune Hospital of Jilin University, Changchun 130021, China

Yuanding Zhang
Department of Otolaryngology, the First Bethune Hospital of Jilin University, Changchun 130021, China

Lili Zhang, Hongyu Li, Shuang Li, Jie Du and Lirong Zhao
Department of Electrical Diagnosis, the First Bethune Hospital of Jilin University, No. 3302, Jilin Road, Changchun 130021, China

Fan Zhang
Department of Hand Surgery, China-Japan Union Hospital of Jilin University, Changchun 130033, China

Yafang Liu
Department of Pathology, the First Bethune Hospital of Jilin University, Changchun 130021, China

Damian Cruse and Davinia Fernández-Espejo
School of Psychology, University of Birmingham, Birmingham B15 2TT, England

Marco Fattizzo
Department of Neurorehabilitation, University Hospital of Ghent, Ghent 9000, Belgium

Adrian M. Owen
The Brain and Mind Institute, University of Western Ontario, London, Ontario N6A 5B7, Canada

Index

www.ingramcontent.com/pod-product-compliance
Lightning Source LLC
LaVergne TN
LVHW080721210926
848485LV00003B/501
* 9 7 8 1 6 3 9 2 7 3 3 4 8 *